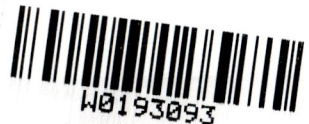

Practical Guide to
Oral and Maxillofacial Surgery

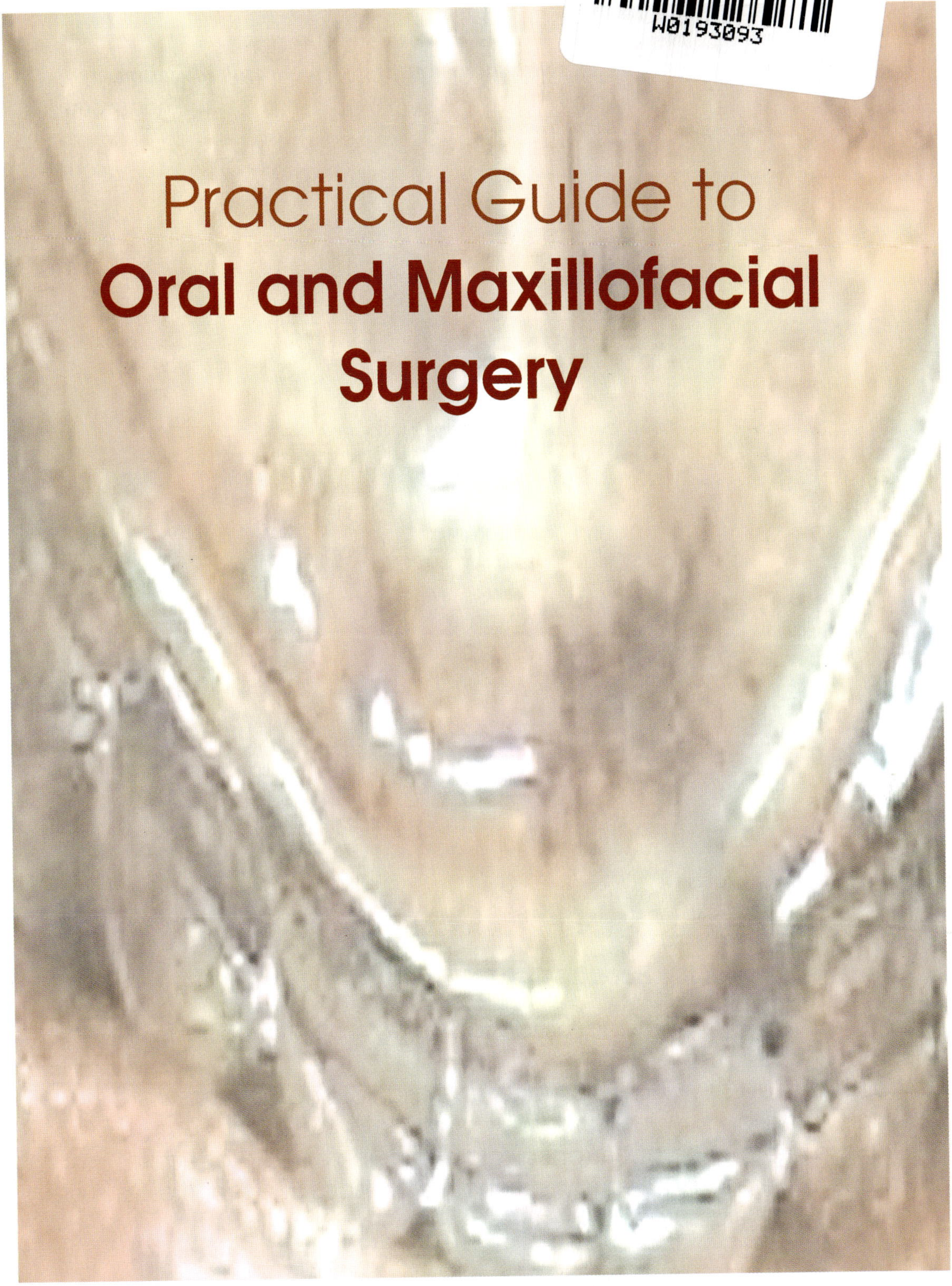

To be conscious of your own ignorance is the first step towards education.

.... Anonymous

Salient Features of the Book

- Excellent coverage of the practical aspects of oral and maxillofacial surgery.
- Well illustrated drawings, diagrams and clinical photographs.
- Simple, lucid and understandable language and text.
- Concise information of current surgical principles and procedures.
- Precise coverage of latest revolutionary advances and techniques in oral and maxillofacial surgery.

Practical Guide to
Oral and Maxillofacial Surgery

CHANDRAKANT P. TAWARE BDS, MDS (Bombay)

Honorary Professor and Postgraduate Teacher,
University of Bombay

Department of Oral and Maxillofacial Surgery,
Government Dental College and Hospital, Mumbai

Joint Director (Dental), Directorate of Medical Education and
Research (DMER), Maharashtra

Ex-Dean, Government Dental College and Hospital, Mumbai

Ex-Director, Directorate of Medical Education and
Research (DMER), Maharashtra

CBS

CBS Publishers & Distributors

New Delhi • Bangalore • Pune (India)

Disclaimer:
Science and technology are constantly changing fields. New research and experience broaden the scope of information and knowledge. The author has tried his best in giving information available to him while preparing the material for this book. Although all efforts have been made to ensure optimum accuracy of the material, yet it is quite possible some errors might have been left uncorrected. The publisher, printer and the author will not be held responsible for any inadvertent errors or inaccuracies.

Practical Guide to
Oral and Maxillofacial Surgery

First Edition 2009

ISBN: 978-81-239-1653-8

Published by Satish Kumar Jain and produced by Vinod K. Jain for
CBS Publishers & Distributors,
CBS Plaza, 4819/XI, Prahlad Street, 24 Daryaganj, New Delhi 110 002
E-mail: cbspubs@vsnl.com; cbspubs@airtelmail.in • Website: www.cbspd.com

Branch Offices:

- Seema House, 2975, 17th Cross, K.R. Road, Banasankari 2nd Stage, Bangalore 70
  Fax : 080-26771680 • E-mail : cbsbng@vsnl.net
- Shaan Brahmha Complex, Basement, Appa Balwant Chowk, Budhwar Peth,
  Next to Ratan Talkies, Pune 411002
  Fax : 020-24464059 • E-mail : pune@cbspd.com

Printed at:
Ajanta Offset and Packagings Ltd.

to

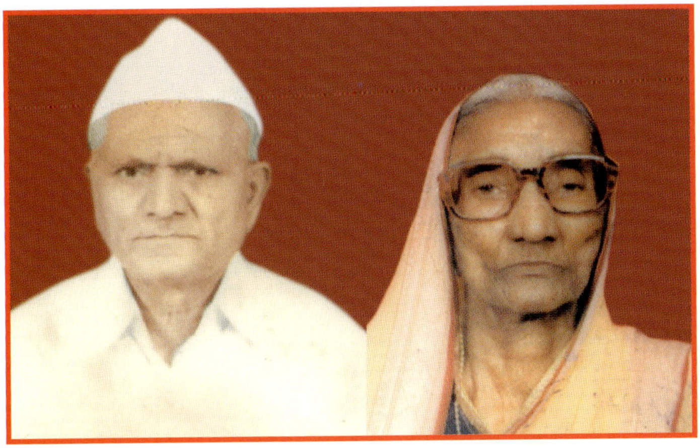

my parents

Late Shri Pandurang

and

Smt. Bhagirathi Taware

who nurtured and cared for me
in true sense

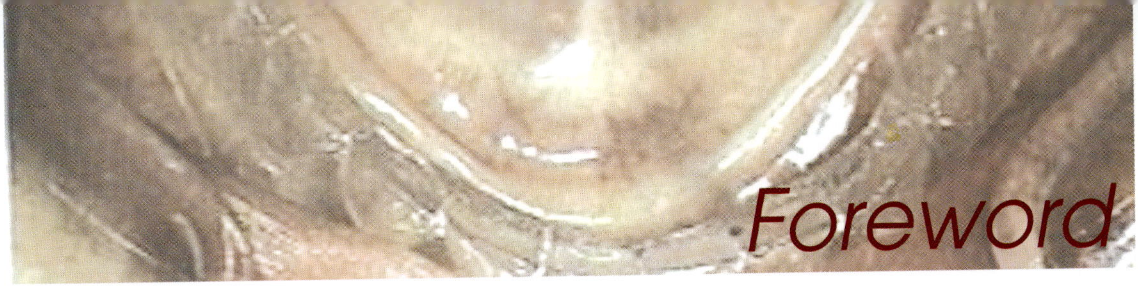

Foreword

महाराष्ट्र आरोग्य विज्ञान विद्यापीठ, नाशिक
Maharashtra University of Health Sciences, Nashik
वणी-दिंडोरी रोड, म्हसरुळ, नाशिक-४२२००४., Vani-Dindori Road, Mhasrul, Nashik-422004
Tel : (0253) 2531835, Fax : (0253) 2539113. Mumbai (off.) Tele Fax : (022) 22653543
Website: www.muhsnashik.com email: vc@muhsnashik.com/ muhsvc@hotmail.com

It gives me immense pleasure to write this Foreword to the book *Practical Guide to Oral and Maxillofacial Surgery* written by Dr. C.P. Taware. Noted philosopher Henry Van Dyke once remarked about teachers, which is so very true even today, "Ah, there you have been the worst paid and best rewarded of all the vocations; dare not to enter it unless you love it; for the vast majority of men and women it has no promise of wealth or fame, but they whom it is dear for its own sake are amongst the nobility of mankind." And, he is one such teacher who has written this book.

Dr. C.P. Taware has held a number of posts during his academic career and has tremendous experience in every walk of life. He has been the postgraduate teacher for a number of students. He has held offices as Joint Director as well as the Director, Medical Education and Research, Maharashtra. In spite of his busy schedule, I always found him very passionate about this subject and he took every effort to educate his students and prepare them to face the challenges in life.

This book provides information on the steps to be followed in the surgical management of a patient. The book gives useful guidelines regarding the patient examination, laboratory investigations, sterilization and the basic principles of surgery. Also with hepatitis and AIDS on the rise, the chapter devoted to "AIDS and its oral manifestations" will prove to be useful to the budding doctors as well as the private practitioners on the necessary steps to be taken in the management of these patients with a humane touch. The book will be useful to the students and teachers.

"Just like a stream, the beginning of all big things is small", and I believe this effort made by Dr. C.P. Taware will enlighten us all. I wish this book a great success and hope that the professionals would await subsequent editions of this book.

Dr (Mrs) Mrudula A. Phadke
Vice-Chancellor
Maharashtra University of Health Sciences, Nashik

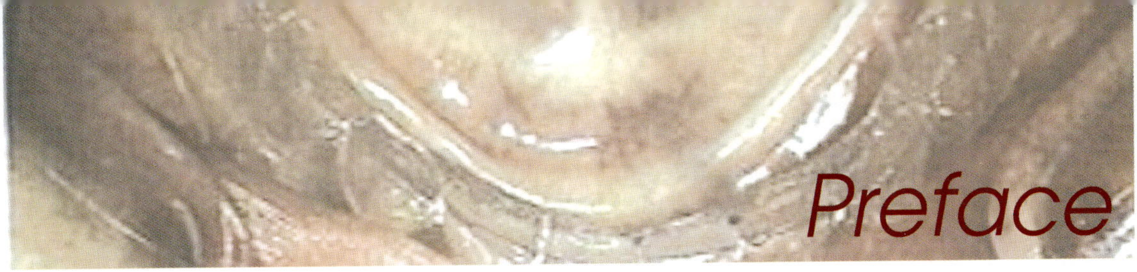

Preface

God spare me sclerosis of the curiosity, for the curiosity which craves to keep us informed about the small things no less than the large, is the main spring, the dynamo, the jet propulsion of all complete living.

.... John Mason Brown

Before penning down the Preface, I would like to express my gratitude to the all powerful, omnipresent God, for it is He who has created us all.

The field of oral and maxillofacial surgery is an ever-changing, ever-refining speciality, which is advancing at a remarkable speed, perhaps more so in the last few decades with advances being made in the fields of orthognathic surgery, bone grafting, distraction osteogenesis, oral cancer surgery, and fields like minimally invasive aesthetic facial surgery, etc.

One of the most important and often neglected aspects of this specialty is hospital or inward management of the patient requiring oral and maxillofacial surgical care. This is an avenue with which the technological boom has progressed in leaps and bounds in regard to various newer methods of investigations, drug administration, sterilization, etc. The crux of the matter is that the surgeons and the trainee residents should keep themselves abreast of these rapid advancements along with certain age-old basic principles of patient's surgical management. Unfortunately during training, generally these basic principles of hospital management are hardly given special importance and many practitioners remain perplexed about the grassroot principles of the hospital management of patients. My book is a humble effort to highlight these principles and considerations of patient care so as to provide the best services for the patients and achieve excellent postoperative outcomes, which is the ultimate goal of any surgeon.

"Knowledge is power when applied."

Prior to commencing any treatment aspect, it is imperative for the practitioner to possess a thorough knowledge of the clinical features, status, severity and possible progress of any ailment along with its possible variants or similar conditions. This axiom holds true for oral and maxillofacial surgery too.

Being a surgical specialty, an oral and maxillofacial surgeon has to be able to manage the patient both surgically and medically. Also, the basic knowledge about the overall anatomy, physiology and pharmacology cannot be overemphasised. Taking a comprehensive history of the patient is an elementary procedure which, if not carefully done, can drastically alter the diagnosis and treatment plan for the patient.

Chapters 1 and 2 deal with an introduction and overview of hospitals in general, their classification and standard protocols for patients' admission to a hospital ward. Chapter 3 enlightens about detailed history-taking and examination. The art of taking case history and recording the patient's details have been elucidated therein. Also I have attempted to orient the reader about various clinical and laboratory investigations which are indispensable in establishing the diagnosis and thus dictating the future treatment. Chapter 4 describes the basic principles of surgery. The invaluable aspects like sterilization, disinfection, asepsis, chemotherapeutic agents, etc. have been comprehensively explained. A detailed discussion on the surgical principles of flap designing, suturing, various armamentarium and surgical techniques has been presented. Chapter 5 discusses HIV/AIDS and its accompanying oral and systemic features and complications. No surgeon should operate on any of his patients without having knowledge about this deadly disease. Chapter 6 describes the management of hospital waste which is an essential aspect of ideal hospital setup, also the segregation and disposal of toxic and hazardous waste. Chapter 7 encompasses the inward management of the patient once admitted in the hospital. It describes the preoperative evaluation, intraoperative management and postoperative care without which the success of any operative procedure will be jeopardised.

Since my days as a student of this specialty, I always found dearth of concise and precise literature on this aspect of oral and maxillofacial surgery and it has been my genuine aspiration for many years to come up with some work which emphasises the readers about this aspect of the speciality.

This book is my modest and unostentatious effort in an easy and interesting language, accompanied by excellent illustrative pictures which would help a beginner to get an equinox of this dynamic subject.

Chandrakant P. Taware

Acknowledgements

I would like to thank Almighty for everything I could ever get and have achieved in life. I am equally indebted to my parents, late Shri Pandurang and Smt Bhagirathi Taware, for their efforts in bringing me up and instilling right principles and values in me.

I would like to thank my wife and my children for standing by me with their endless love, support and inspiration.

I would like to thank all my teachers, especially my mentor Dr. J.N. Khanna, Dr. Dudhani, Dr. S.S. Khera, Dr. Wadkar, Dr. A.P. Chitre, Dr. Vandekar, Dr. Kali Kapadia, and all my teacher colleagues for inspiring me over the years in this subject. I would like to thank all my postgraduate students who have always supported me, inspired me, and were of great help to me.

I must thank my postgraduate student and my assistant Dr. Abdul A. Khan, now working as a Lecturer in Department of Oral and Maxillofacial Surgery at Government Dental College, Aurangabad, who strived hard and helped me very sincerely to bring this work to completion. I also acknowledge the efforts put in by my other postgraduate students Dr. Samir D. Khaire, Dr. Sagar Vaishampayan, and also all the staff in the Department of Oral and Maxillofacial Surgery, Government Dental College, Mumbai.

I express my sincere thanks to all those sources for permitting us to use figures mentioned in references.

I thank CBS Publishers & Distributors, New Delhi, for their efforts and support to publish my book.

The most important are my patients, who allowed me to serve them over the years and enriched my knowledge and experience not only in the speciality but also in my life too.

Chandrakant P. Taware

About the Author

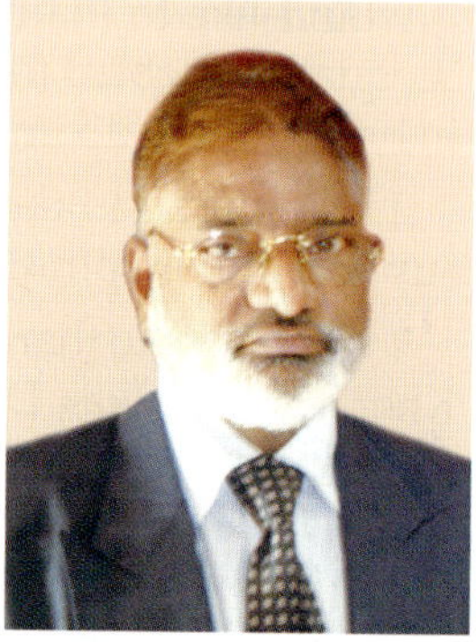

Dr. Chandrakant P. Taware has been in academics since 1976, and has worked in various capacities at Government Dental College, Mumbai, and Government Dental College, Aurangabad (Maharashtra). He has been a postgraduate teacher in the subject of oral and maxillofacial surgery under Mumbai University, since 1991. He was Professor and Head, Department of Oral and Maxillofacial Surgery, and Dean at Government Dental College, Mumbai. He was Director, Directorate of Medical Education and Research, Government of Maharashtra, Mumbai (Jan 2003–June 2004). He has been working as Joint Director (Dental), Directorate of Medical Education and Research (DMER), Maharashtra, since 2001.

Dr. Taware has been examiner for undergraduate, postgraduate and DNB courses in the subject of oral and maxillofacial surgery for Mumbai University and various universities across India. He has worked as ex-officio member of various advisory committees for Mumbai University and Maharashtra University of Health Sciences (MUHS), Maharashtra State Dental Council, and Dental Council of India in the capacities of Professor and Head, Dean, Joint Director and Director (DMER). He has presented many research papers at various state and national conferences. Besides these, he has made contributions to many national and international publications. He is truly a seasoned teacher, academician and administrator.

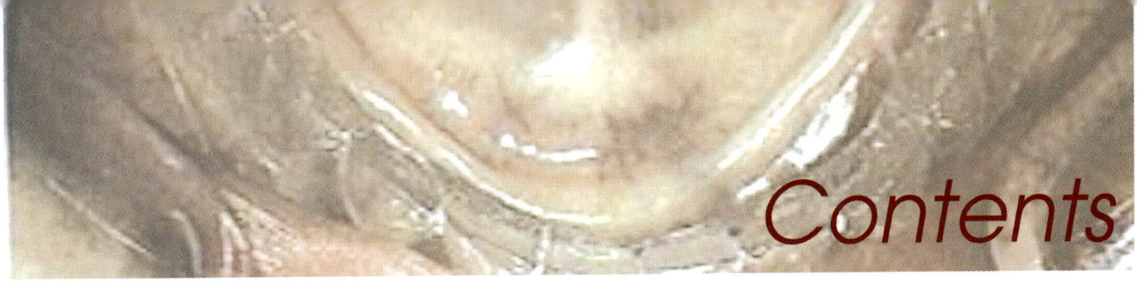

Contents

Chapter 1

Preamble

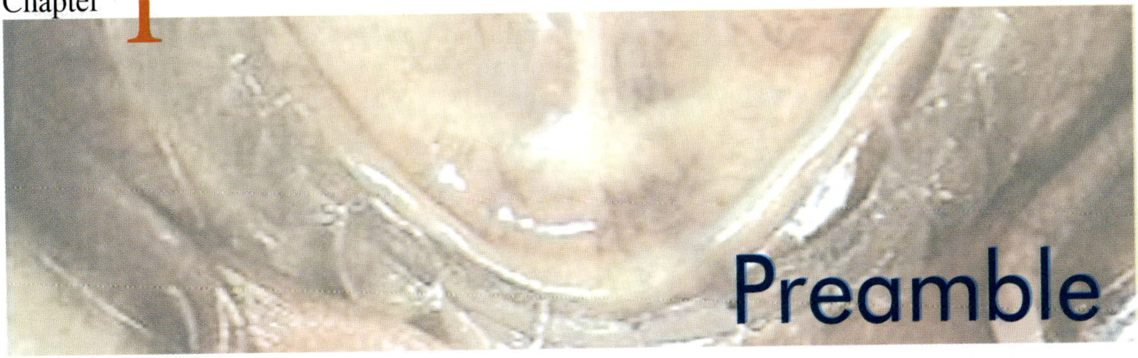

Oral and maxillofacial surgery is the specialty of dentistry that includes the diagnosis, surgical and adjunctive treatment of diseases, injuries and defects, including both the functional and aesthetic aspects of the hard and soft tissues of the oral and maxillofacial region.

The scope of oral and maxillofacial surgery for the general practitioner is defined by the individuals desire to perform surgical procedures, his/her training in performing complex surgical procedures, skill level and the availability of specialists in the vicinity. During the completion of their course, the dental trainees are under the protection of their institution and can seek their senior's opinion and guidance when they encounter with any problems. However, when they setup their own practice then every decision has to be self-made and during such a time this book can serve as a useful guide with important hints from practical point of view.

It is said that "habits work more constantly and with greater force than reason, which when we have most need of it, is seldom fairly consulted and rarely obeyed."

It is very important for a general practitioner or a specialist to develop good habits and abide by them whenever consulting a case. It is very important to take a complete case history of the patient. The complete aseptic precautions need to be taken even though one may just be examining a patient. Also it is very important to plan the execution of treatment right from the necessary armamentarium needed till the postoperative care of the patient and the expected result. This helps to deliver good treatment and to gain patient's confidence which in turn gives the surgeon a feeling of satisfaction.

"The beauty of life does not depend on how happy you are, but on how happy others can be because of you." To be excellent a surgeon must be technically skilled but also have strong components of humanism, kindness and compassion. It is important that he or she have a great deal of personal insight into the patient's concerns regarding the upcoming surgical procedure. This humanistic approach will be the most important factor in the patient's judgement of the surgeon's overall skill. A surgeon must have great respect for soft as well as hard tissues.

"A strong and positive attitude creates more miracles than any other thing, because life is 20% how you make it and 80% how you take it." Success in life does not come with the absence of failures. A determined person will look upon his failures as stepping stones towards success and improvise on them every time he encounters such a situation.

"When moving ahead in time it is important to acknowledge the efforts of seniors and not bypass them." Thus this book is a sincere attempt to present an insight into the subject of oral and maxillofacial surgery. The principles outlined by the senior members in the field of surgery have been mentioned along with innovative contributions from our side.

Chapter 2

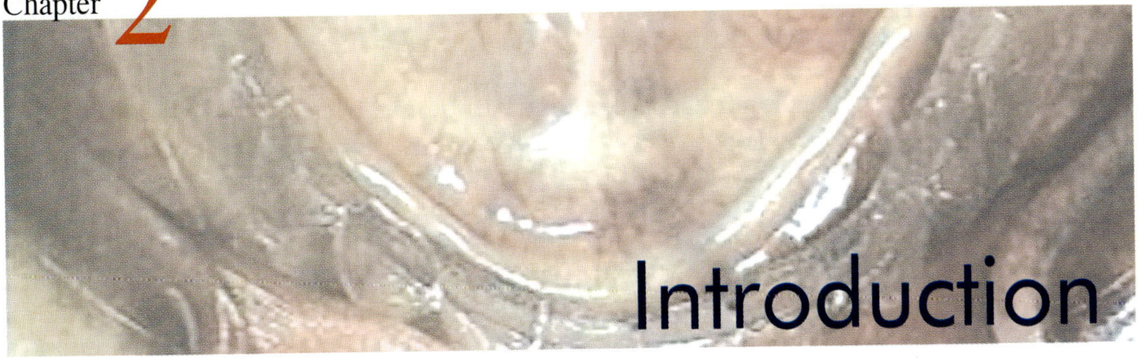

Introduction

> "The patient is the centre of the medical universe around which all our works revolve and towards which all our efforts trend."
>
> *J.B.Murphy 1857-1916*
> *Professor of Surgery, Northwestern University, Chicago, Illinois, USA.*

Oral and maxillofacial surgery is a rapidly changing and expanding area of health care and a multidisciplinary approach is necessary to meet the needs of many patients. Cooperation and coordination of care between general dentists and medical and dental specialists are more important today than ever before. In order to render the best oral and maxillofacial surgery care for a patient, the dental surgeon must have a good understanding of the basic fundamentals and a comprehensive view of the scope of the specialty.

Surgical diagnosis is based on a sound knowledge of anatomy, physiology and pathology, a specific history and examination with confirmation by imaging and invasive diagnostic procedures as the case warrants. Studying surgery concerns defining the basic facts on which the consequences of a disease process can be built.

With the presumption that the freshly passed graduates are aware of the subject of oral and maxillofacial surgery, elaborate description of the text has been avoided to keep the matter limited. The main objective of this book is to present a model practical guide with stepwise description of the basic oral surgical procedures that the fresh graduates and professional learners intend to attempt at their respective establishments. It aims to provide a guideline to the practicing dentist on how to plan the treatment for a patient seeking oral and maxillofacial surgery care, the necessary investigations to be done and the postoperative care of the patient. It also aims to provide illustrated examples wherever necessary for better understanding.

The surgical process starts with the patient from whom a careful history is taken. The chapter "General Considerations" gives a comprehensive description of history taking and physical examination. Extraoral and intraoral examination is described along with illustrative examples and explanations. It also gives an exhaustive coverage of differential diagnoses. After the patient's history has been taken and physical examination carried out pointing to a differential diagnoses, we advise certain investigations in particular pertaining to the case to reach a probable diagnosis. Laboratory investigations have been exhaustively covered giving the normal ranges for the tests along with the changes seen in pathological conditions. Next in sequence is the 'Radiological investigation' which covers the principles of radiographic interpretation along with the radiographic features of different conditions affecting the maxillofacial region.

The chapter "Basic principles of surgery" has thoroughly covered the principles of sterilization and asepsis, the surgical techniques including 'extraoral and intraoral incisions', principles of flap design and reflection, haemostasis and suturing techniques. In the 'Surgical armamentarium' an attempt has been made to explain about the instruments most commonly used in routine procedures. 'Operating room decorum' provides an insight into the design of an operating room, the equipment planning , air changes and air distribution within the room, microbiological contamination of hospital environment, management of clinical waste and used linen, categories of used linen, and electrical hazards posed in the operating room.

"Exodontics" has been covered under three headings of 'uncomplicated exodontia', 'complicated exodontia' and 'impacted teeth.' The protocol for the extraction or surgical removal of teeth has been outlined along with the necessary postoperative care to be taken. "Odontogenic infections" highlights the microbiology of odontogenic infections, principles of therapy of odontogenic infections, principles of prevention of metastatic infections and antibiotic regimen for prophylaxis of bacterial endocarditis.

"Oral and maxillofacial trauma" describes the clinical presentation of the patient following trauma, the necessary investigations to be carried out and the protocol for management of such patients. The illustrated photographs and schematic diagrams help in better understanding.

Pathological lesions have been covered taking only a few cases as representatives of the variety of lesions reported. Describing all the pathological lesions would have been beyond the scope of this practical guide as the permutations and combinations would enlist several conditions and also newer inventions. Hence an attempt has been made to outline a general protocol for the management of these pathological conditions. "Dental implantology" has gained widespread popularity in recent years and a separate chapter has been devoted for the same.

Acquired immunodeficiency syndrome (AIDS) has been a matter of concern right from the day the first case was reported. There has been an alarming increase in the number of seropositive cases reported globally. The chapter on "Oral manifestations of AIDS" outlines the nature of the disease, the possible causes and modes of transmission with illustrated photographs.

Treating a pathological condition without paying attention to the patient as a whole may sometimes be the cause of failure because one may miss a very important systemic condition that the patient may be suffering from and which carries the potential to influence the treatment plan. Thus it is very important that every practitioner reviews the systemic condition of the patient as well. The chapter on "Oral manifestations of systemic diseases" has been exclusively devoted to point out the various systemic conditions which present with signs and symptoms affecting the oral cavity.

Thus this book describes the biological foundation and surgical techniques necessary for the general practitioners.

Chapter 3

General Considerations

CLINICAL HISTORY AND PHYSICAL EXAMINATION

Patients present themselves to the oral and maxillofacial surgeons with a large variety of problems involving both emergency and elective care. In every case, whether the patient has facial trauma, is in need of orthognathic or preprosthetic management, or is coming to the office for any of the multitude of procedures that are performed by the oral and maxillofacial surgeon, a systematic history should be taken and a careful examination be performed to define and delineate the clinical problem and help establish a rational treatment plan.

HISTORY TAKING

The history consists of two parts—the history of presenting complaint (onset and course) and the general history, which provides information about medical, surgical, psychological, social, occupational and family background. The areas covered and the extents of questions asked in this portion of history are governed by their relevance to the clinical situation.

It is preferable to begin the history with questioning about the present problem because this permits easier interpretation of the significance of more general findings. The patient should be encouraged to provide information in the chronological order. Given the opportunity, most patients are eager to discuss the history of their problem and their symptoms. The clinician should guide them through the use of both open and closed ended questions, allowing patients to freely relate their complaints while still keeping to the subject at hand. Would you tell me more about the pain?

Identification and General Information

Record the patient's complete name including the maiden name for a married woman. Other data include age, sex, race, occupation and marital status.

Source of Data and Qualitative Reliability

At times the medical history will not be obtained from the patient because of age or general condition. For example, in a head injury patient it is important to note the details of the person who has accompanied the patient and who was an eyewitness to the incident which caused the injury to the patient. Occasionally an interpreter may be necessary for a patient interview in another language. Thus the importance of this record.

Chief Complaint

The chief complaint are usually recorded in the patients own words but at times medical terminology is used. All symptoms should be recorded in the order of importance to the patient. The duration of each symptom should be recorded. Symptoms should be attended in the order of urgency. For example, the pain of the patient should be attended first rather than the removal of dental calculus.

History of Present Illness

It is the most important part of patient interview as it contains the basic diagnostic data. It's purpose is to furnish the interviewer with a clear, chronologic order of symptoms beginning with the appearance of initial symptom, the circumstances surrounding the initial symptom and how the patient has been affected by the course of the illness. Past treatments for the condition and results should be noted. It is also customary to include the review of that major system affected by the illness in this section.

Past Medical History

It contains the information that summarises the patient's health status prior to the present illness. It can be divided into several sections:

Childhood Diseases

A few childhood diseases such as scarlet fever, rheumatic fever, and glomerulonephritis have the potential to cause serious functional and organic impairments.

Adult Illnesses

Infectious diseases such as tuberculosis and hepatitis as well as parasitic, fungal and bacterial infections may have debilitating or generalized systemic effects that will alter the treatment plan for even minor procedures. Diseases that affect the endocrine system, such as those of thyroid or pancreas, will modify the patient's response to anaesthetic agents and surgical stress and influence post operative healing and medication. Anaemias, coagulation defects, agranulocytosis and other haematologic disorders will affect the course of anaesthesia and surgery. Diseases of respiratory and cardiovascular system may affect patient tolerance to anaesthesia and surgery.

Previous Hospitalization, Operation, Anaesthetics

A record of the patients prior hospitalization can be useful, not only to establish the cause of hospitalization, but in some instances to obtain laboratory and radiographic data. Moreover future problems in patient care can be anticipated from knowledge of patient's response to prior operations and anaesthetics.

Accidents and Injuries

Not every injury is serious enough to require hospitalization, but the history of such an occurrence may be significant in establishing a diagnosis and appropriate plan of treatment.

Allergies

Existing allergies and their manifestations as well as allergic tendencies are elicited.

Immunization Record

Knowledge of patient's immunization record, especially for tetanus, is essential.

Present and Recent Medications

There are a large number of drug effects, side effects and interactions. The patient's present and recent medication history can have important implications in differential diagnosis and determining the course of therapy.

Habits

Questions about the use of tobacco, drugs, alcohol, tea and coffee can elicit information that may not be significant in relation to patients presenting complaint but may also be important in consideration of their general physical condition. Sleeping and eating habits should also be considered.

Social History

Information in social history is intended to summarise the patient's life with respect to how the environment may be contributing to the disease. It may include questions about the patients marital status, social and economic status, birth place and areas of residency.

Family History

It involves information about the present state of parents, siblings and offspring. Certain diseases have a familial tendency and others have a hereditary basis.

Review of Systems

- *Integument:* Important symptoms include pruritis and urticaria. These may involve an allergic reaction, a viral infection such as herpes zoster or idiopathic conditions such as erythema multiforme, psoriasis or lichen planus.
- *Endocrine system:* Fatigue, dry skin, weight gain, heat or cold intolerance, tremors, nervousness or exophthalmos can suggest thyroid disease.
- *Head:* Important symptoms involving the head include headaches, their location, duration, periodicity, type and prodromal symptoms.
- *Eyes:* Symptoms such as icterus suggest liver disease. Other symptoms include inflammation, ocular pain, diplopia. Oedema of the lower eyelids may suggest congestive heart disease.
- *Ears:* Important symptoms include decreased hearing, earache, tinnitus, vertigo and discharge.
- *Nose and sinuses:* Symptoms involving the nose and sinuses are anosmia, discharge, obstruction, trauma, epistaxis, frequency of colds and sinusitis.
- *Jaws:* Information about jaw fractures, dislocation, and subluxation, pain on opening or closing movements, trismus and joint noises should be obtained.
- *Oral cavity:* The oral cavity has many structures that need to be examined properly. The normal colour of the oral mucosa is coral pink with deeper shades in some region and lighter shades in others. The thickness of the epithelium and the vascularity of the sub epithelial tissues are responsible for the colour differences. The gingivae should be inspected for colour, stippling, width of attached gingival. Cheek mucosa should be checked for any traumatic lesions, blanching, palpable fibrous bands, and parotid duct papillae openings. The soft palate should be checked for its movement, position of uvula. The tonsillar region should be inspected for the palatoglossus and palatopharyngeal folds, enlargement of the tonsils. The tongue should be checked for its normal mucosal covering, papillae, movement of tongue, and ventral surface for varicosities. Finally teeth should be checked for caries, malalignment, impactions.
- *Pharynx and larynx:* Tumors in throat can produce symptoms of hoarseness, difficulty in swallowing, progressive dysphagia. Other symptoms include pain, swelling and haemorrhage.

- ***Neck:*** Limitation of motion, swelling and pain are major symptoms of diseases involving the neck.
- ***Respiratory system:*** Important symptoms include dyspnoea on exertion, haemoptysis, cough, pain, wheezing.
- ***Cardiovascular system:*** Important findings include a history of hypertensive heart disease, angina pectoris, congenital heart disease, rheumatic heart disease, heart failure, heart murmurs.
- ***Gastrointestinal system:*** Symptoms include loss of weight, haematemesis, epigastric pain, anorexia, and change in bowel habits, nausea, vomiting, and diarrhea.
- ***Genitourinary system:*** Polyuria, haematuria, pyuria, dysuria, oliguria, nocturia, lumbar pain and urethral discharge.
- ***Gynaecologic considerations:*** A discussion about missed menstrual period may lead to recognition of an unknowingly pregnant patient.
- ***Haematopoietic and lymphatic system:*** Symptoms of dysfunction of the haematopoietic and lymphatic systems include anaemia, bleeding problems, swollen lymph nodes, petechiae and purpura.
- ***Orthopedic system:*** Symptoms such as pain, limitation of motion and swelling of the joints are present in diseases involving the extremities.
- ***CNS status:*** Important symptoms include orientation, level of consciousness, convulsions, anaesthesia and paraesthesia, ataxia, paresis or paralysis, tremors.
- ***Psychiatric status:*** Findings include a history of psychiatric treatment, insomnia, behavioural changes, nervousness, anxiety and depression.

PHYSICAL EXAMINATION

Once the complete medical history and review of systems have been completed, the clinician can then proceed with the physical examination. The extent of this examination is guided by the symptoms that were elicited by prior questioning.

The actual clinical examination of the patient begins from the first moment of contact between the clinician and the patient. Observations about the patient's physical and emotional status can be made during the initial questioning. Skin condition, facial configuration, eye contact and movements, voice quality, speech habits and a myriad of other objective as well as subjective qualities are appreciated by the astute clinician before the final examination begins.

Vital Signs

They include temperature, pulse, respiration and blood pressure.

Temperature

It is generally measured orally or rectally. Oral route is considered the standard and a value of 98.6° F (37° C) is considered normal. Rectal values average 0.5 to 1.0 degree higher than oral.

Pulse

The pulse is a pressure wave travelling through the arterial system. It may be palpated at any accessible artery, but it is most commonly taken at the radial, brachial or temporal arteries. When palpating the artery, the rhythm and quality as well as the rate should be determined. The character and compressibility of the vessel wall are also significant observations. The normal pulse appears at regular intervals and has a rate between 60–100 per minute.

Respiration

In evaluating respiration, the rate, depth and rhythm are observed. Respiratory rate varies with age. In the young child the rate may be up to 30 per minute. The rate for the average adult is 14–18 per minute.

Blood Pressure

Normal blood pressure varies with age being lowest in the infant and increasing with age. It varies from moment to moment with respiration, emotion, exercise, meals, alcohol, tobacco, bladder distension, temperature and pain. It is also influenced by the circadian rhythm, age and race. Shortly after Scopine Riva-Rocci had invented the sphygmomanometer, the Russian surgeon Korotkoff suggested that by placing a stethoscope over the brachial artery at the ante-cubital fossa distal to the sphygmomanometer cuff, sounds could be heard. The phases are:

Phase 1: The first appearance of faint clear tapping sounds (thud) which gradually increases in intensity.

Phase 2: The softening of the sounds which may become swishing or blowing.

Phase 3: The return of sharper, softer sounds which may become crisper, but never regain the intensity of phase 1 sounds.

Phase 4: Distinct, abrupt muffling of sounds, which become soft and blowing.

Phase 5: The point at which all sounds disappear completely.

EXTRAORAL EXAMINATION

The clinical examination of the patient should begin with a general overall evaluation of the individual. Observe the patient as s/he walks to the dental chair. Attitude may be readily ascertained as in the patient who will not make eye to eye contact and who may look the other way. On shaking hands, a patient with extremely large hands may have the disease acromegaly. Swollen ankles may indicate edema due to a kidney or a heart problem. The medical and dental history should be reviewed before the examination begins. On viewing and palpating the face, the examiner should observe whether or not there is basic symmetry.

Although most faces have some asymmetry, an obvious asymmetry may be due to a dental problem, particularly if associated with pain. An abscess of a tooth or the periodontal tissues is a common cause for facial swelling, once trauma is ruled out (Fig. 3.1).

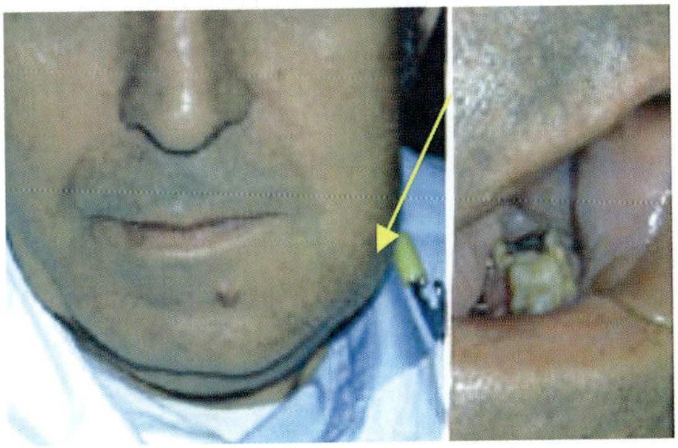

Fig. 3.1: Facial view of patient in distress with face showing swelling on the left side (as shown by the arrow). The swelling is a cellulitis and is related to a broken-down molar tooth with an abscess.

Pigmented lesions such as moles and age spots and ulcers such as with skin cancers are readily observable and should be questioned (Fig. 3.2).

A rash on the skin of the face may be due to an allergy which can lead to more knowledge

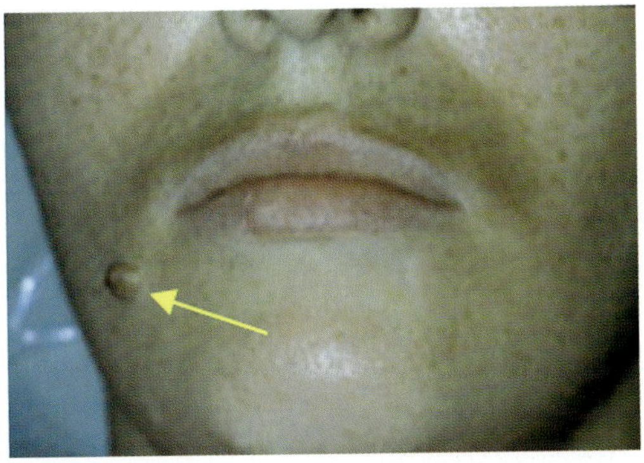

Fig. 3.2: Facial view of patient with a large, pigmented mole on the right side of her face (as pointed by the arrow). The mole has melanin pigment. Extra melanin pigment (chloasma or melasma) is noted particularly over the patient's upper lip due to the taking of oral contraceptives.

about the history of the patient and about future treatment plans. Some asymmetries may be due to swollen lymph nodes or glands. On doing the facial and head and neck examination, the examiner should palpate all of the areas of known lymph nodes regardless of swellings since a swollen gland may be only palpable and not visible. Lymph nodes are concentrations of lymphatic tissue with T cells, B cells and macrophages which recognize antigens and mount a response. When a lymph node responds, it undergoes a hyperplasia with an increase in the numbers of cells. This causes the gland or tissue to enlarge so that it may become palpable. A major component of the immune surveillance system, lymphatic tissue responds to inflammation, infections and malignant tumors. Any of these may cause an enlargement. For inflammation and infection, the nodes may be swollen and tender and movable. After the insult or injury subsides, then, within weeks or months, the node will return to a more normal size. However, sometimes, as when there is scar tissue or calcification in the node, it will not return to normal size and will stay enlarged. When a tumor grows within a lymph node (lymphatic metastasis), the node will be enlarged, usually, non-tender, and may not be movable, especially if the tumor has invaded to the outside of the node. Thus, exactly what palpating a lymph node (positive lymphadenopathy) means cannot readily be known. Other findings must be used to determine the significance. For example, a patient with an upper respiratory infection, such as a cold, may have several enlarged, tender nodes due to the drainage from the affected tissue sites to the nodes. They will get smaller some time after the infection has passed. Tumor bearing nodes on the other hand will not regress but will continue to expand. The patient would need a medical workup to find the tumor. Lymph nodes are oval or bean-shaped structures found along lymphatic vessels that drain body parts. Normally, they are non-tender, soft and cannot be felt even though they are present. Therefore, one uses the knowledge of anatomical location of the nodes to perform the palpation to find them. The examiner kneads just beneath the skin with a rotating motion in the areas that nodes would be expected to be found. In most circumstances they will not be felt. However, in young children, with response to so many new antigens, it is easy to palpate nodes in the head and neck. A logical place to start palpating for nodes is in the submental area, below and lingual to the chin, against the mylohyoid muscle. This node is significant because it is the one node that is easy to discover the site of drainage. The lower lip, lower anterior gingivae, corners of the mouth, and skin and tissue of the chin drain to the submental node. Thus, palpating a node there, one should look for a possible lesion in those sites. All of the other lymph nodes do not have as direct a relationship to the area that they may drain as there are interconnections with other nodes and lymphatic vessels. The submandibular nodes are bilateral and can be palpated by pressing the tissue below the jaw against the medial side of the mandible or by bimanual palpation with

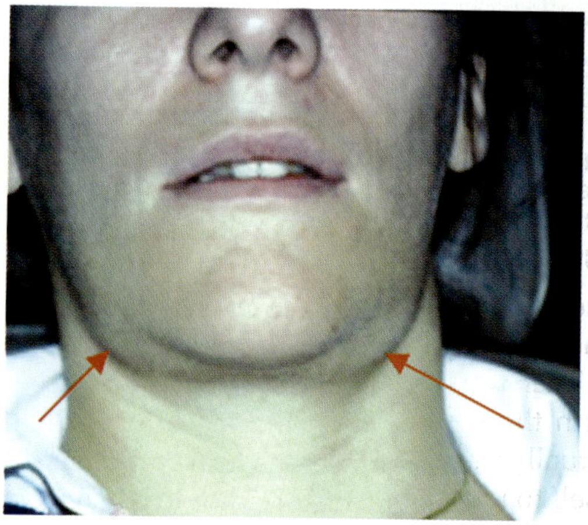

Fig. 3.3: Bilaterial submandibular gland swellings (as pointed by the arrows) due to reactive lymph nodes in a 24-year-old female with primary herpetic gingivostomatitis.

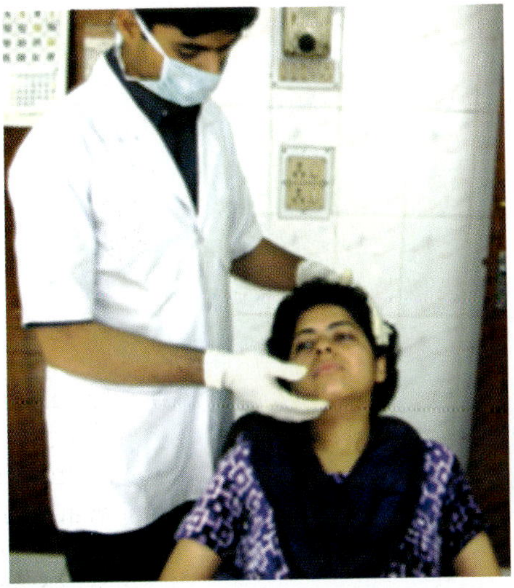

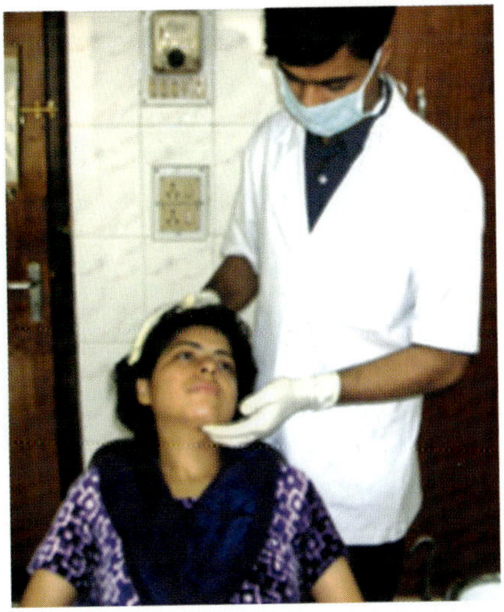

Fig. 3.4: Examination of the submandibular lymph nodes. Patient turns head to ipsilateral side and flexes the neck. The surgeon stands by the side of the patient and examines with one hand, the other hand gently supporting the head.

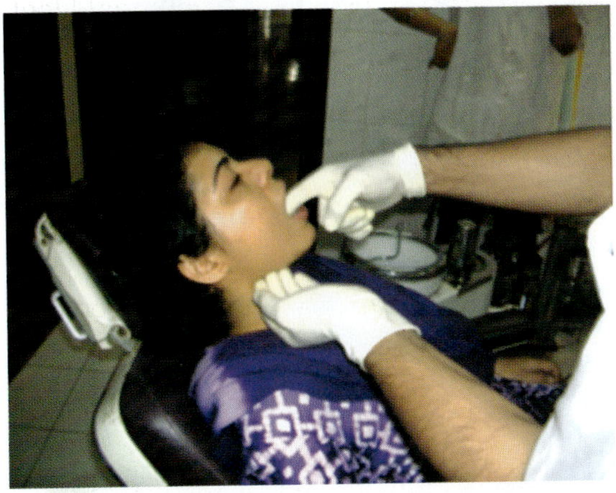

Fig. 3.5: Bimanual palpation to differentiate between swellings of the submandibular gland and enlargement of the submandibular lymph node in the submandibular region.

one finger in the mouth and the other externally pushing up (Figs 3.3, 3.4, 3.5).

There are three groups of nodes associated with the submandibular gland. What one is actually palpating is the submandibular gland itself to identify these nodes. Next are a group of nodes associated with the parotid gland. It is helpful to have the patient clench the teeth together to make the masseter muscle firm, against which one can palpate for any swellings. Then, one should move the ear lobe aside and look and feel behind the ear for post auricular nodes. At the same time as looking for nodes, one is looking for any other deviation of normal. Skin tumors may be found behind the ears. While at the ear, one can palpate the temporomandibular joint by having the patient open and close while the fingers are in the canal or near the tragus of the ear. Any clicking or deviation should be noted (Figs 3.6 and 3.7).

Next the cervical chains should be palpated. The posterior cervical chain is along the back of the neck and the anterior is along the front of the neck (Fig. 3.8).

A landmark for tracing the anterior superficial and deep nodes is the sternocleidomastoid muscle. One can start behind the ear and trace the muscle to the clavicle. Nodes generally are deep and medial to the muscle, which is kneaded to try to find the nodes. Then, when reaching the clavicle, one palpates behind the clavicle and along it in the neck. These supraclavicular nodes may be enlarged from disease in the mediastinum or from the thyroid gland. The thyroid gland may be palpated by putting the

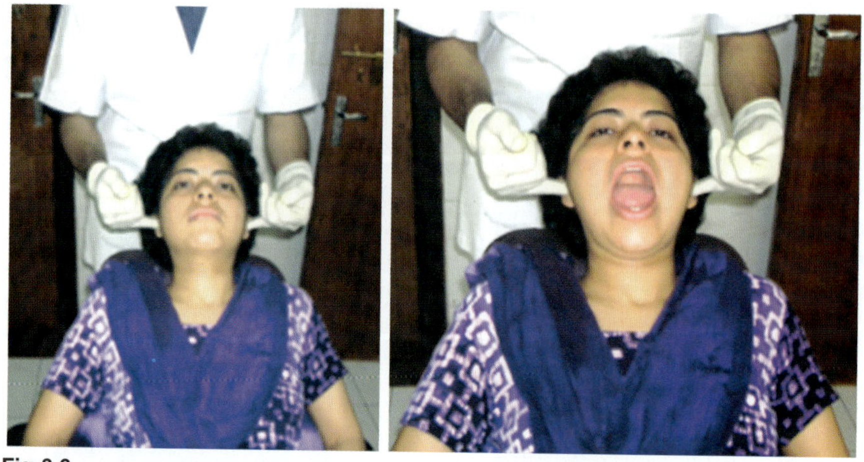

Fig. 3.6

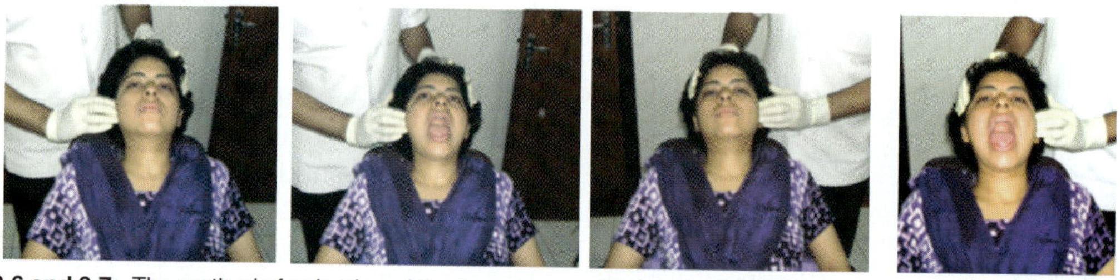

Figs 3.6 and 3.7: The method of palpation of the temporomandibular joints at the tragus of the ear as the patient opens and closes the mandible.

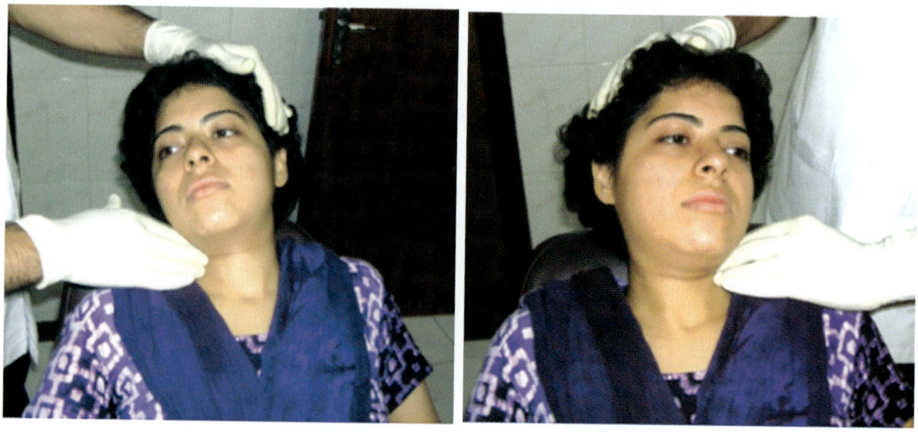

Fig. 3.8: Palpation and gentle squeezing of the sternocleidomastoid muscle to locate the cervical chain of nodes just medial and deeper to the muscle.

fingers gently over the area and having the patient swallow. The oral examination can start with the lips. One should observe the vermilion border and the corners of the mouth for any deviation. For instance, patients who have been overexposed to the sunlight frequently have a loss of the vermilion line and whitish lesions and may have a premalignant lesion. Next, have the patient bring the teeth together to relax the lip muscles. Drape the upper and the lower lips and look at the mucous membrane sides down to the vestibule. On the upper lip, one should see a maxillary labial frenum as a normal structure. Often, there is a small tab or tag of normal appearing tissue hanging from this frenum. This is a mucosal tag and may get irritated if caught between the upper teeth. It is a variation of normal. Also noted in some patients along the upper lip near the vermilion are clusters of yellow-white submucosal pinhead glands that are called Fordyce's glands. These are ectopic sebaceous glands that are not associated with any hairs (Fig. 3.9).

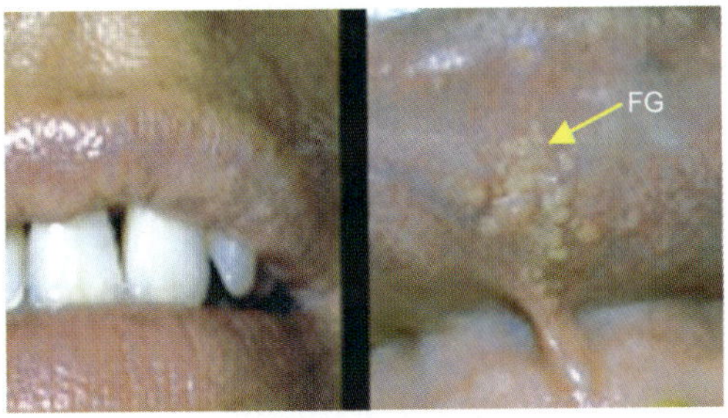

Fig. 3.9: Fordyce's glands (as pointed by the arrow) on inner aspect of upper lip. Ectopic sebaceous glands appear as submucosal yellowish, pinhead-sized papular lesions, often gathered together in clusters as seen here in two patients. FG = Fordyces glands

On retracting the lower lip one may see fine white, slightly depressed lines, which are scars, usually from falling as a youngster. Also, if the lower lip is held for a while and dried, one can test the minor salivary glands of the lip by noting whether or not mucus is expressed from the many glands of the lower lip. One can also note the vestibule area, the gingivae and the anterior teeth. Next, retract the corners of the mouth to reveal the buccal mucosae. Here, there are two normal landmarks. One is the papilla and opening of the parotid duct (Stenson's) (Figs 3.10, 3.11).

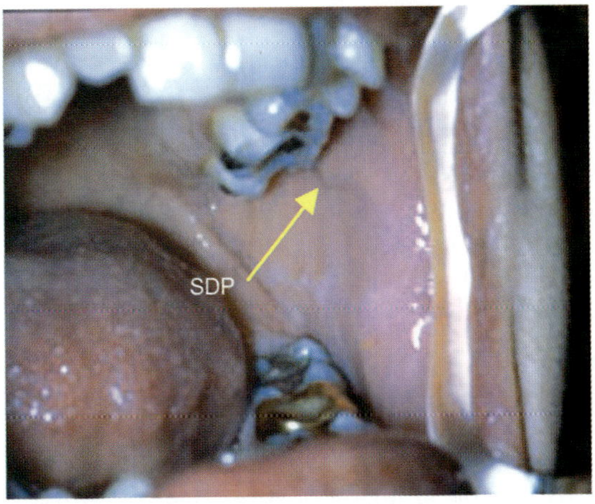

Fig. 3.10: Retraction of the cheek to view the buccal mucosa which includes the papilla of Stenson's duct (as pointed by the arrow) opposite the maxillary second molar and the occlusal or bite line opposite where the teeth occlude.
SDP = Stenson's duct papilla

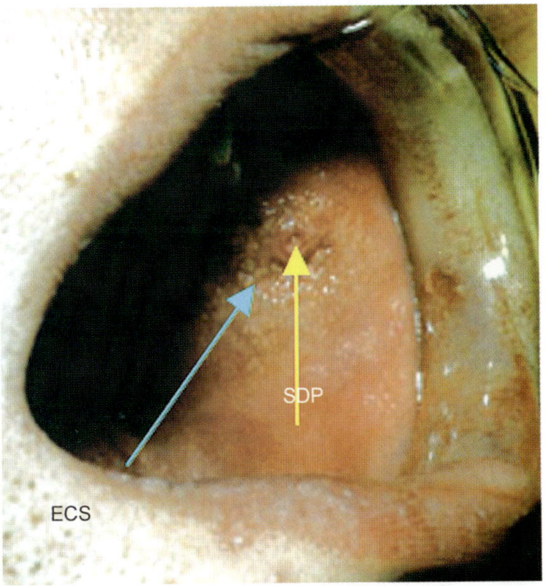

Fig. 3.11: Buccal mucosa with a prominent papilla of the Stenson's duct (as shown by the yellow arrow) with an expression of clear, watery saliva from the parotid gland. Also note a large cluster of ectopic sebaceous glands (as shown by the blue arrow), a common location.
SDP = Stenson's duct papilla; ECS = ectopic sebaceous glands

A lack of flow or sluggish flow may indicate a dry mouth (xerostomia). Causes may be medication induced or radiation therapy, amongst others. A yellowish salivary flow usually indicates a bacterial infection in the parotid gland, requiring treatment. The other landmark on the buccal mucosa is a white line known as the occlusal or bite line, a horizontal line running from the corner of the mouth posteriorly where the teeth meet the mucosa (Fig. 3.13). It can be much exaggerated in some patients and mimic disease. The hard palate can be viewed next either directly of using a dental mirror. The anterior portion has prominent, firm folds called rugae that can be large in some patients (Fig. 3.12). Posteriorly, the hard palate is whitish due to the keratinized surface. Laterally, where there are numerous minor salivary glands and blood vessels, there is a bluish hue. There are pin-sized, pink, ductal openings from minor glands. In smokers, they may be reddened and prominent against a whiter than normal background. There is also a linea alba or white line seen in the midline running anteriorly to posteriorly. At the

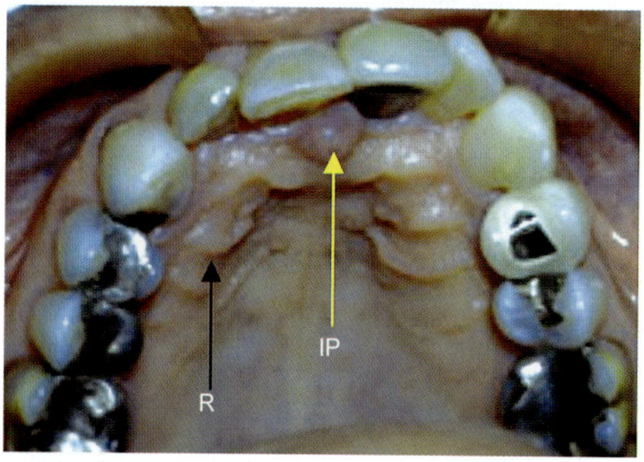

Fig. 3.12: Examination of the hard palate showing the incisive papilla (shown by the yellow arrow), rugae (as pointed by the black arrow), a whitened color due to the keratinized surface, the bluish color bilaterally due to the mucous glands and prominent blood vessels, and the linear alba or white line running down the center.
IP = incisive papilla; R = palatine rugae

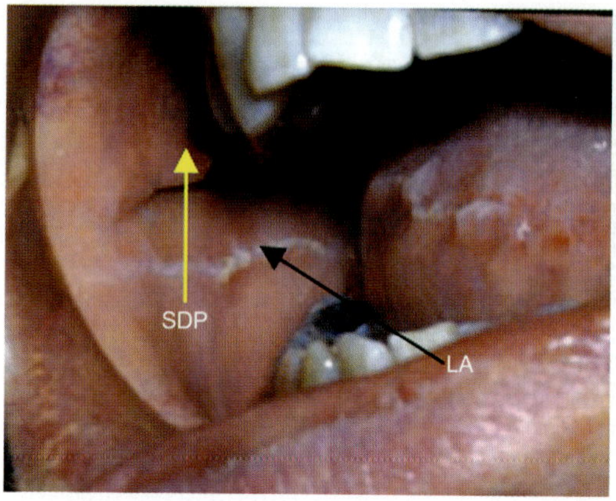

Fig. 3.13: Buccal mucosa with a prominent, white occlusal line (as shown by the black arrow) and a prominent papilla of Stenson's duct (as pointed by the yellow arrow).
SDP = Stenson's duct papilla; LA = linea alba

posterior segment, in the midline, may be small depressions called fovea palatini, just anterior to the vibrating line of the palate.

In the midline of the hard palate extra bone may be found. Called a torus, it may be minimal or very enlarged. It will feel bony hard and will appear opaque on a radiograph confirming that it is composed of extra, but normal bone. Moving posteriorly with the examination; one envisions the soft palate which ends at a pendulous structure, the uvula (Fig. 3.14). One may ask the patient to say "ah" or "eh" and see that the soft palate vibrates, also confirming the intactness of cranial nerve VIII.

In this posterior aspect of the soft palate is a circle of lymphoid tissue Waldeyer's ring, including the tongue. The major tonsillar tissues are readily identifiable. The palatine tonsils are located on each side situated between the palatoglossal and the palatopharyngeal folds (Figs 3.14 and 3.15). They may be very large in children, appearing to close off the airway, but in adults they are usually receded between the folds. If only one palatine tonsil is enlarged and pushed toward the midline, then one should consider tumor, lateral pharyngeal abscess or other condition.

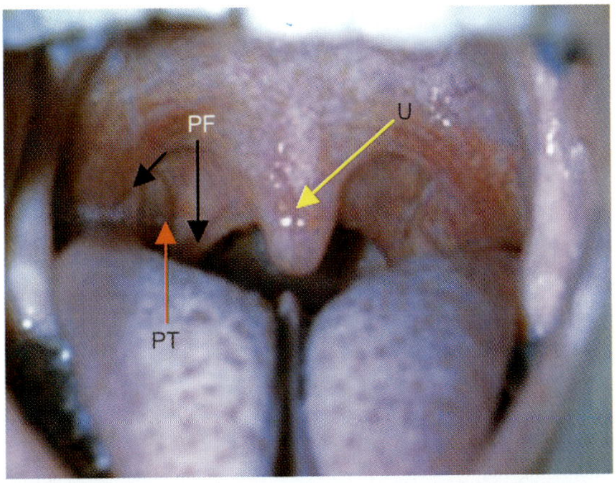

Fig. 3.14: Soft palate viewed with the tongue depressed by a dental mirror. Note the pink color, the uvula at the base, the bilateral fauces which enclose the palatine tonsils. The posterior pharyngeal wall is farthest posterior.
PF = palatine fauces; PT = palatine tonsils; U = uvula

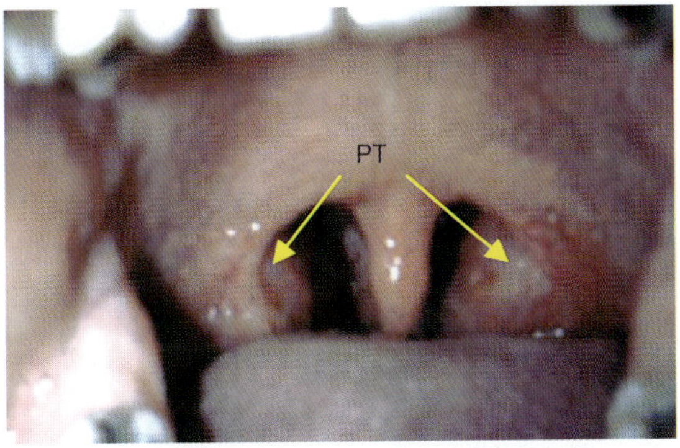

Fig. 3.15: Enlarged palatine tonsils with some crypts showing at the surface.
PT = palatine tonsils

Tonsillar crypts are indentations that can become filled with bacteria. A large accumulation of bacteria in a crypt is a bacterial plug. It can cause a tickle in the throat and malodor. The bacterial plug is best diagnosed by expressing the yellow mass from the tonsil. Another lesion that may be noted in tonsillar tissue is the pseudocyst of the tonsil. It is formed by the closing over of the opening of the tonsillar crypt which then allows desquamating epithelial cells to accumulate, causing a raised, yellow lesion. Diagnosis is usually made by trying to express the yellow. In pseudocysts, there is a covering and the yellow cannot be readily expressed as in the bacterial plug. Eventually, the contents spontaneously are expressed.

The lesion is one that need not be removed although they can be confused with a fatty tumor (lipoma).The accessory tonsils may be noted at the posterior part of the soft palate, often near the base of the uvula (Fig. 3.16). They may resemble a small tumor. However, they do get smaller after reacting to a stimulus and this gives a clue to their tonsillar origin.

If the palatine tonsils have been removed, two findings may be present. One is a band of white that represents scar tissue. The other is a mass of tonsillar tissue called residual tonsil (Fig. 3.17). These fleshy masses may become reactive and remain enlarged.

They represent foci that were not totally removed at the tonsillectomy. More tonsillar tissue can be noted by depressing the tongue

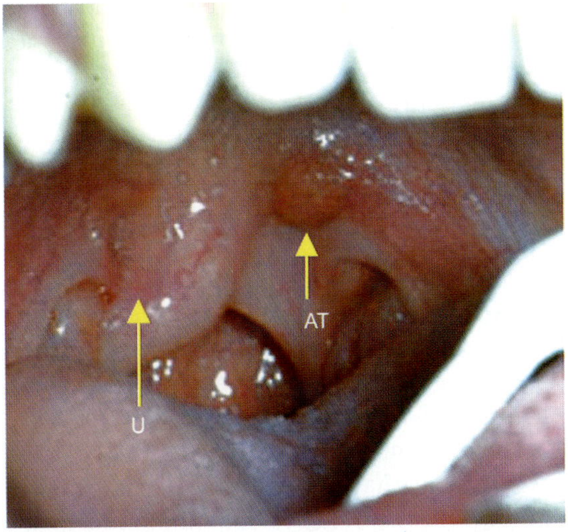

Fig. 3.16: Accessory tonsil at the base of the uvula. It is pink, salmon colored, and may react and become bigger and smaller. It has a smooth surface in contrast to a papilloma which has a pebbly surface and can appear in this location.
AT = accessory tonsil; U = uvula

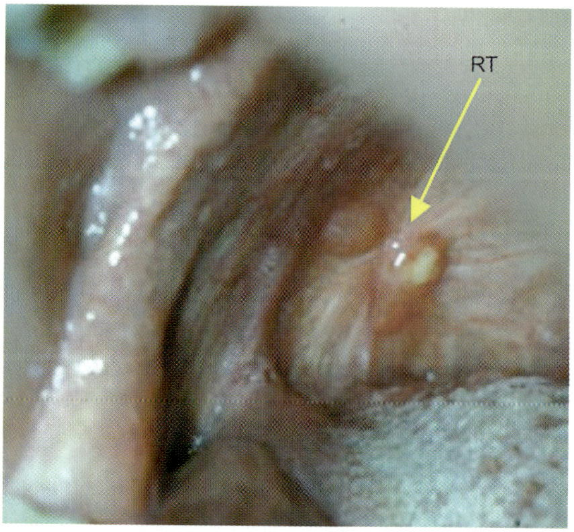

Fig. 3.17: Residual tonsils (as pointed by the arrow) in the palatine tonsillar area. Scar tissue from the removal of the palatine tonsils is white. The lower residual tonsil has a pseudocyst.
RT = residual tonsils

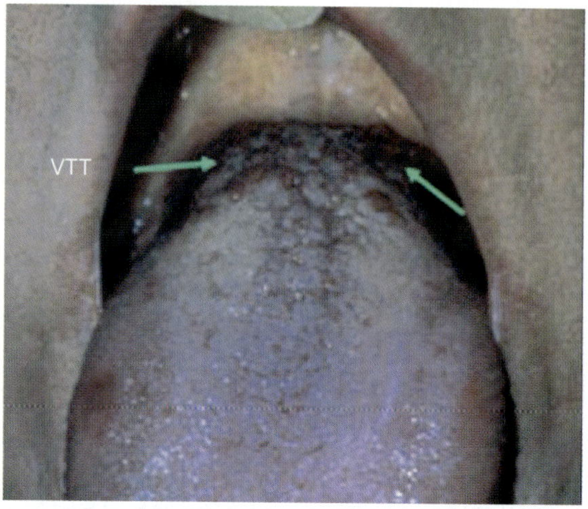

Fig. 3.18: Vascular tonsillar tissue at the base of the tongue (green arrows). VTT = vascular tonsillar tissue.

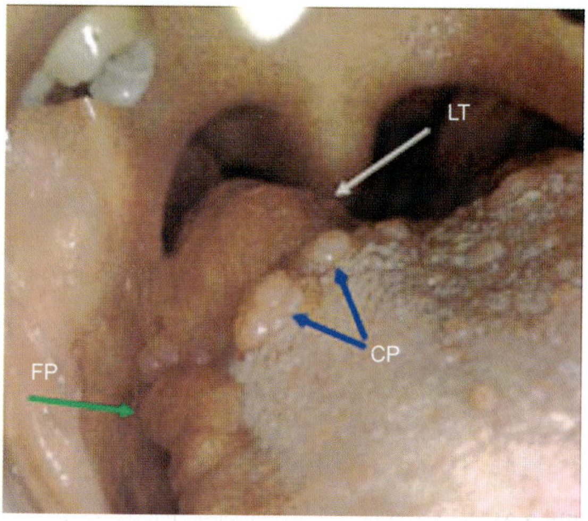

Fig. 3.19: An enlarged lingual tonsil, Grey arrow. Also, a prominent foliate papilla (tonsillar tissue) at the posterior lateral surface of tongue, green arrow, and some circumvallate papillae, blue arrows.
LT = lingual tonsils; FP = foliate papilla;
CP = circumvallate papilla.

down and having the patient say "ah". In the posterior pharyngeal wall are tissues that are tonsillar and can become reactive and then noted as bright pink, fleshy masses. Sometimes pseudocysts are noted in them. Also noted in some patients in this area is a yellow, white, sticky mucus plug (postnasal drip) (Fig. 3.20).

Tonsillar tissue is prominent at the very base of the tongue but is usually hard to visualize (Figs 3.18 and 3.19).

Other tonsillar tissue in the tongue is noted on the lateral surfaces, most posteriorly, in the foliate papillae bilaterally.

These are small reddened areas with small bumps and indentations. They may be very enlarged in smokers and do undergo reactive hyperplasia that may mimic a tumor. One should follow a reactive foliate papilla to see that it regresses. Bacterial plugs and pseudocysts may occur here also.

The tongue can be viewed next, by holding it with a gauze and gently moving it (Fig. 3.21), or by having the patient move it from side to side, while holding the buccal mucosa to the side, and forward while opening wide. (This also checks cranial nerve XII.) Several anatomical entities can be checked. The filiform papillae (Figs 3.22, 3.23) are the most numerous ones.

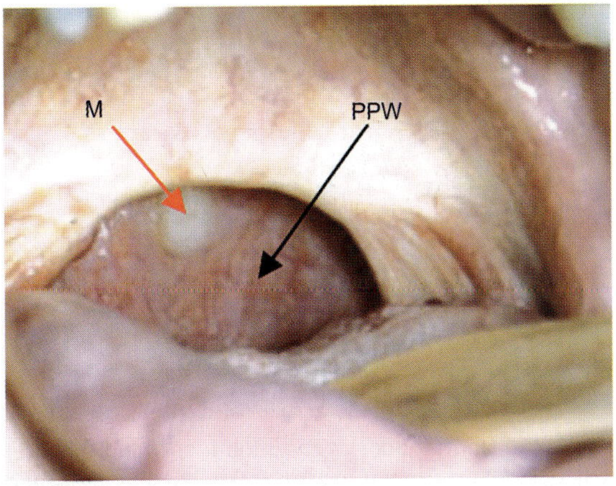

Fig. 3.20: A white removable mass of mucus (as pointed by the red arrow)on the posterior pharyngeal wall in a patient who had removal of the palatine tonsils.
M = mass of mucous; PPW = posterior pharyngeal wall as well as the uvula.

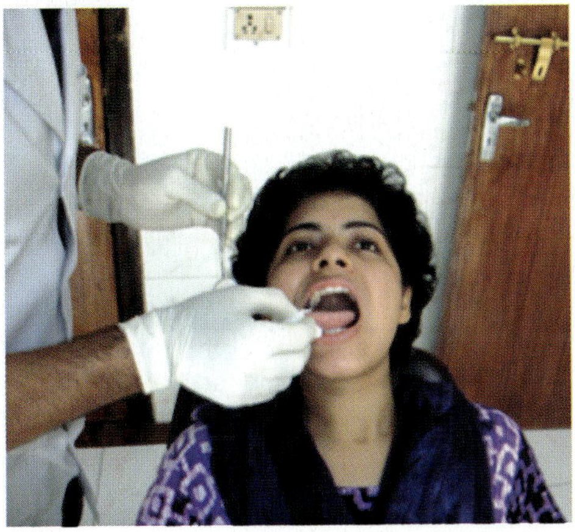

Fig. 3.21: The method of examination of the tongue.

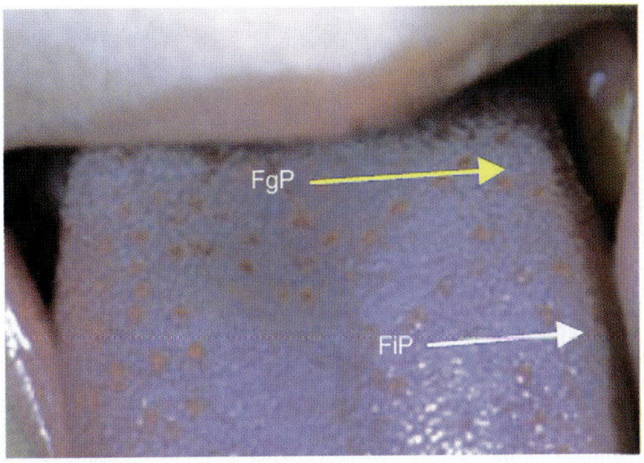

Fig. 3.22: Dorsal surface of the tongue showing the white filiform papillae (as pointed by the white arrow) and the red fungiform papillae (as pointed by the yellow arrow). FgP = fungiform papilla; FiP = filiform papilla.

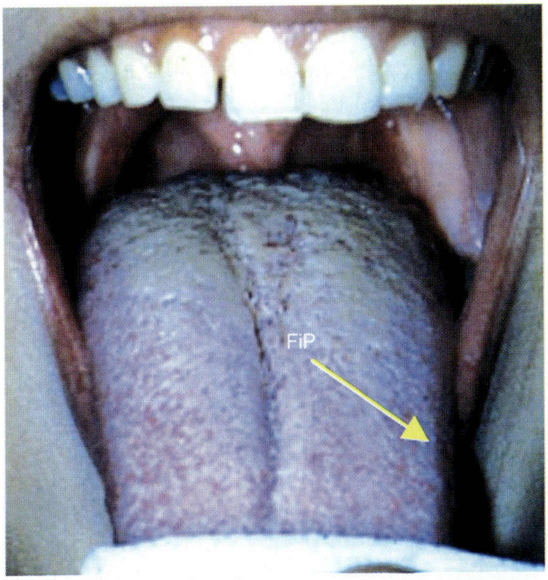

Fig. 3.23: Extension of the tongue with a gauze, showing the dorsal surface with elongated filiform papillae (as pointed by the yellow arrow).
FiP = filiform papilla

Interpersed among the filiform papillae are small, pink, dome-shaped fungiform papillae, which may or may not have taste buds. The circumvallate papillae, the largest of the papillae, are present in the most posterior part of the tongue as two rows of structures forming an upside down "V", with pointing toward the throat (Fig. 3.24). Sometimes they extend beyond the surface and can mimic small tumors.

The true lingual tonsils are beyond the circumvallate papillae and usually are seen only with a mirror reflecting light on them. The foliate papillae are bumps or grooves of tonsillar tissue on the lateral borders of the tongue at its most posterior segment where the tongue meets the floor of the mouth.

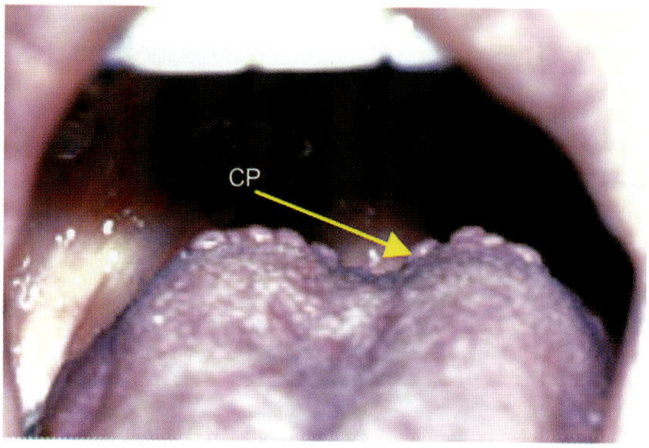

Fig. 3.24: Dorsal surface of tongue showing a double row of circumvallate papillae (as pointed by the arrows) running posteriorly to form a "V" shape. These are raised above the surface and mimic small "tumors."
CP = circumvallate papilla.

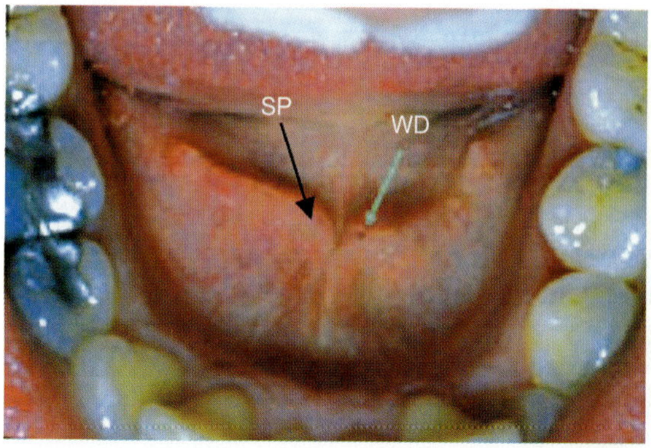

Fig. 3.26: Normal floor of the mouth showing bilateral sublingual plicae or carunculae (as pointed by the black arrow). At the medial aspect of each is the opening of Wharton's duct (as pointed by the green arrow).
SP = sublingual plica; WD = Wharton's duct orifice

Next, have the patient open the mouth and try to touch the hard palate with the tongue (Figs 3.25, 3.26, 3.27). Some patients cannot perform this maneuver and it indicates a short lingual frenum in a condition called ankyloglossia or tongue-tie. In addition to noting the lingual frenum in the midline of the ventral surface of the tongue, one should visualize the large blue veins running lateral to it on each side. These can become prominent and in older patients there can be other, deeply blue veins that are prominent (varicose veins). Varicosities are common and can mimic a vascular lesion such as a hemangioma, a benign tumor composed of blood vessels.

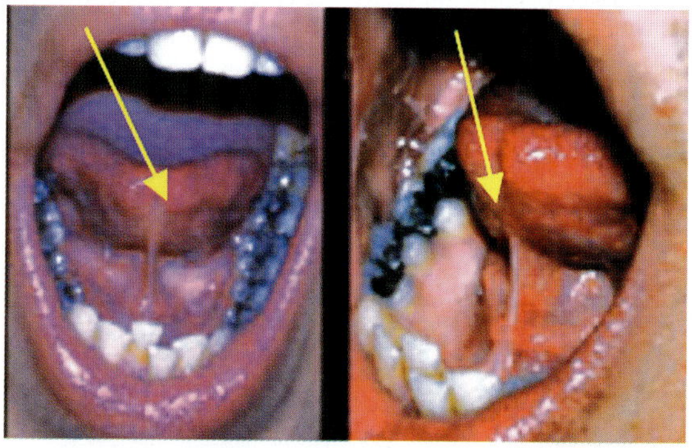

Fig. 3.27: Ventral surface of the tongue and the floor of the mouth in a patient with ankyloglossia or "tongue-tie." The lingual frenum is attached too far forward toward the tip of the tongue (as pointed by the arrow) and the patient cannot touch the hard palate with the mouth open.

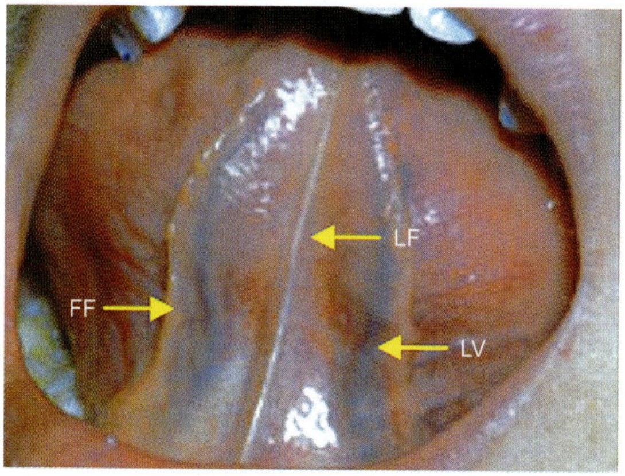

Fig. 3.25: Normal ventral surface of the tongue showing the midline lingual frenum, and the two prominent lingual veins running on each side. Also, note the fimbriated folds or lines running parallel to the veins.
LF = lingual frenum; LV = lingual veins; FF = fimbriated folds

The floor of the mouth is examined next. In the anterior portion on each side are the sublingual plicae or carunculae, slightly raised, cylindrical structures running from the midline to each side and housing openings of the

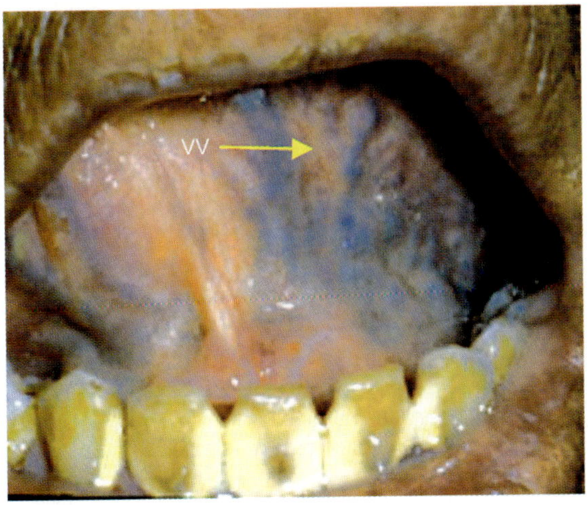

Fig. 3.28: Varicose veins (as pointed by the arrow), ventral surface of the tongue in an older patient. These are dilated veins due to loss of elasticity and do not reflect any systemic condition. VV = varicose veins.

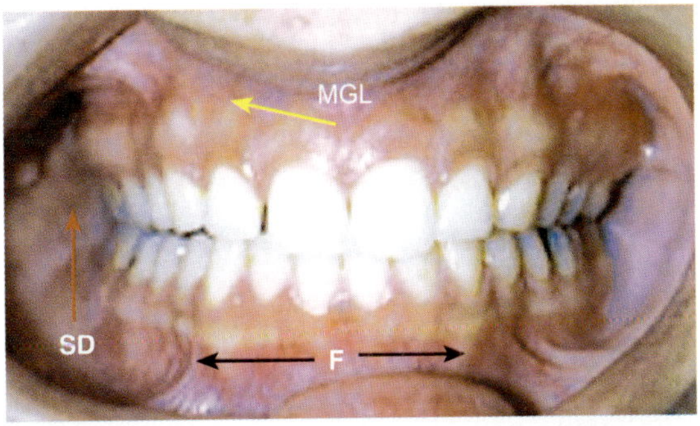

Fig. 3.29: View of the labial and buccal vestibules, gingivae and the teeth. Note the mucogingival line (as pointed by the yellow arrow), the freni (as pointed by the black arrow), and the slight melanin pigmentation of the gingivae. The papilla of Stensen's duct (as pointed by the red arrow) is also visible.
MGL = mucogingival line; F = freni; SD = Stenson's duct papilla.

sublingual glands. At the most anterior portion of each is a more raised nodule with an opening to the submandibular gland (Wharton's duct). The submandibular gland can be milked to see a less clear but not milky solution expressed from the duct. A stone in the duct can prevent the saliva from exiting. If the patient is edentulous and the mandible is greatly resorbed, then the floor of the mouth can appear dome-shaped as a tumor-like mass rising above the mandible and mimicking disease. Sometimes, hyperplastic, reactive oral tonsillar tissue may be noted in the floor of the mouth. These may be associated with lymphoepithelial cysts or pseudocysts of tonsillar tissue.

With a dental mirror and by direct viewing, the unattached and attached gingivae should be noted. The mucogingival line (Fig. 3.29) should be seen and the amount of attached tissue noted.

In some patients, particularly in the earlier years, retrocuspid papillae may be seen (Figs 3.30, 3.31). They are found on the attached gingivae of the mandible, often bilaterally, lingual to the cuspid or canine teeth as raised, nodules, usually 0.5 mm, with a broad base (sessile) or a pedunculated base (emanating from a stalk). Normal structures in these individuals, they may regress with age, require no treatment, but may be mistaken for disease.

On the anterior gingivae, usually of the mandible, a similar condition may be found at the mucogingival line. Called gingival fibrous nodules or gingival nodules, they are small,

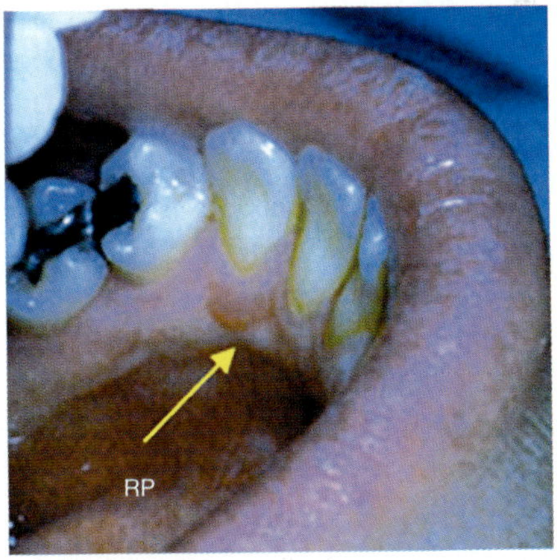

Fig. 3.30: Retrocuspid papilla (as pointed by the arrow); here, a reddish, slightly-raised sessile small nodule behind or lingual to the lower cuspid tooth.
RP = retrocuspid papilla

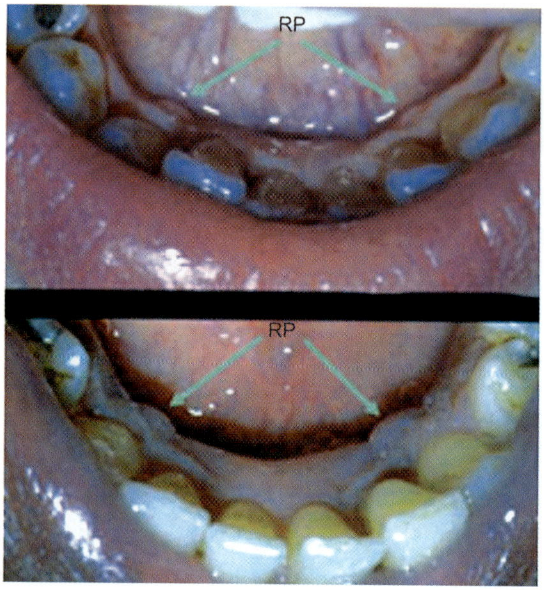

Fig. 3.31: Retrocuspid papillae in two patients. They are bilateral, (green arrows). They may be mistaken for disease.

RP = retrocuspid papilla

pink, nodules with a sessile base composed of normal collagen. They may be single or multiple and, if removed, may recur. But they are normal structures that can mimic disease.

Another condition to be found on the gingiva is gingival mandibular ridges. Found on the molar attached gingivae, they appear as small, white to pink, linear slightly raised lesions. With a similar histology to the retrocuspid papilla and the gingival nodule, they also are normal structures that can be mistaken for disease. Next, the teeth can be examined. One checks for any dental defect, malocclusion (Figs 3.32, 3.33), or missing teeth.

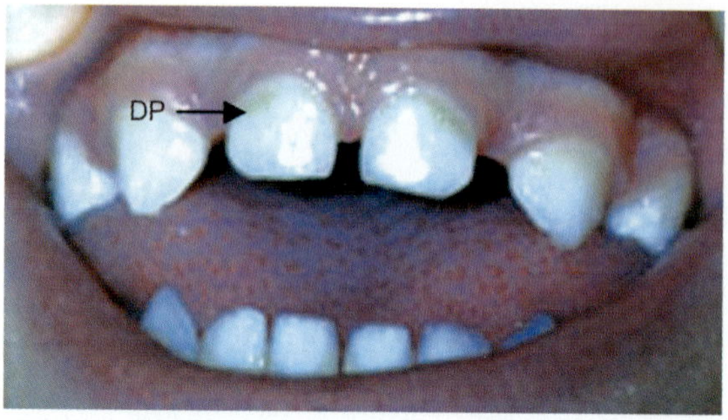

Fig. 3.32: Missing maxillary lateral incisors in a youngster. Also note the stained dental plaque (as pointed by the black arrow) at the cervical margins.

DP = dental plaque (stained)

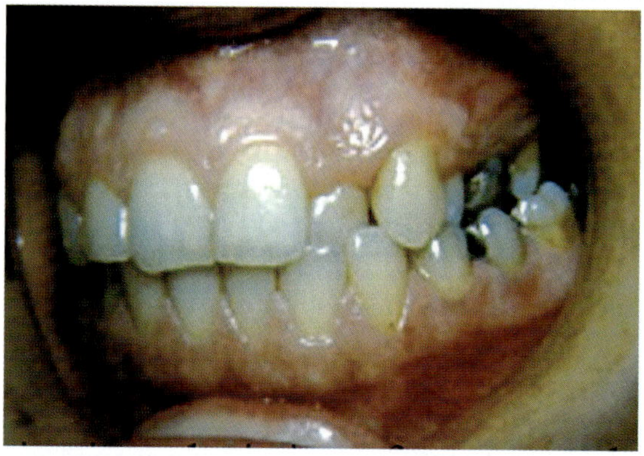

Fig. 3.33: Malocclusion with the maxillary left lateral and the posterior maxillary teeth in crossbite.

By doing a routine, methodical, systematic oral examination, deviations from normal should be observed. Astute observations lead to proper diagnosis and treatment.

DIFFERENTIAL DIAGNOSIS

Conditions which may Cause Pain

Pulpal disease, gingival and periodontal disease, tongue condition, salivary gland infection or inflammation, lesions of jaw bone, lymph node infections, myofascial pain disease, maxillary sinus disease are a few conditions which may cause pain.

Conditions which may Cause Burning Sensation in Oral Cavity

Burning mouth syndrome, neuroses, viral infections, vitamin deficiencies, xerostomia, anaemia are few of the conditions which may cause burning sensation in oral cavity.

Conditions which may be Associated with Bleeding

Gingivitis and periodontal disease, traumatic incidents including surgery, tumours, and deficiencies in haemostasis are few of the examples which may cause bleeding.

Conditions which may be Associated with Loose Teeth

Periodontal disease, trauma, normal resorption of deciduous teeth, malignant tumours, AIDS are few of the examples which may cause loosening of teeth.

Conditions Associated with Delayed Tooth Eruption

Malposed or impacted teeth, cysts, odontomes, sclerosed bone are few of the examples which may delay the eruption of teeth.

Conditions Associated with Dry Mouth

Local inflammation, infections and fibrosis of major salivary glands, drug therapy, autoimmune diseases, post radiation changes are few of the examples which may cause drying of the mouth.

Conditions which Present as a Swelling

Inflammations and infections, cysts, inflammatory hyperplasias, benign and malignant tumours may present as a swelling.

Conditions which Cause Bad Taste

Aging changes, heavy smoking, poor oral hygiene, dental caries, periodontal disease, ANUG, diabetes, uraemia are few of the conditions which may cause a bad taste.

Conditions which may Cause Halitosis

Poor oral hygiene, periodontal disease, decayed teeth, ANUG, oral cancer, spicy food, nasal infection, sinus infection, pharyngeal infection, uraemia are few of the examples which may cause halitosis.

Conditions which may Cause Paraesthesia and Anaesthesia

Injury to regional nerves, malignancies, medications, diabetes are few of the examples which may cause either paraesthesia or anaesthesia.

GENDER PREDILECTION OF SOFT TISSUE LESIONS

Male

Lymphoma, melanoma, metastatic carcinoma to cervical nodes, squamous cell carcinoma, verrucous carcinoma, erythema multiforme, leukoplakia, median rhomboid glossitis are few of the conditions which are more commonly seen in males.

Female

Geographic tongue, lichen planus, peripheral giant cell granuloma, pyogenic granuloma, recurrent aphthous ulcers are few of the conditions which are more commonly seen in females.

GENDER PREDISPOSITION OF BONY LESIONS

Male

Cancer of the alveolus, cherubism, eosinophilic granuloma, incisive canal cyst, osteoblastoma, osteoid osteoma, osteomyelitis, traumatic bone cyst are few of the conditions which are more commonly seen in males.

Female

Central giant cell granuloma, central haemangioma, periapical cemental dysplasia, secondary hyperparathyroidism are few of the conditions which are more commonly seen in females.

JAW BONE AND REGIONAL PREDILECTION OF BONY LESIONS

Mandible and Predominant Region

Ameloblastic fibroma, ameloblastoma, aneurysmal bone cyst, benign non odontogenic tumours, cancer, cementifyingfibroma, cherubism, odontogenic keratocyst, odontogenic myxoma, Pindborgs tumour, osteomyelitis are more commonly seen in the mandibular molar-ramus area.

Maxilla and Predominant Region

Adenomatoid odontogenic tumour is more commonly seen in the anterior maxillary region.

LABORATORY INVESTIGATIONS

Hematology

The routine blood examination consists of a hemoglobin and hematocrit determination and complete blood count (CBC), which includes the red blood cell count, white blood cell count, differential white cell count, an estimation of platelet number, and a description of the blood smear. Other determinations are performed when specifically indicated.

Hemoglobin (Hb)

Hemoglobin is the oxygen-carrying material found in red blood cells. In females, it is normally in the range of 12–16 gm/100 ml of blood and in males 14–18 gm/100 ml of blood.

Anaemia is present when there is a decrease in the normal amount of circulating haemoglobin. This reduction in haemoglobin may result from:

a. Blood loss; as is common in iron-deficiency anaemia.

b. From increased destruction of RBCs; as seen in haemolytic anaemias.

c. From decreased production of RBCs; as seen in pernicious and folic acid deficiency anaemias.

d. From combination of these three mechanisms.

Anaemias may be classified according to their pathophysiologic basis:

i. Size of RBCs; microcytic, macrocytic or normocytic.

ii. Haemoglobin concentration of the RBCs; normochromic, hyperchromic, hypochromic.

General symptoms of all anaemias include:

a. Pallor of the skin, palpebral conjunctiva and nail beds.
b. Dyspnoea
c. Easy fatiguability.[1]

Hematocrit (HCT)

Hematocrit is a measurement of the packed red cell volume in a volume of blood. It is a simple laboratory test and is easily reproducible. The normal value is between 37% and 47% for females and between 40% and 52% for males. The hematocrit is valuable in evaluating polycythemia, anemia, and blood loss. A rule of thumb is that a four point loss or gain in hematocrit is roughly equal to the loss or gain of one unit or 500 ml of blood.

Red Blood Cell Count (RBC)

The red blood cell count in adult males varies between 4.5 and 6.2 million cells/cu mm and in adult females between 4.5 and 5.5 million cells/cu mm. The red cell count provides a gross estimate of the body's oxygen carrying capacity and is used in figuring the red cell indices, which are important in the diagnosis of various types of anemia.

Red Cell Morphology

A well-prepared smear of the peripheral blood, usually stained with a poly-chrome stain such as Wright's stain, can give a vast amount of information concerning the morphology of the red blood cells. Some terms to describe alterations in size, shape and staining characteristics are as follows.

Normocytic: normal size red blood cell.

Macrocytic: large size red blood cell.

Microcytic: small size red blood cell.

Normochromic: normal haemoglobin content.

Hyperchromic: greater than normal haemoglobin content.

Hypochromic: smaller than normal haemoglobin content.

Anisocytosis: abnormal size of the red blood cells.

Poikilocytosis: abnormal shapes of the red blood cells and include such descriptive terms as burr cells, sickle cells, target cells, spherocytes and ovalocytes.

Target cells: they have a central area of haemoglobin with a pale zone around this and a normal staining periphery; found in sickle cell anaemia and iron deficiency anaemia.

Sickle cells: red blood cells are crescent shaped owing to the presence of abnormal haemoglobin S.

Burr cells: They have spiny crenated borders; usually result from technical problems in slide preparation but can be associated with advanced uremia.

Nucleated red blood cells: They are normally found in the peripheral blood of the newborn; beyond this age, abnormal finding in the peripheral blood representing an abnormally large demand on the bone marrow to produce red blood cells; associated with infections and hypoxic conditions.

Polychromasia: Describes the staining quality of some young, mature red blood cells and is due to a mixture of haemoglobin and retained nuclear material.

White Blood Cell Count (WBC)

The white blood cell count is an extremely valuable laboratory study when dealing with infections or other diseases such as leukemia that affect the white cell series. The normal white count is between 5000 and 10,000 white cells/cu mm. Values above 10,000 are referred to as a leukocytosis, and values below 5000 are referred to as a leucopenia.

Differential White Cell Count

The white blood cells are the mobile units of the body's protective system. They are formed partially in the bone marrow (the granulocytes and the monocytes and a few lymphocytes) and partially in the lymph tissue (lymphocytes and plasma cells). The real value of the white blood cells is that most of them are specifically transported to areas of serious inflammation, thereby providing a rapid and potent defence against any infectious agent. Six different types of white blood cells are normally found in the blood. These are polymorphonuclear neutrophils, polymorphonuclear eosinophils, polymorphonuclear basophils, monocytes, lymphocytes and plasma cells.

The differential white cell count is a cell type distribution of the total white blood cell count. On a well-prepared, Wright stained slide, 100 to 200 white cells are counted and the percent of each kind of cell is reported. The normal distribution of white cells is as follows: neutrophils 50% to 70%; lymphocytes 25% to 40%; monocytes 3% to 8%; eosinophils 1% to 4%; basophils 0% to 1% (Fig. 3.34).

Platelet Count

The normal platelet count is between 1,50,000 and 4,00,000 cells/cumm.

Platelet disorders may be divided into[1]:

a. Two categories by aetiology
   i. congenital
   ii. acquired
b. Two categories by type
   i. thrombocytopenias
   ii. thrombocytopathies.

Red Cell Indices

Red cell indices are very useful laboratory tools for measuring the size, shape, and hemoglobin content of the red cells. They utilize the hematocrit, hemoglobin, and red cell count determinations as a basis.

Mean Corpuscular Volume (MCV)

The mean corpuscular volume uses the hematocrit and red cell count to estimate the volume of the average red cell as shown by the following equation.

$$MCV = \frac{HCT \times 10}{RBC}$$

The normal range is 82 to 98 cuμ (cubic micron) values below the normal indicate microcytic anemias and values above indicate macrocytic type anemias. Normocytic anemias fall in the normal range.

Mean Corpuscular Hemoglobin (MCH)

The mean corpuscular hemoglobin uses the hemoglobin content and red blood cell count to estimate the hemoglobin content of the individual red blood cell, as shown by the following equation.

$$MCH = \frac{Hb \times 10}{RBC}$$

The normal range is 27 to 32 picograms with values above this being suggestive of

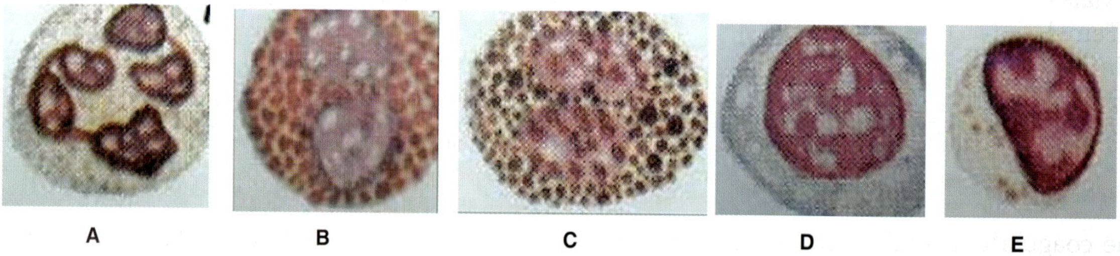

Fig. 3.34: Morphology of white blood cells. (A) Polymorphonuclear neutrophil, (B) Eosinophil, (C) Basophil, (D) Monocyte (E) Lymphocyte.

the microcytic anemias and values above being suggestive of the macrocytic type anemias.

Mean Corpuscular Hemoglobin Concentration (MCHC)

The mean corpuscular hemoglobin concentration estimates the average amount of hemoglobin in 100 ml of packed red blood cells by using the hemoglobin and hematocrit determinations, as shown by the following equation.

$$MCHC = \frac{Hb \times 10}{HCT}$$

The normal range is 32 to 38 gm/100 ml. The MCHC is only elevated in hereditary spherocytosis and decreased in the microcytic type anemias.

Reticulocyte Count

Reticulocytes are an immature form of red blood cell that represent a stage between the nucleated red blood cell and the mature red blood cell.Normally they account for 0.5 % to 1.5% of red blood cells counted. Reticulocytes are found in large numbers when red cell formation is increased and are associated with the treatment of various anemias and blood loss.

Sedimentation Rate (SR)

It is a nonspecific test. It can be measured by the Westergren's method or the Wintrobe's method.

Westergren's method

Males	0–15 mm/hr
Females	0–20 mm/hr

Wintrobe's method

Males	0–9 mm/hr
Females	0–20 mm/hr

COAGULATION TESTS

The coagulation mechanism originates from two pathways, the extrinsic and intrinsic, which then lead to the conversion of prothrombin to thrombin through the common pathway. Thrombin, in turn, activates fibrinogen to fibrin.

The following is a list of coagulation factors:

Factor I	Fibrinogen
Factor II	Prothrombin
Factor III	Tissue thromboplastin
Factor IV	Calcium
Factor V	Accelerator globulin (AcG), Proaccelerin
Factor VII	Serum prothrombin conversion accelerator (SPCA)
Factor VIII	Antihemophilic globulin (AHG)
Factor IX	Plasma thromboplastin component (PTC; Christmas factor)
Factor X	Stuart-Prower factor
Factor XI	Plasma thromboplastin antecedent (PTA)
Factor XII	Hageman factor
Factor XIII	Fibrin stabilizing factor (FSF)

In order to evaluate the competency of these various pathways, a coagulation profile, including a prothrombin time, partial thromboplastin time, platelet count, bleeding time, and fibrinogen concentration, is ordered.

Prothrombin Time (PT)

The prothrombin time measures the extrinsic and common pathways. It also measures the metabolic aspects of protein synthesis in the liver.[1] The normal values are reported in either seconds or percentages. If the values are reported in seconds, the laboratory will give the patient's prothrombin time over the control time, with the normal range being between 11 and 15 seconds. If it is reported in percentages the normal range is between 70% and 100%.The prothrombin time is prolonged in factor I, II, V, and VII and X deficiencies.

INR (international normalized ratio)[1]: Because of individual laboratory reagent variability and the desire to be able to reliably compare the PT from one laboratory to that of another, the PT is now commonly reported with it's INR. The INR, introduced by the World Health Organisation in 1983, is the ratio of PT that adjusts for the sensitivity of thromboplastin reagents, such that the normal coagulation profile is reported as an INR of 1.0.

Partial Thromboplastin Time (PTT)

The partial thromboplastin time measures the intrinsic and common pathways. The normal values are between 25 and 40 seconds.The partial thromboplastin time is prolonged in factor VIII IX, XI and XII deficiencies and in deficiencies of those factors necessary for the common pathway I, II, V, and X. The partial thromboplastin time is also prolonged in patients undergoing heparin therapy.

The aPTT is considered normal if the control aPTT and the test aPTT are within 10 seconds of each other. The unactivated PTT was originally described by Langdell and associates in 1953 as a simple one-stage assay for measuring factor VIII. Since the addition of the activator (a rare earth), the test no longer measures factors XI and XII.[1]

Platelet Count

The normal platelet count is between 150,000 and 400,000 cells/cu mm. Bleeding from thrombocytopenia rarely occurs until the count is below 60,000/cu mm.

Bleeding Time

The bleeding time, although difficult to standardize and reproduce, nevertheless gives some information concerning vascular and platelet interaction. Bleeding time can be checked by the Ivy's method and the template method.

Ivy's method	2–7 min.
Template method	2.5–9.5 min.

Bleeding time is usually prolonged in thrombocytopenia, von Willebrand's disease, and disorders of platelet function.

Fibrinogen

The normal level of fibrinogen is between 200 and 400 mg%.

However bleeding does not usually ensue until a level of 100 mg% is reached.

Tourniquet Test (Rumpel-Leede)

The tourniquet test is a crude test used to study the capillary-platelet interphase. Classically the study consists of placing a blood pressure cuff on the upper arm and leaving it inflated for 5 minutes halfway between the patient's systolic and diastolic pressures. A positive test shows more than five petechiae in a 2.5 cm circle on the forearm in males and more than 10 petechiae in females. The test is not used routinely because of its poor correlation with the platelet count and the fact that petechiae are usually present in thrombocytopenia.

Clot Retraction

Clot retraction represents a complex interaction between platelets, fibrin and trapped red blood cells. The normal range for clot retaction is 48% to 64%. Clot retraction is deficient with thrombocytopenia and circulating fibrinolysins.

Clotting Time

If the blood sample is drawn cleanly and there is no tissue thromboplastin contamination, the clotting time should measure the intrinsic and common pathways.The chief use for the clotting time is in the management of heparin therapy. The normal range for the clotting time is 4 to 10 minutes.

Thromboplastin Generation Time

The thromboplastin generation test is used to differentiate specific factor deficiencies in the intrinsic and common pathways , namely, factors VIII, IX, XI, XII, V and X.The normal range is 12 seconds or less.

Prothrombin Consumption Test

The prothrombin consumption test measures the same factors as the thromboplastin generation test but it is less sensitive and will not pick up mild factor deficiencies.The normal value is 20 seconds or longer.

BLOOD CHEMISTRY

The SMA-12 (Sequential Multiple Analyzer-12) is a biochemical survey of 12 blood constituents that help in screening patients for a variety of diseases. The tests vary somewhat in different hospitals. Some substitute the electrolytes for uric acid, phosphorus, cholesterol, and glutamic pyruvic transaminase, and include a bilirubin determination. In screening for specific diseases or following their clinical course individual tests should be ordered.

Albumin

The normal value for albumin is between 3.5 and 5 gm/100 ml. Increase in serum albumin is most often associated with dehydration. Decreases in serum albumin are associated with kidney diseases such as nephrosis and chronic glomerulonephritis, gastrointestinal diseases such as ulcerative colitis and protein losing enteropathy, and liver diseases such as Laennec's cirrhosis and hepatocellular damage secondary to hepatitis. Decreases are also found in some of collagen diseases and in lymphatic and myelogenous leukemia.

Calcium

The normal value for serum calcium is between 8.5 and 10.5 mg/100 ml. Increased levels are associated most commonly with excessive osteolysis such as occur in hyperparathyroidism and malignancy with bone metastasis. Decreased levels are associated with hypoparathyroidism, tetany, hypoalbuminemia, acute pancreatitis, renal failure, and starvation. *Since one-third to one-half of serum calcium is bound to protein- the total protein and serum albumin levels must be known before serum calcium levels can be interpreted.*

Phosphorus

The normal value for serum phosphorus is between 2.5 and 4.5 mg/100 ml.Increased levels are associated with hypoparathyroidism, secondary hyperparathyroidism caused by chronic renal failure, and metabolic acidosis. Decreased levels are associated with primary hyperparathyroidism, vitamin D deficiency, malabsorption diseases, and chronic antacid usage. A high phosphorous and low glucose level may be an artifact associated with an unrefrigerated sample.

Cholesterol

The normal cholesterol value is between 150 and 300 mg/100 ml. Increased levels are associated with idiopathic hypercholesterolaemia and secondary hypercholesterolaemia caused by nephrosis, chronic obstructive biliary disease, hypothyroidism and diabetes. Decreased levels are associated with hyperthyroidism, malnutrition and severe liver damage.

Recent data emphasize the advantage in knowing the concentrations of lipid subfractions such as low-density lipoprotein (LDL) and high density lipoprotein (HDL) in addition to total cholesterol. The concentration of serum HDL concentration is inversely related with coronary heart disease (CHD) incidence. Data from the Framingham Heart study suggest that the risk for myocardial infarction (MI) increases by about 25% for every 5mg/dL decrement below median values for men and women.[1]

Glucose

The normal glucose value is between 65 and 110 mg/100 ml. Increased levels are associated with diabetes mellitus, Cushing's disease, acromegaly, stress that increases the endogenous output of epinephrine and glucocorticoids, pheochromocytoma, acute and chronic pancreatitis, pancreatectomy, and hyperthyroidism. Decreased levels are associated with hypoglycemic medications, islet cell tumors of the pancreas, advanced cirrhosis or hepatitis, early diabetes mellitus, Addison's disease, functional hypoglycemia, and certain inborn errors of metabolism such as hereditary fructose intolerance, galactosemia, and maple syrup urine disease.

Uric Acid

The normal uric acid value is between 2.5 and 8 mg/100 ml. Increased levels are associate with gout, renal failure, diets high in nucleoproteins, and diseases associated with increased breakdown of nucleoproteins such as leukemia, multiple myeloma, lymphoma, and haemoltic anaemia.When hyperuricemia is associated with hypercholesterolemia, the incidence of myocardial infarction secondary to coronary artery disease is increased.

Creatinine

The normal value is between 0.7 and 1.4 mg/100ml. Increases are associated with impaired kidney function and muscle diseases. Serum creatinine varies inversely with the glomerular filtration rate and is a more sensitive indicator of this rate than blood urea nitrogen test.

Creatinine clearance test: The glomerular filtration rate assesses the amount of functioning renal tissue and can be calculated indirectly by the endogenous creatinine clearance test. Creatinine is a breakdown product of muscle, liberated from muscle tissue and excreted from urine at a constant rate of 0.7–1.5 mg/dL. Creatinine is 100% filtered by the glomerulus and is not reabsorbed by the tubules. Although a very small amount is secreted by the tubule, the creatinine clearance test is an effective way to estimate the glomerular filtration rate (GFR). The creatinine clearance test is performed by collecting a 24-hour urine specimen and a blood sample in the 24 hour period. *The most accurate way to measure the GFR is the inulin clearance test.*

Alkaline Phosphatase

The normal adult alkaline phosphatase value is between 20 and 48 I mU/ml (1.5 to 4.5 Bodansky units; 4 to 13 King-Armstrong units). In the child the values are higher (5 to 14 Bodansky units; 15 to 30 King-Armstrong units). Increases in this enzyme are associated with hepatic obstruction, either intrahepatic or extrahepatic secondary to infection or tumor. The enzyme is also elevated as a result of osteoblastic activity associated with Paget's disease, hyperparathyroidism, osteoblastic tumors of bone, and osteogenesis imperfecta. The differentiation of hepatic and bone origin of alkaline phosphatase can be accomplished by analysis of the isoenzymes. Decreases are associated with hypophosphatasia, hypothyroidism, and malnutrition.

Lactic Dehydrogenase (LDH)

The normal value of lactic dehydrogenase is between 90 and 200 mU/ml. Serum lactic dehydrogenase is a ubiquitous enzyme found in many tissues, including kidney, heart, skeletal muscle, liver, red and white blood cells, and skin. It is increased in various malignancies, inflammations, necrotic processes, and infections. Some of the most common diseases that are associated with increases in the enzyme are myocardial infarction, where the enzyme may remain elevated for 10 to 14 days, pulmonary embolus and pulmonary infarction, hepatitis, leukemia, lymphoma, and congestive heart failure. The enzyme has been divided into five isoenzymes that often can be used to identify the tissue of origin.

Glutamic Oxaloacetic Transaminase (SGOT)

The normal serum value of SGOT is between 10 and 50 mU/ml. Like LDH,SGOT is found in many tissues, including heart, kidney, liver, skeletal muscle, and pancreas. The enzyme remains elevated in myocardial infarction from about 12 hours to 3 to 5 days. High elevations are also found in hepatitis, with moderate elevations occurring in cirrhosis and liver neoplasms. Slight elevations are seen with muscular trauma and after surgery.

Glutamic Pyruvic Transaminase (SGPT)

The normal serum value of SGPT is between 6 and 36 mU/ml. The values generally parallel those for SGOT but are more elevated in liver damage than myocardial damage.

OTHER BLOOD DETERMINATIONS

Blood Urea Nitrogen (BUN)

The normal value is between 10 and 20 mg/100 ml. Increases are associated with a decrease in the glomerular filtration rate (GFR); however, an approximately 30% to 40% decrease in GFR is needed before the BUN becomes elevated. Increases can also be associated with pre- and postrenal azotemia. Decreased levels are associated with advanced liver disease and low protein diets.

Bilirubin

Bilirubin is a breakdown product of hemoglobin. Its measurement is therefore important in evaluating for hemolytic anemias. Since it is removed from the blood by the liver through a process of conjugation to protein, it is also an important measure of hepatic function.

Bilirubin is measured in two forms: direct (conjugated) and total (conjugated and unconjugated). The difference between total and direct bilirubin represents the unconjugated form (indirect). Determining the type responsible for elevation of total bilirubin helps distinguish between hepatocellular and obstructive forms of liver disease.

The normal serum contains less than 0.8 mg of total bilirubin/100 ml. Of this, no more than 0.3 mg is unconjugated.

The hyperbilirubinemia may affect the developing teeth during the neonatal period. The two most common causes are *erythroblastosis fetalis* and *biliary atresia.*

The extent of dental changes correlates with the period of hyperbilirubinemia, and most patients' exhibit involvement limited to the primary dentition. Occasionally the cusps of the permanent first molars may be affected. In addition to enamel hypoplasia, the affected teeth frequently demonstrate a green discolouration *(chorodontia).*[2]

Acid Phosphatase

The normal value of acid phosphatase is between 0.5 and 11 mU/ml (0.13 to 0.63 Sigma units). The prostate is rich in acid phosphatase and small amounts are also found in red blood cells, bone, kidney, liver and spleen. An increase in acid phosphatase usually indicates that a carcinoma of the prostate has metastasized, especially to bone.

Amylase

The normal value of amylase is between 60 and 150 Somogyi units/100 ml. Increases are most often associated with diseases of the pancreas, such as acute pancreatitis, recurrent bouts of chronic pancreatitis, pancreatic duct obstruction secondary to a carcinoma, or spasm resulting from the use of opiates. Increases may also occur with salivary gland disease, bowel obstruction and upper gastrointestinal surgery.

Glucose Tolerance Test (GTT)

When elevated glucose levels are found in

the blood and/or urine, the glucose tolerance test (GTT) may be used to diagnose diabetes mellitus. This test is started with a patient who has been fasting overnight. After the patient ingests a glucose load, blood and urine specimens are taken at 30 minutes, 1 hour, $1^1/2$ hours, 2 hours, and 3 hours. Specimens are also taken prior to glucose ingestion.

The normal value for fasting blood sugar is between 65 and 110 mg/100 ml, with the fasting urine negative for glucose. From here the glucose level will climb to 160 mg/100 ml or less within 30 minutes to 1 hour, with a gradual decrease and return to fasting levels or slightly below at the 2 hour interval and a leveling off at the 3 hour interval. Urine samples are negative for glucose at the same time intervals. The diabetic curve may show the fasting blood level at or near the upper limits of normal. Following the test dose, blood values do not come back to normal before the 2 hour interval. The 1 and 2 hour values are over 160 mg/100 ml,with the urine samples also positive for glucose at these intervals.

Creatine Phosphokinase (CPK)

The normal values range between 5 and 50 I mU/ml. Like other tissue enzymes, CPK is found in striated muscle, heart, and brain. Elevation of CPK with myocardial infarction generally parallels that of SGOT, rising quickly and peaking in 1 to 2 days. Increases are also associated with cerebral infarction. An association between increased CPK levels and malignant hyperthermia has been described.

Serologic Tests for Syphilis

A number of screening tests for syphilis are available, which, if positive, must be further tested against more specific antigens. Examples of screening tests are the Venereal Disease Research Laboratory (VDRL), Kahn, and Hinton tests. These tests. may give false positive results with lupus erythematosus, leprosy, malaria, infectious mononucleosis, hepatitis A, rheumatoid arthritis, and in narcotic addicts. More specific tests are the Reiter, *Treponema pallidum immobilization* (TPI), and fluorescent treponemal antibody absorption (FTA-ABS) tests. The last is the most sensitive test.

Viral Hepatitis

Viral hepatitis is of particular concern to the dental practitioner because of the potential for infection of the dentist and dental staff. Consequently, the practitioner must fully understand the epidemiologic and clinical courses of the various types of viral hepatitis so that each patient who gives a positive history of hepatitis A, B, C, D, E, F, or G can be fully assessed.

Hepatitis A

Hepatitis A (infectious hepatitis) is caused by an RNA virus known as hepatitis A virus. Transmission occurs via faecal-oral route usually through contaminated food or water. Although HAV is usually not detectable in the serum, shortly after the appearance of clinical symptoms, there is a rising titer of hepatitis A antibody (anti-HAV). The anti-HAV initially consists mainly of immunoglobulin M (IgM), but after approximately 6 months it is replaced by immunoglobulin G (IgG). Thus the presence of anti-HAV IgM indicates acute HAV infection.

Hepatitis B

Hepatitis B (serum hepatitis) is caused by a DNA virus known as hepatitis B virus. The major mode of transmission of HBV is the parenteral route (e.g. blood, blood products, and contaminated needles). The HBsAg is accompanied by anti-HBc; anti-HBc is more likely present in chronic persistent hepatitis and HBeAg in chronic active hepatitis. The former is more common than the latter, but a liver biopsy is often necessary to make the diagnosis.

Hepatitis C

It was formerly known as *blood-borne* non-A, non-B *hepatitis.* An RNA virus causes this disease and has been coded as *hepatitis C virus.* At least four different strains of the hepatitis C virus have been identified in different countries. The principal mode of transmission for HCV is the parenteral route. Type C disease thus occurs frequently in many of the same groups as hepatitis B: recipients of blood or blood products, patients on renal dialysis, certain health care professionals, and intravenous drug users. As in hepatitis B, another route is through sexual contact. The clinical features of acute hepatitis C are usually less severe than those of hepatitis A or hepatitis B. After the incubation period (which averages 6 to 8 weeks for posttransfusion hepatitis), acute hepatitis C often has insidious prodromal and icteric phases. First- and second-generation serologic antibody tests are available for identification of HCV infections. These include enzyme immunoassays (EIA-1 and EIA-2) and recombinant immunoblot assays (RIBA-1 and RIBA-2).Unfortunately, because of problems with sensitivity or selectivity, none is diagnostic by itself; a second type of test must confirm the diagnosis. The polymerase chain reaction test is specific for HCV RNA and can positively identify HCV infection, but this test is complicated and not routinely available.

Delta Hepatitis/Hepatitis D

A potential complication of HBV infection is the development of delta hepatitis.It is caused by a RNA agent that requires the presence of HBsAg to replicate. The combined effects of HBV infection and acute delta hepatitis are associated with fulminant hepatitis 10 times more frequently than with HBV infection alone and results in an increased mortality rate. This may be associated with severe, progressive liver disease. Recovery from hepatitis B, with loss of HBsAg, also signals recovery from delta hepatitis. Individuals with anti-HBs are also immune to HDV infection.

Hepatitis E

The virus formerly recognized as causing enterically transmitted non-A, non-B hepatitis has been isolated and coded as hepatitis E virus (HEV), an RNA virus. Transmission commonly occurs through fecally contaminated drinking water, and outbreaks have occurred in developing countries. The disease usually follows a benign pattern like HAV, with a mortality rate of 1% to 2%, which increases to 20% to 40% in pregnant women. Serologic tests such as EIA and polymerase chain reaction assays of RNA are now available for HEV.

Hepatitis F and G

There is some evidence of the existence of other unidentified hepatitis viruses, perhaps other enterically transmitted non-A, non-B agents, and these have been arbitrarily assigned as F and G.

Iron

The normal value for iron range between 50 and 175 pg/100 ml, with males being slightly higher than females in this range. Serum iron is available for the formation of hemoglobin. Increases are associated with hemolytic anemias, hemochromatosis, and pernicious anemia. Decreased levels are found in iron deficiency anemias and anemias secondary to chronic infections

Total Iron Binding Capacity (TIBC)

The normal value is between 250 and 410 µg/100 ml. Increases are found in iron deficiency anemias and anemias secondary to blood loss. Decreased levels are associated with chronic infection and liver disease.

Serum Osmolality

The normal values for serum osmolality range between 275 and 295 mOsm/L. Serum osmolality measures the total concentration of all particles in solution whether they are electrolytes or not. Increases are associated with excessive water loss, chronic renal disease with a rising BUN, increasing serum glucose levels secondary to diabetes mellitus, and diabetes insipidus. Decreases are associated with inappropriate antidiuretic hormone secretion (IADH) and Addison's disease.

Carbon Dioxide (CO_2)

The normal value is between 24 and 32 mEq/L and reflects the amount of carbonic acid and bicarbonate in the blood. In acid-base balance, the CO_2 level must be evaluated in light of the other electrolytes and blood gases. In general, the bicarbonate level will be decreased in metabolic acidosis and respiratory alkalosis and increased in metabolic alkalosis and respiratory acidosis. This will be reflected by similar changes in CO_2 content of the blood.

SERUM ELECTROLYTES

Sodium (Na)

The normal values of sodium range between 135 and 145 mEq/L. Hyponatremia is associated with cirrhosis, congestive heart failure, adrenal insufficiency, nephrosis, excessive use of diuretics, inappropriate antidiuretic hormone secretion, and water intoxication. Hypernatremia is usually caused by excessive loss of water in vomiting, diarrhea, severe sweating, and diabetes mellitus.

Potassium (K)

The normal value of potassium is between 3.2 and 5.5 mEq/L. Hypokalemia is usually associated with inadequate intake or losses from the gastrointestinal or the urinary tracts. The latter include vomiting, diarrhea, nasogastric suction, and use of diuretic medications. Hyperkalemia is associated with release of cellular potassium secondary to surgery, crush injuries, hemolysis of red blood cells, renal failure, and acidosis.

Chloride (Cl)

The normal value of chloride is between 95 and 105 mEq/L. Serum chloride levels usually follow those for serum sodium; however, chloride will be reduced in vomiting.

Magnesium (Mg)

The normal value of magnesium is between 1.5 and 2 mEq/L. Increases can be associated with renal failure and large doses of antacids that contain magnesium. Decreases are associated with alcoholism, diabetic acidosis, malabsorption, hypocalcemia, and hypokalemia.

LIPID PROFILE

Hyperlipoproteinemias can be subdivided into five types. In order to clinically distinguish these five types, a serum cholesterol, serum triglyceride level, and lipoprotein electrophoresis should be obtained.

Cholesterol

The normal cholesterol value is between 150 and 300 mg/100 ml. Increased levels are associated with idiopathic hypercholesterolaemia and secondary hypercholesterolaemia caused by nephrosis, chronic obstructive biliary disease, hypothyroidism and diabetes. Decreased levels are associated with hyperthyroidism, malnutrition and severe liver damage.

Triglycerides

The normal value of triglycerides ranges between 35 and 150 mg/100 ml of blood. Increased levels are associated with congenital hyperlipidemia, nephrotic syndrome, diabetes mellitus, and myocardial infarction.

Lipoprotein Electrophoresis

The electrophoretic pattern consists of an alpha band, a prebeta band, and a beta band. Chylomicrons are not present on electrophoresis in normal patients but are present in type I and II hyperlipoproteinemias.

IMMUNOGLOBULINS

IgG

The normal value of IgG is between 800 and 1500 mg/100 ml of blood. IgG forms about 73% of the immunoglobulins in normal serum. Increased levels are found in cirrhosis of the liver. Decreased levels are found in the nephrotic syndrome and in the antibody deficiency syndromes.

IgM

The normal value of IgM is between 50 and 120 mg/100 ml of blood. IgM forms about 7% of the total immunoglobulins in normal serum and is efficient in stimulating agglutination and phagocytosis.

IgA

The normal value of IgA is between 40 and 120 mg/100 ml of blood. IgA forms about 19% of the total immunoglobulins. IgA is found mainly in external secretions such as saliva, intestinal tract secretions, respiratory tract secretions, and lacrimal and nasal secretions. It appears that its main role is in the prevention of infections in various mucosal membranes.

BLOOD GASES

Blood gas determinations help in evaluation of acid-base balance and the degree of oxygenation. The studies are usually done on an arterial blood sample, but venous blood may be used. In addition to measurement of actual blood gases, determination of related factors such as pH and CO_2 combining power and calculation of blood bicarbonate and base excess permit identification of the clinical cause of acid-base disturbances and monitoring of subsequent treatment.

pH

The normal value for arterial pH is 7.40 with a range of 7.35 to 7.45. With venous blood the normal value is 7.36 with a range of 7.31 to 7.41. The acidity or alkalinity of the blood is measured by the pH. Values less than 7.35 indicate acidosis and those greater than 7.45 indicate alkalosis.

PCO_2

The normal value for arterial blood ranges between 35 and 45 mm Hg and for venous blood between 41 and 51 mm Hg. PCO_2 refers to the pressure of dissolved CO_2 in the blood and is influenced by the lungs; increases secondary to hypoventilation represent respiratory acidosis and decreases secondary to hyperventilation represent respiratory alkalosis.

Actual Bicarbonate (HCO_3)

Bicarbonate can be calculated from the Henderson-Hasselbalch equation if the pH and PCO_2 are known. The normal values for both arterial and venous blood are 22 to 26 mEq/L. HCO_3 is not regulated by respiratory processes but is controlled by metabolic processes. Increases in the HCO_3 level are therefore associated with metabolic alkalosis and decreases are associated with metabolic acidosis.

Carbon Dioxide Combining Power (CCP)

The carbon dioxide combining power of the blood is an indicator of the state of acid-base balance. Since all but about 5% of the CO_2 derived from bicarbonate, it is actually a measure of alkaline reserve. The normal range is from 55 to 75 ml of CO_2/100 ml of plasma (24 to 29 mEq/L). Acidosis is shown by a decrease in CO_2 combining power and alkalosis by an increase.

Base Excess

Base excess is another calculated value used to determine the state of acid-base balance. It represents the difference between theoretical and actual total CO_2 content of the blood. Normally it should be 0 with a range of ± 2 mEq/L for either arterial or venous blood. A negative value below this signifies bicarbonate deficit and a positive value indicates bicarbonate excess. Therefore positive numbers represent metabolic alkalosis and negative values represent metabolic acidosis.

PO_2

The normal value for arterial PO_2 is between 80 and 100 mm Hg and for venous blood between 35 and 40 mm Hg. Decreased level of PO_2 is associated with various degrees of hypoxia and may be associated with respiratory acidosis secondary to impaired diffusion or shunting. Normal levels of PO_2 may be present in metabolic acidosis and alkalosis.

O_2 Saturation

The normal value for arterial O_2 saturation is between 95% and 98% and for venous blood between 60% and 85%.

URINALYSIS

The urine analysis consists of a gross, chemical, and microscopic examination.

Gross Examination

Color

The color of urine varies with its dilution and endogenous and exogenous pigment content. The normal color of urine is straw to amber; dilute urine is almost colorless, and concentrated urine is yellow to dark yellow. Examples of abnormal endogenous pigments are hemoglobin, which turns urine a red or reddish brown color; bilirubin, which turns it a greenish orange; urobilin, which turns it an orange-brown; and homogentisic acid, which turns it a brown to black color on standing. Red blood cells will give urine a smoky red to brown color. Examples of exogenous pigments that change the color of urine are beets, which turn urine red, and rhubarb, which turns it a yellow-brown.

Appearance

Normal urine is usually clear; however, amorphous phosphates and urates may form a whitish sediment. Bacteria can cause cloudy urine and pus will usually give a white mucoid-like sediment.

Odor

Normal urine has a faint aromatic odor that is not unpleasant. If urine is allowed to stand without being refrigerated, the odor becomes heavy and unpleasant secondary to bacterial overgrowth. Odors from asparagus and fecal contamination are also characteristic.

Specific Gravity

The specific gravity of urine depends on the state of hydration of the patient. In a dilute sample from a well-hydrated patient, the specific gravity will be under 1.010. In a concentrated sample (dehydrated patient), the specific gravity is usually above 1.020. Solutes such as protein and glucose will also elevate the specific gravity and should be suspected when there are high values.

Chemical Examination

pH

Normal urine is usually acid, being in the range of 4.8 to 7.5. Acid urine results from the normal ability of the renal tubules to exchange hydrogen ions for sodium ions. Urine allowed to stand may become alkaline secondary to the liberation of ammonia by bacteria that split urea.

Protein

Normally the kidney tubules will reabsorb most of the protein in the glomerular filtrate. Approximately 30 to 100 mg of protein are lost in 24 hours. Increased transient losses of protein normally occur after strenuous exertion, in orthostatic proteinuria, and with fevers. Pathologic conditions that cause a constant proteinuria are hypertension, congestive heart failure, glomerulonephritis, pyelonephritis and the nephrotic syndrome.

Glucose

The normal renal threshold is approximately 180 mg/100 ml of blood sugar. When this level is exceeded, glucose will appear in the urine. Glucosuria associated with hyperglycemia is usually secondary to diabetes mellitus but will also be seen with dextrose infusion, Cushing's disease, pheochromocytoma, ingestion of large amounts of glucose, stress, and increased intracranial pressure.

Ketone

Acetone, acetoacetic acid, and betahydroxybutyric acid are known as ketone bodies and are the breakdown products of fat metabolism. Increased ketone levels are found in diabetic ketoacidosis; starvation; fever; high fat, low carbohydrate diets; and dehydration.

Hemoglobin

Hemoglobinuria is the result of red cell hemolysis in the blood or in the urine specimen. Hemoglobinuria is found with hemolytic anemias and incompatible blood transfusions.

Bilirubin

Bilirubin in the urine is an indication of liver disease. Conjugated, direct acting bilirubin, when present in the urine, is usually associated with extrahepatic and intrahepatic obstruction and hepatocellular disease.

Urobilinogen

The normal value of urobilinogen is 1 Ehrlich unit or less in 2 hours or 0.5 to 4 units (0.05 to 2.5 mg) in 24 hours. Increased levels are associated with hepatocellular disease, whereas decreased levels are associated with obstructive jaundice.

Bence-Jones Protein

Bence-Jones protein is an abnormal protein that is found 20% to 50% of the time in the urine of patients with multiple myeloma. It is also seen in patients with polychythemia vera and leukemia.

Microscopic Examination

White Blood Cells

Occasionally white blood cells are found in the urinary sediment, with 1 to 5 white cells per high-power field being considered within normal limits. An increased urinary WBC count is usually suggestive of urinary tract infection.

Red Blood Cells

The normal range is from 0 to 1 cell per high power field. An increased red cell count, when not associated with menstrual flow, is usually associated with glomerulonephritis, renal infarction, nephrolithiasis, urethritis, prostatitis, blood dyscrasias, anticoagulant therapy, or excessive physical exertion.

Epithelial Cells

Renal cells are indicative of kidney damage, whereas transitional cells indicate possible pathologic conditions in the renal pelvis, ureter, or bladder. Squamous cells originate from the superficial layers of the urethra and vagina and are of little diagnostic importance.

Casts

Casts are composed of protein material alone or a combination of protein material and cells. They are called casts because their shape is a replica of the internal diameter of the distal and collecting renal tubules where they are formed. There are three types: hyaline, blood, and epithelial. Hyaline casts occur with intrinsic renal disease, heart failure, shock, fever, and excessive exercise. The presence of red blood cell casts indicates glomerular damage or ruptured tubules. White blood cell casts are associated with renal infections. Epithelial cell casts usually indicate heavy metal poisoning, advanced glomerulonephritis pyelonephritis, or malignant nephrosclerosis.

Crystals

The significance of crystals in the urine is not great—depending on the urinary pH, various crystals may be precipitated. Their main importance is when one suspects nephrolithiasis or gout.

FECAL EXAMINATION

Occult Blood

Blood in the stool is abnormal. The guaiac test is used to reveal blood that is not visible on gross examination. Usually bleeding from the upper gastrointestinal tract will produce black "tarry" colored stools, whereas bleeding from the lower gastrointestinal tract will usually show gross blood in the stool. The guaiac test is particularly useful in examining for asymptomatic lesions of the gastrointestinal tract.

Urobilinogen

The normal value of urobilinogen is between 40 and 300 mg/24-hour sample. Increased levels are due to hemolytic anemias, while decreased levels are associated with hepatic obstruction or hepatocellular disease and antibiotics that destroy, the intestinal flora.

MICROBIOLOGIC EXAMINATIONS

Specimens from the oral cavity must be taken very carefully so as not to contaminate them with extraneous oral flora. For aerobic cultures, the swab must be placed directly in the lesion, wound, or fluid. Specimens from an abscess that are to be cultured anaerobically can be taken by cleaning the oral mucosa or skin, placing a needle into the abscess and withdrawing some material, then corking the needle and sending the needle and syringe to the laboratory.

Smears

The material being submitted should be smeared on a glass slide and stained in an attempt to identify the type of organism. The routine stains include Gram stain, acid-fast stain, and stains for fungus.

Cultures

Routine cultures are done for aerobic, anaerobic, and acid-fast organisms as well as for fungi.

Antibiotic Sensitivity Test

The most widely used technique is the disc method; in which the organism(s) cultured from the original specimen are grown in the presence of antibiotic-impregnated disc. The discs that develop a wide zone of bacterial inhibition around them indicate that the organism is sensitive to that antibiotic.

RADIOLOGICAL INVESTIGATIONS

The face and jaws present unusual difficulties in radiographic examination. To overcome these problems a great many special projections have been devised with which the oral and maxillofacial surgeon should be familiar. The radiographic examination is of great value in diagnosis. It gives evidence of abnormalities of the anatomic structure of the bones and discloses changes in their architecture and alterations in their radiability. Its diagnostic value, however, is often considerably overestimated because it does not show disease-radiographs only portray the effects of pathologic processes on the bone.

The relationship of lesions to other structures, such as foramina, nerve canals, the roots of the teeth, and the nasal cavity and accessory sinuses, is easily determined by radiographic examination.

It should be remembered, however, that radiographs are two-dimensional pictures and that a structure may appear involved by a lesion when actually it lies in front or behind; likewise a highly calcified structure, normal or abnormal, may hide a smaller defect.

PRINCIPLES OF RADIOGRAPHIC INTERPRETATION

Radiographs are advised when the surgeon thinks that they are likely to offer useful diagnostic information that will influence the treatment plan. Often some clinical sign or symptom from the patients history indicates the need for a radiologic examination. This clinical information should be used first to select the type of radiographs and later to aid in their interpretation.

An insufficient number or inadequate quality of the radiographs limits the information available for diagnostic imaging. As the surgeon is responsible for both prescribing and interpreting radiographs, inadequate films should be recognized and supplemental images obtained before proceeding with the analysis.

VIEWING CONDITIONS

Ideally viewing conditions should include the following characteristics:

a. Ambient light in the viewing room should be reduced.
b. Intraoral radiographs should be mounted in a film holder.
c. Light from the view box should be of equal intensity across the viewing surface.
d. The size of the view box should accomodate the size of the film.If the viewing area is larger than the film, an opaque mask should be used to eliminate all light from around the periphery of the film.
e. An intense light source is essential for evaluating dark regions of the film.
f. A magnifying glass allows detailed examination of small regions of the film.

The first step in image analysis is to use a systematic approach to identify all the normal anatomy present in an image or set of images.

First examine the bone. Identify all anatomic landmarks appropriate for the region. Also examine the character of the trabecular bone. Compare the same areas on adjacent images and with the corresponding area on images of the other side.

Next make a second visual circuit through all the images, examining the bone of the alveolar process. Examine in particular the height of the alveolar crest relative to the teeth and its cortication. Examine the trabecular pattern of the alveolar process. The lamina dura may be examined later together with the periodontal membrane space and tooth roots. Finally make a third visual circuit, examining the dentition and the associated structures. Note the way the tooths appearance and root structure change with different orientations of the X-ray beam. Count the teeth looking for missing or supernumerary teeth. Examine the roots for shape and form to detect developmental or acquired abnormalities such as external resorption.

Extraoral Radiograph

Two basic approaches can be used to analyze images of a lesion. One is the picture matching or 'Aunt Minnie' method. This involves trying to match the radiographic image with a mental picture.

The preferred method is a step-by-step analysis of all the radiographic characteristics of the abnormality and production of a radiographic interpretation based on these findings.

Localize the Abnormality

Attempt is made to describe the lesion on the basis of following points: localized or generalized, position in the jaws, single or multifocal, and the size.

Assess the Periphery and the Shape

A well defined lesion is one in which most of the periphery is well-defined.In contrast it is difficult to draw an exact delineation around most of an ill-defined periphery.These two types of peripheries can be further broken down under two sub-categories: well-defined borders and ill-defined borders.The lesion may have a particular shape or it may be irregular.

Analyze the Internal Structure

The internal appearance of a lesion can be classified into one of the three basic categories: totally radiolucent, totally radiopaque or mixed radiolucent and radiopaque (mixed density).

Analyze the Effects of the Lesion on the Surrounding Structures

The effects of the lesion on the teeth, lamina dura, and periodontal membrane space should be studied. Also the surrounding bone density and trabecular pattern should be noted. Changes in the dimensions of the inferior alveolar canal and the mental foramen region should be noted. Outer cortical bone and periosteal reactions should be noted.

Formulate a Radiographic Interpretation

Avoid making an interpretation from a single observation. In the analysis, all the accumulated characteristics point the way to the diagnosis.

Decision 1: Normal versus abnormal.
Decision 2: Developmental versus acquired.
Decision 3: Classification
Decision 4: Ways to proceed

GENERAL RADIOLOGIC FEATURES OF THE INFLAMMATORY LESIONS OF THE JAWS

With periapical inflammatory lesions, which are pathologic conditions of the pulp, the epicenter typically is located at the apex of a tooth. However, lesions of pulpal origin also may be located anywhere along the root surface because of accessory canals or perforations caused by root canal therapy or root fractures. Periodontal lesions have an epicenter that is located at the alveolar crest. If periodontal bone loss is severe, the bone inflammatory changes may extend to the root furcation level or even the root apex. Figure 3.35 is a representative figure for studying the radiographic changes in inflammatory conditions of the jaw bones.

Periphery

Most often the periphery is ill-defined, with a gradual blending of normal trabecular pattern

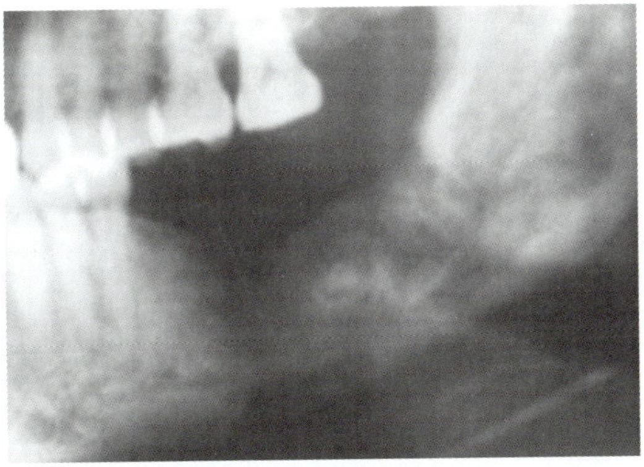

Fig. 3.35: The radiographic appearance of an inflammatory lesion affecting the body of the mandible.

into a sclerotic pattern, or the normal trabecular pattern may gradually fade into a radiolucent region of bone loss.

Internal Structure

The internal structure of inflammatory lesions presents a spectrum of appearances. Cancellous bone may respond to an insult by tipping the bone metabolic balance either in favour of resorption (giving the area a radiolucent appearance) or toward bone formation (resulting in a radiopaque or sclerotic appearance). Usually there is a combination of these two reactions. The radiolucent regions may show no evidence of previous trabeculation or a very faint pattern of trabeculation. The increased radiopacity is caused by an increase in bone formation on existing trabeculae. Radiographically these trabeculae appear thicker and more numerous, replacing marrow spaces. In acute disease, resorption typically predominates; with a chronic disease, excessive bone formation leads to an overall radiopaque, sclerotic appearance. In cases of osteomyelitis, careful examination of the x-ray films may reveal sequestra, which appear as ill-defined areas of radiolucency containing a radiopaque island of non-vital bone.

Effects on Surrounding Structures

The effects of inflammation on surrounding cancellous bone include stimulation of bone formation, resulting in a sclerotic pattern, or bone resorption, resulting in radiolucency. The periodontal ligament space involved in the lesion will be widened; this widening is greatest at the source of the inflammation. For example, with periapical lesions the widening is greatest around the apical region of the root; in periodontal disease the widening is greatest at the alveolar crest. With chronic infections, root resorption may occur and cortical boundaries may be resorbed. The periosteal component of bone, whether on the surface of the jaws or lining the floor of the maxillary sinus, also responds to inflammation. The periosteum contains a layer of pluripotential cells that under the right conditions, differentiate into osteoblasts and lay down new bone. Inflammatory exudate from infection within the bone can penetrate the cortex, lift up the periosteun, from the surface of the bone, and stimulate the periosteum to produce new bone. Because inflammatory exudate is a fluid, the periosteum is lifted from the surface of bone in a manner that positions the periosteum almost parallel to the surface of the bone: thus the layer of new bone is almost parallel to the bone surface.

GENERAL RADIOGRAPHIC FEATURES OF THE CYSTS OF THE JAWS

Location

Cysts may occur centrally (within bone) in any location in the maxilla or mandible but are rare in the condyle and coronoid process. Odontogenic cysts are found most often in the tooth-bearing region (Fig. 3.36). In the mandible, they originate above the inferior alveolar nerve canal. Odontogenic cysts may grow into the maxillary antrum. Some non-odontogenic cysts also originate within the antrum. A few cysts arise in the soft tissues of the orofacial region.

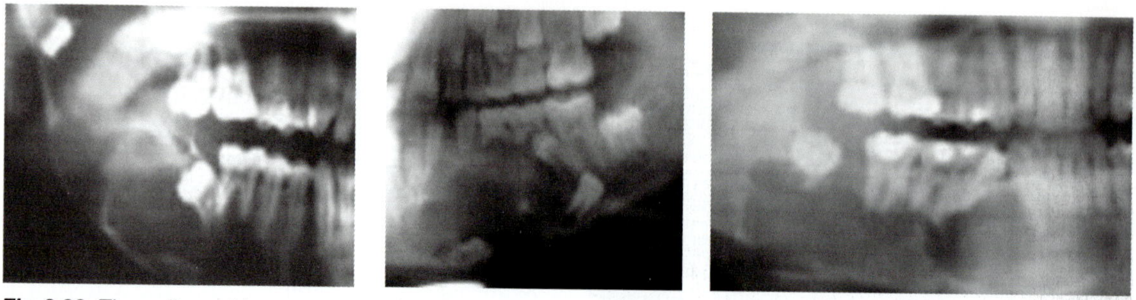

Fig. 3.36: The radiographic appearance of cystic conditions affecting the jaws.

Periphery

Cysts that originate in bone usually have a periphery that is well defined and corticated (characterized by a fairly uniform, thin, radiopaque line). However, a secondary infection or a chronic state can change this appearance into a thicker, more sclerotic boundary.

Shape

Cysts usually are round or oval, resembling a fluid-filled balloon. Some cysts may have a scalloped boundary.

Internal Structure

Cysts often are totally radiolucent. However, long-standing cysts may have dystrophic calcification, which can give the internal aspect a sparse, particulate appearance. Some cysts have septa, which produce multiple loculations separated by these bony walls or septa. Cysts that have a scalloped periphery may appear to have internal septa. Occasionally the image of structures that are positioned on either side of the cyst may overlap the internal aspect of the cyst, giving the false impression of internal structure.

Effects on Surrounding Structures

Cysts grow slowly, sometimes causing displacement and resorption of teeth. The area of tooth resorption often has a sharp, curved shape. Cysts can expand the mandible, usually in a smooth, curved manner, and change the buccal or lingual plate into a thin cortical boundary. Cysts may displace the inferior alveolar nerve canal in an inferior direction or invaginate the maxillary antrum, maintaining a thin layer of bone that separates the internal aspect of the cyst from the antrum.

GENERAL RADIOGRAPHIC FEATURES OF THE BENIGN TUMOURS OF THE JAWS

Location

Because many tumors have a specific anatomic predilection, the location of a particular neoplasm is important in establishing the differential diagnosis. For example, odontogenic lesions occur in the alveolar processes above the inferior alveolar nerve canal, where tooth formation occur (Fig. 3.37). Vascular and neural lesions may originate inside the mandibular canal, arising from the neurovascular tissues. Cartilaginous tumors occur in jaw locations where residual cartilaginous cells lie, such as around the mandibular condyle.

Periphery and Shape

Benign tumors enlarge slowly by formation of additional internal tissue. Because of this, the radiographic borders of benign tumors appear relatively smooth, well defined and sometimes corticated. If the tumor produces a calcified product, for example, abnormal tooth material or abnormal bone, the most

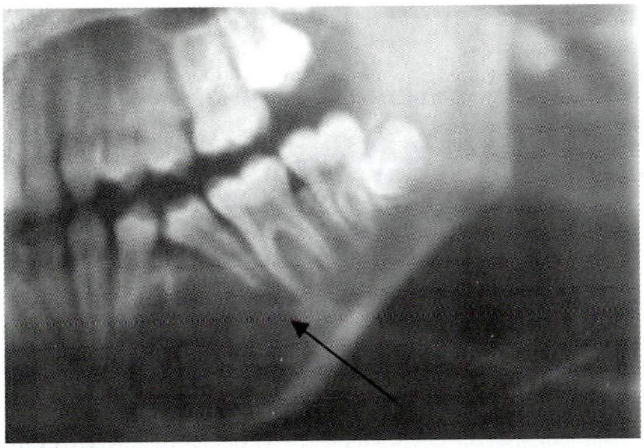

Fig. 3.37: A benign tumour affecting the premolar region of the left side of the mandible causing displacement of the roots of the premolars and the inferior alveolar canal.

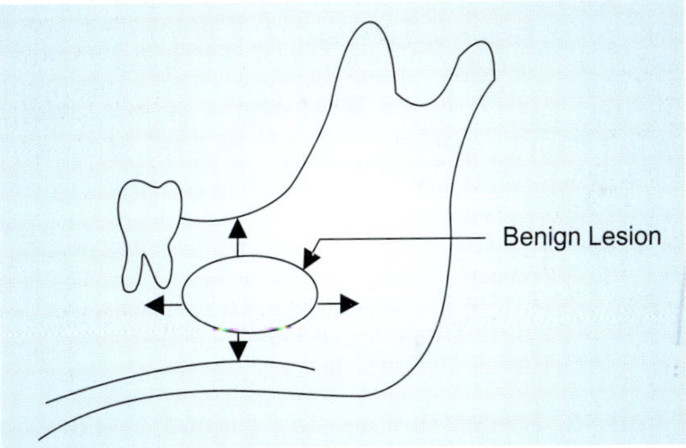

Fig. 3.38: Growth of benign lesion.

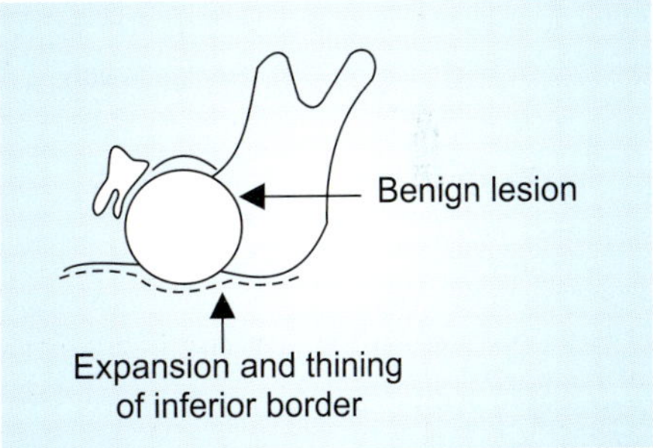

Fig. 3.39: Benign lesions growing in bone tend to be round.

mature part of the tumor will be in the central region with the most immature aspect at the periphery. This sometimes results in a radiolucent band of soft tissue or capsule at the periphery where the calcified product has not yet formed; this band separates the more mature internal radiopaque portion from the surrounding normal bone.

Internal Structure

The internal structure may be completely radiolucent or radiopaque or may be a mixture of radiolucent and radiopaque masses. If the lesion contains radiopaque elements, these structures usually represent either residual bone or a calcified material that is being produced by the tumour.

Effects on the Surrounding Structures

The manner in which a tumour affects adjacent tissues may suggest it's behaviour. A benign tumour exerts pressure on neighbouring structures, resulting in the displacement of teeth or bony cortices (Figs 3.38 and 3.39). If the growth is slow enough, there will be adequate time for the outer cortex to remodel in response to the pressure, resulting in an appearance that the cortex has been displaced by the tumor.

This is caused by simultaneous resorption of bone along the inner surface (endosteal) of the cortex and deposition of bone along the outer cortical surface by the periosteum.

Through this remodeling process, the cortex maintains its integrity and resists perforation (Fig. 3.48). Benign tumors may also cause bodily displacement of nearby teeth. The movement of teeth adjacent to benign tumors is slow because these lesions grow slowly (Fig. 3.41).

The roots of teeth may be resorbed by either benign or malignant tumours, but root resorption more commonly is associated with benign processes. The benign tumours especially likely to resorb roots are ameloblastomas ossifying fibromas, and central giant cell granulomas. Benign tumours tend to resorb

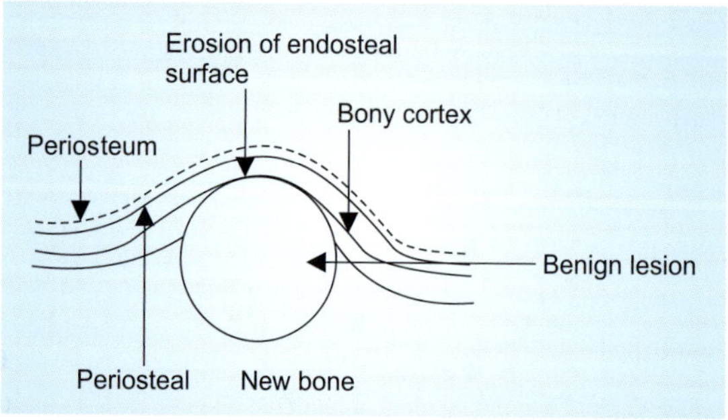

Fig. 3.40: Benign tumour may expand by outward remodeling of its cortical borders.

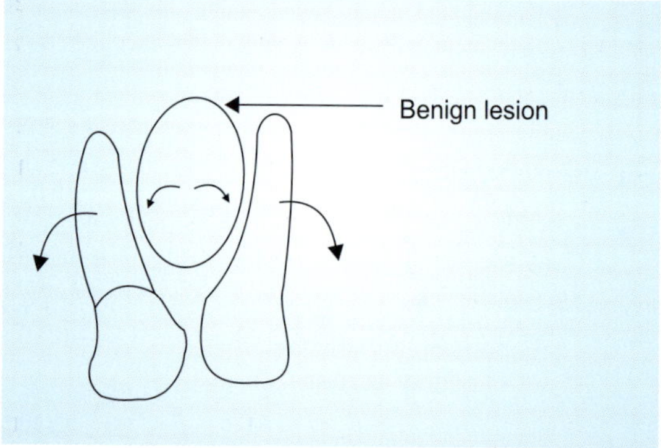

Fig. 3.41: Benign tumour grows slowly by causing displacement of adjacent teeth.

the adjacent root surfaces in a similar fashion. Bone dysplasias such as fibrous dysplasia do not usually resorb teeth.

GENERAL RADIOGRAPHIC FEATURES OF THE MALIGNANT TUMOURS OF THE JAWS

Radiology plays a number of important roles in the management of the patient with cancer. First, diagnostic images may aid in the establishment of an initial diagnosis of the tumor. Diagnostic imaging also aids in the appropriate staging of disease from early small cancers to large cancers that have spread. Appropriate radiologic investigations assist the surgeon or radiation oncologist to determine the anatomic spread of the tumour so that it can be excised or irradiated adequately. Radiologic investigation has the potential to determine the presence of osseous involvement from soft tissue tumours and allow the practitioner to assess the involvement of lymph nodes and treatment outcome. Finally a thorough radiographic dental examination plays a part in the management of cancer survivor who often is rendered xerostomic, neutropenic, and susceptible to dental caries, periodontal disease and systemic infection.

Location

Primary and metastatic malignant tumors may occur anywhere in the oral and maxillofacial region. Primary carcinomas are more commonly seen in the floor of mouth, tonsillar area, lip, soft palate, or gingiva and may invade the jaws from any of these sites. Sarcomas are more common in the mandible and in posterior regions of both jaws. Metastatic tumours are most common in the posterior mandible and maxilla. Some metastatic lesions grow at the apices of teeth or in the follicles of developing teeth.

Periphery and Shape

The typical appearance of the periphery of a malignant lesion is an ill-defined border with lack of cortication and absence of encapsulation. This infiltrative border has uneven extensions of bone destruction. Finger like extensions of the tumour occur in many directions; this extension is followed by osseous destruction producing a region of radiolucency. Evidence of osseous destruction with adjacent soft tissue mass is highly suggestive of malignancy. The shape of the malignant tumour of the jaw is irregular.

Internal Structure

Because most malignancies do not produce bone or stimulate the formation of bone, their internal aspect is radiolucent in most instances. Occasionally residual islands of bone are present resulting in a pattern of patchy destruction with some scattered residual internal osseous structure. Some tumours such as metastatic prostate or breast lesions can induce bone formation resulting in an abnormal appearing internal osseous structure, whereas others such as osteogenic sarcomas produce abnormal bone giving the involved bone a sclerotic appearance.

Effects on Surrounding Structures

Malignancy is destructive, often rapidly so. The effect on surrounding structures mirrors this behaviour. Slower growing benign tumours or cysts may resorb tooth roots or displace them in a bodily fashion without causing loose teeth. In contrast, rapidly growing malignant lesions generally destroy supporting alveolar bone so that teeth may appear to be floating in space. Occasionally root resorption is present: this is more common in sarcomas. Internal trabecular bone is destroyed as are cortical boundaries such as the sinus floor, inferior border of the mandible, follicular cortices, and the cortex of the inferior alveolar neurovascular canal. Because malignant tumours tend to grow rapidly they invade by means of easiest routes such as through the maxillary antrum or through the periodontal ligament space around the teeth resulting in irregular widening with destruction of the lamina dura: they also may spread through the inferior alveolar neurovascular canal causing similar widening. Where the tumour has destroyed the outer cortex of bone usually no periosteal reaction occurs, however some tumours stimulate unususal periosteal new bone formation. Lesions such osteosarcoma and metastatic prostatic lesions can stimulate the formation of thin straight spicules of bone giving a 'hair-on-end'or sunburst appearance. If there is a secondary inflammatory lesion coexisting with the malignancy, a periosteal reaction normally associated with an inflammatory lesion (onion-skin like) may be seen.

GENERAL RADIOGRAPHIC FEATURES OF THE SYSTEMIC DISEASES MANIFESTED IN THE JAWS

Because systemic disorders affect the entire body, the radiographic changes manifested in the jaws are generalized. In most cases it is not possible to identify diseases based on radiographic characteristics. Figure 3.42 shows the changes seen in multiple myeloma as seen on a true lateral view of the skull. The general changes include the following.

1. A change in size and shape of the bone.
2. A change in the number, size and orientation of the trabeculae.
3. Altered thickness and density of cortical structures
4. An increase or decrease in overall bone density

Changes in the first three elements can result in a decrease or increase in bone density. Because many parameters in the production of a radiograph influence the density of the image, it is difficult to detect genuine changes in the

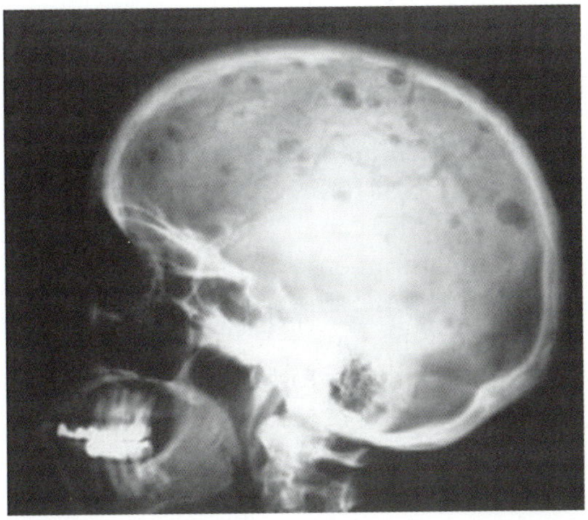

Fig. 3.42: Multiple punched out lesions as seen in multiple myeloma.

density of bone. Systemic conditions that result in a decrease in bone density do not affect the teeth; therefore the image of the teeth may stand out with normal density against a generally radiolucent jaw. In severe cases the teeth may appear to be bereft of any bony support. Also, cortical structures appear thin and less defined and occasionally disappear. On the other hand, a true bone density may be detected by a loss of the inferior cortex of the mandible as the radiopacity of the cancellous bone approaches that of cortical bone. Changes to the teeth and associated structures include the following.

1. Accelerated or delayed eruption.
2. Hypoplasia
3. Hypocalcification
4. Loss of a distinct lamina dura.

IMAGING IN TRAUMA

The response of the skeleton to trauma changes both with the nature and force of the injury and with the maturity and strength of the skeleton. In children the physis or growth plate provides the weakest link and therefore epiphyseal injuries or apophyseal displacements are common. The skeleton is less brittle, resulting in buckling of the cortex or incomplete *'green-stick'* fractures. In the mature adult skeleton the soft tissue ligaments and muscular insertions are the weakest link, and sprains and strains occur more commonly than fractures. The elderly osteopenic skeleton is brittle and susceptible to fracture often with minimal force.

Fracture radiographs should be performed in two planes and where possible should include the adjacent joint. When a fracture is strongly suspected but not demonstrated, a repeat X-ray 5-10 days after the injury may identify the fracture line when bone absorption has begun.

'Stress fractures,' either *'fatigue fractures' (normal bone)* or *'insufficiency fractures' (abnormal bone)* can be difficult to diagnose. Radionuclide bone scanning and more recently MRI are useful additional investigations if stress fractures are strongly suspected.

RADIOLOGICAL DIFFERENTIAL DIAGNOSIS

ANATOMIC RADIOLUCENCIES

Structures peculiar to the mandible are:

- Mandibular foramen.
- Mandibular canal
- Mental foramen
- Lingual foramen
- Airway shadows
- Submandibular fossa
- Mental fossa
- Midline symphysis
- Medial sigmoid depression
- Anterior buccal mandibular depression
- Cortical plate mandibular defects

Structures peculiar to the maxilla are:

- Intermaxillary suture
- Incisive foramen, incisive canal and superior foramina of incisive canal.
- Nasal cavity
- Naris
- Nasolacrimal duct or canal
- Maxillary sinus
- Greater palatine foramen

Structures common to both the jaws:

- Pulp chamber and root canal
- Periodontal ligament space

- Marrow space
- Nutient canal
- Developing tooth crypt

PERIAPICAL RADIOLUCENCIES

- Pulpoperiapical radiolucencies are:
  - Periapical granuloma
  - Radicular cyst
  - Surgical scar
  - Chronic and acute dentoalveolar abscess
  - Osteomyeli
- Dentigerous cyst
- Periapical cemento-osseous dysplasia
- Periodontal disease
- Traumatic bone cyst
- Malignant tumours
- Rarities
  - Ameloblastic variants
  - Ameloblastoma
  - Aneurysmal bone cyst

PERICORONAL RADIOLUCENCIES

- Pericoronal or follicular space
- Dentigerous cyst
- Ameloblastoma
- Adenomatoid odontogenic tumour
- Calcifying odontogenic cyst or tumour
- Ameloblastic fibroma
- Rarities
  - Calcifying epithelial odontogenic tumour
  - Ewing's sarcoma.

INTERRADICULAR RADIOLUCENCIES

- Anatomic radiolucencies
  - Primary tooth crypt
  - Mental foramen and mental canal
  - Maxillary sinus
  - Incisive foramen
  - Bone marrow pattern
  - Nutrient canal
- Pathologic radiolucencies
  - Periodontal pocket
  - Furcation involvement
  - Lateral radicular cyst
  - Traumatic bone cyst
  - Primordial cyst
  - Incisive canal cyst
  - Lateral periodontal cyst
  - Median mandibular cyst
- Rarities
  - Adenomatoid odontogenic tumour
  - Histiocytosis X.

SOLITARY CYST-LIKE RADIOLUCENCIES NOT NECESSARILY CONTACTING THE TEETH

- Anatomic patterns
  - Marrow spaces
  - Maxillary sinus
  - Early stage of tooth crypts
  - Median sigmoid depression
- Post-extraction socket
- Residual cyst
- Traumatic bone cyst
- Lingual mandibular bone defect
- Odontogenic keratocyst
- Ameloblastoma
- Focal osteoporotic defect of the jaws
- Surgical defect
- Giant cell granuloma
- Giant cell lesion
- Focal cemento-osseous dysplasia
- Incisive canal cyst
- Mid-palatine cyst
- Cementifying and ossifying fibroma
- Rarities
  - Adenomatoid odontogenic tumours.

MULTILOCULAR RADIOLUCENCIES

- Anatomic patterns
- Multilocular cyst
- Ameloblastoma

- Central giant cell granuloma
- Giant cell lesion of hyperparathyroidism
- Cherubism
- Odontogenic myxoma
- Odontogenic keratocyst
- Aneurysmal bone cyst
- Metastatic tumours to the jaws
- Central haemangioma of bone
- Rarities
  - Ameloblastic variants
  - Arteriovenous malformations
  - Burkitt's lymphoma.

MULTIPLE SEPARATE WELL-DEFINED RADIOLUCENCIES

- Anatomic variations
- Multiple cysts or granulomas
- Basal cell nevus syndrome
- Multiple myeloma
- Metastatic carcinoma
- Langerhan's cell disease
- Rarities
  - Ameloblastomas
  - Cherubism
  - Craniofacial dysostosis.

GENERALIZED RAREFACTIONS OF THE JAW BONES

- Hyperparathyroidism (primary, secondary and tertiary)
- Osteoporosis
- Osteomalacia
- Hereditary haemolytic anaemia (thalassaemia and sickle cell anaemia)
- Leukemia
- Langerhan's cell disease
- Pagets disease
- Multiple myeloma
- Rarities
  - Acromegaly
  - Agranulocytosis
  - Burkitt's lymphoma.

MIXED RADIOLUCENT-RADIOPAQUE LESIONS ASSOCIATED WITH TEETH

- Periapical mixed lesions
  - Calcifying crown of developing teeth
  - Tooth root with rarefying osteitis
  - Rarefying and condensing osteitis
  - Periapical cemento-osseous dysplasia
  - Cemento-ossifying fibroma
  - Rarities
    i. Calcifying odontogenic cyst
    ii. Cementoblastoma-intermediate stage
- Pericoronal mixed lesions
  - Odontoma-intermediate stage
  - Adenomatoid odontogenic tumour
  - Calcifying odontogenic cyst
  - Ameloblastic fibroodontoma
  - Calcifying epithelial odontogenic tumour
  - Rarities
    i. Ameloblastic fibrodentinoma
    ii. Central odontogenic fibroma.

MIXED RADIOLUCENT-RADIOPAQUE LESIONS NOT NECESSARILY CONTACTING TEETH

- Healing surgical site
- Chronic osteomyelitis
- Osteoradionecrosis
- Focal cemento-osseous dysplasia
- Fibrous dysplasia
- Paget's disease—intermediate stage
- Cemento-ossifying fibromas
- Osteogenic sarcoma
- Osteoblastic metastatic carcinoma
- Chondroma and chondrosarcoma
- Desmoplastic ameloblastoma
- Rarities
  - Adenomatoid odontogenic tumour
  - Ameloblastic fibrodentinoma
  - Ameloblastic fibroodontoma

ANATOMIC RADIOPACITIES OF THE JAWS

- Radiopacities common to both the jaws
  - Teeth
  - Bone
  - Cancellous bone
  - Cortical plates
  - Lamina dura
  - Alveolar process
- Radiopacities peculiar to the maxilla
  - Nasal septum and boundaries of the nasal fossa
  - Anterior nasal spine
  - Canine eminence
  - Walls and floor of the maxillary sinus
  - Zygomatic process of the maxilla andzygomatic bone
  - Maxillary tuberosity
  - Pterygoid plates and the pterygoid hamulus
  - Coronoid process
- Radiopacities peculiar to the mandible
  - External oblique ridge
  - Mylohyoid ridge
  - Internal oblique ridge
  - Mental ridge
  - Genial tubercles
- Superimposed radiopacities
  - Soft tissue shadows
  - Mineralized tissue shadows.

PERIAPICAL RADIOPACITIES

- True periapical radiopacities
  - Condensing osteitis
  - Periapical or focal cemento-osseous dysplasia
  - Unerupted succedaneous teeth
  - Foreign bodies
  - Hypercementosis
  - Rarities
- False periapical radiopacities
  - Anatomic structures
  - Impacted teeth, supernumerary teeth
  - Foreign bodies
  - Mucosal cyst of the maxillary antrum
  - Ectopic calcifications
- Rarities
  - Calcifying odontogenic cyst
  - Mineralized tumours

SOLITARY RADIOPACITIES NOT NECESSARILY CONTACTING TEETH

- True intrabony radiopacities
  - Tori, exostoses, and peripheral osteomas
  - Unerupted, impacted and supernumerary teeth
  - Retained roots
  - Idiopathic osteosclerosis
  - Condensing or sclerosing osteitis
  - Fibrous dysplasia
  - Focal sclerosing osteomyelitis
  - Diffuse sclerosing osteomyelitis
  - Mature complex odontoma
  - Rarities
    i. Chondromas
    ii. Mature osteoblastoma
- Projected radiopacities
  - Anatomic structures
  - Foreign bodies
  - Pathologic soft tissue masses
  - Ectopic calcifications
  - Rarities
    i. Calcified acne lesion
    ii. Calcified haematoma
    iii. Calcinosis cutis.

GENERALIZED RADIOPACITIES

- Florid cemento-osseous dysplasia
- Paget's disease
- Osteopetrosis
- Rarities
  - Albright's disease
  - Caffey's disease
  - Diffuse sclerosing osteomyelitis
  - Fluorosis

REFERENCES AND BIBLIOGRAPHY

1. Oral and Maxillofacial Surgery: Daniel M.Laskin
2. Differential Diagnosis of Oral and Maxillofacial Lesions; Fifth edition; Norman K.Wood, Paul W. Goaz.
3. Burket's Oral Medicine; Diagnosis and Treatment; Tenth edition; Martin S. Greenberg and Michael Glick.
4. Oral and Maxillofacial Pathology; Second Edition; Neville, Damm, Allen, Bouquot.
5. Oral Radiology; Principles and Interpretation; Fifth edition; Stuart C.White, Michael J.Pharoah
6. Bailey and Love's Short Practice of Surgery; 23rd edition.

Chapter 4

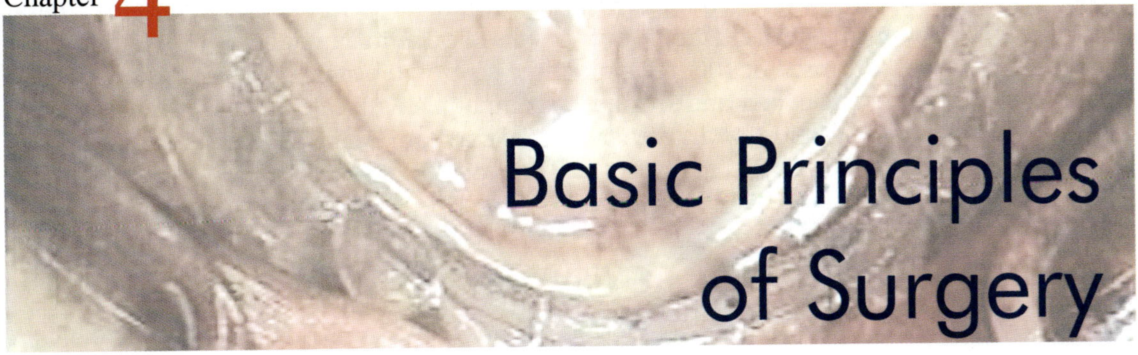

Basic Principles of Surgery

STERILIZATION AND ASEPSIS

The discovery of the importance of asepsis in the prevention of infection may be the single most important advance in the history of surgery. According to Maki (1976), the concept was advocated decades before bacteria were conclusively implicated in wound suppuration and even before contagion was generally accepted. It was not until Joseph Lister's studies on the prevention of wound infection, made between 1865 and 1891, that these principles were accepted. Lister initially applied dilute carbolic acid (phenol) to contaminated wounds and then progressed to its application in all surgical wounds, as well as in the operating room by nebulization of the solution. Further developments in Listerian asepsis occurred rapidly in the 1890's with the advent of steam sterilization, surgical masks, sterile gloves, sterile gowns, sterile drapes, and sterile sponges for the surgical wound.

Despite modern methods of sterilization and the use of aseptic techniques, microorganisms are introduced into surgical sites.

Although it is probable, as suggested by Elek and Conen (1957), that most postoperative infections today result from faulty surgical technique, the importance of disinfection, asepsis, and sterility in minimizing the patient's exposure to pathogenic bacteria cannot be overemphasized.

DEFINITIONS

Antiseptic

A chemical that is applied to living tissues such as skin or mucous membrane to reduce the number of microorganisms present through inhibition of their activity or destruction.

Disinfectant

A chemical used on nonvital objects to kill surface vegetative pathogenic organisms, but not necessarily spore forms or viruses.

Sterilization

A process by which all microbial forms are destroyed.

Unfortunately, living tissue cannot withstand sterilization by known methods without irrevocable damage or loss of its own vitality.

Therefore, while it would be advantageous to have the surgeon, operating room, patient, instruments, nurses, anesthetic equipment, and operating room air sterile, this is not practical by present means. For this reason, each of the preceding is cleaned and treated with antiseptics or disinfectants, or draped, or sterilized by means applicable to that object.

CLEANSING INSTRUMENTS

According to Lawrence and Block (1968), protein and other polymolecular structures, particularly when dry, can serve as a protective covering for microorganisms and prevent penetration of a sterilizing medium. Therefore, to allow penetration by heat or chemicals, surgical instruments must first be scrupulously cleaned of all debris including blood, saliva, and necrotic material.

Time-consuming and careful scrubbing by hand may be necessary to clean certain instruments such as bone burs or bone files, where solid particles are wedged into small crevices. Usually a stiff wire brush will facilitate the cleaning. However, the greatest portion of the cleaning procedure can be managed by ultrasonic cleaning devices. These devices act by converting electrical energy into vibratory sound waves, which then pass through a soap solution containing the instruments to be cleaned.

Cavitation

Microscopic bubbles rapidly form and then collapse on the instrument surfaces, creating a suction that removes the debris.

Soaps and detergents are commonly used to aid in the removal of debris from instruments. Soaps are the salts of fatty acids and detergents are synthetic compounds. Both groups act by reducing surface tension along the instrument surface, allowing emulsification of the contaminants, which can then be removed in the rinsing phase. According to Accepted Dental Therapeutics (1975), soaps are only effective at pH 9 or higher, and even in a weakly acidic environment or in one containing the soluble salts of calcium or magnesium, precipitation of the soap will occur. Detergents, however, are compatible with calcium and magnesium ions and maintain their efficacy in neutral or slightly acidic solutions.

DISINFECTANTS

Alcohols

Ethanol and isopropyl (Fig. 4.1) alcohols are overused as disinfectants. They are more

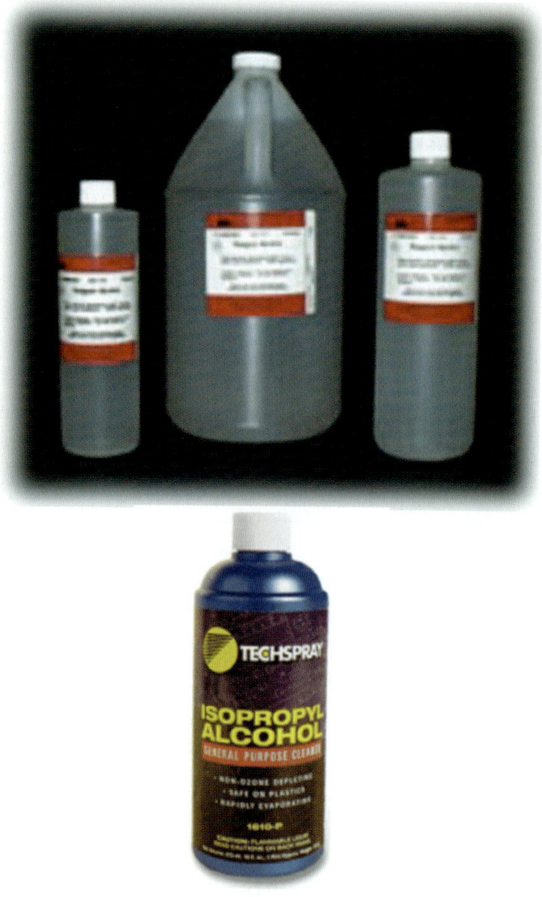

Fig. 4.1: Ethanol and isopropyl alcohol used as disinfectants.

frequently and correctly used as antiseptics. They act by denaturing protein. Spores and viruses are generally unaffected by the alcohols. Spaulding (1939) found that to reach maximum effectiveness, the alcohol must have at least a 10-minute contact with the organisms.

They are corrosive to carbon steel, and instruments of this composition should not be soaked in alcoholic solutions. Rubber articles absorb alcohol, and prolonged soaking can cause a reaction when the article subsequently comes in contact with living tissue.

Aqueous Quaternary Ammonium Compounds

Benzalkonium chloride (Zephiran) is one of the most common aqueous quaternary ammonium compounds and is used both as an antiseptic and as a disinfectant (Fig. 4.2).

Benzalkonium chloride (Zephiran)

a. This molecule is a strong surfactant that increases the permeability of the bacterial wall and permits the escape of phosphorous and nitrogen.
b. It also denatures intracellular protein.

Phenolic Compounds

Phenolic compounds are one of the oldest groups of disinfectants, having been used by Joseph Lister in the form of carbolic acid. Phenol itself is toxic to the skin and bone marrow. Substituted phenolic compounds (Amphyl, O-Syl, Staphene, Ves-Phene) have been developed to reduce these side effects, but they are still toxic to living tissues (Fig. 4.3).

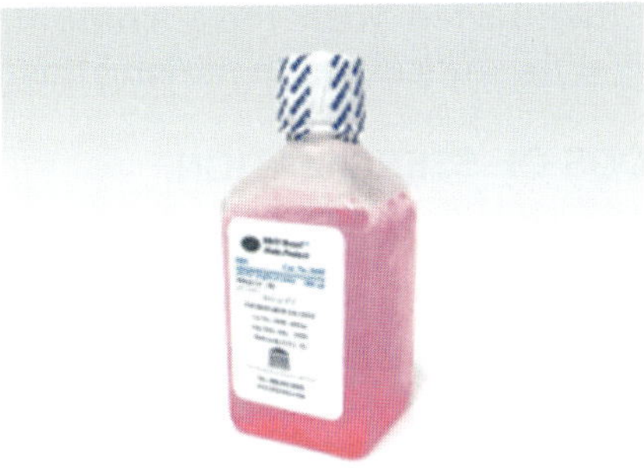

Fig. 4.3: Phenolic compounds.

None of these compounds are sporicidal at room temperature, but they are active against many viruses, fungi, and bacteria (Lawrence and Block, 1968).

Aldehyde Compounds

Aldehyde compounds such as aqueous formaldehyde (formalin) (Fig. 4.4) and glutaraldehyde (Cidex) are very effective disinfectants. Formalin is not popular because of its noxious odor and because contact of 18 to 30 hours is necessary for cidal action.

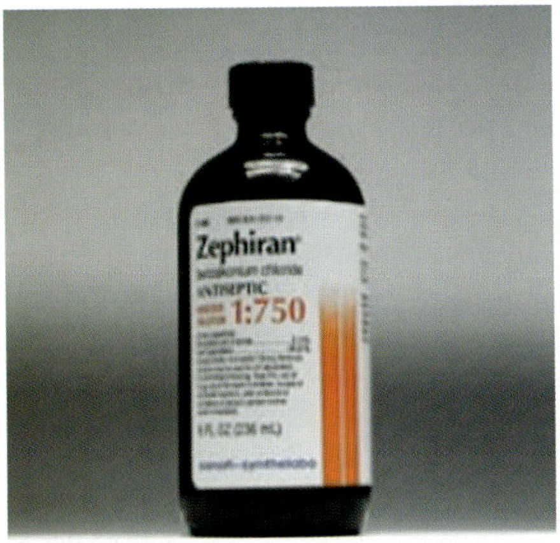

Fig. 4.2: Benzalkonium chloride (Zephiran)

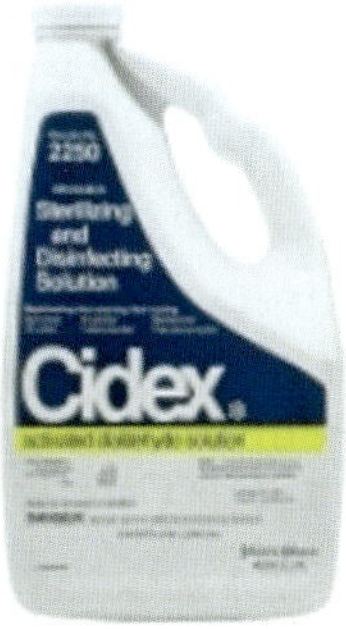

Fig. 4.4: Cidex is an effective disinfectant.

Glutaraldehyde will kill vegetative bacteria, spores, fungi, and perhaps all viruses by alkylation on 10-hour contact prior to patient exposure, the instruments must be thoroughly rinsed with sterile water or alcohol to remove the compound. Therefore porous object that come in contact with patient should probably not be disinfected with these compounds because of the difficulty in removing them.

METHODS OF STERILIZATION

Heat is the most common and one of the most effective methods of sterilization. Heat may be transmitted through the air, water, or oil. Factors affecting sterilization when using heat as the means of sterilization are:

- The temperature reached by these modalities.
- It's penetration ability.
- The heat of vaporization.

Boiling Water

Water maintains and conducts heat extremely well. Moist heat kills microorganisms by coagulation of their protein. Boiling water at normal atmospheric pressure will produce a temperature of 100° C. While exposure to this temperature for 10 minutes will kill many bacteria, time periods of up to 24 hours may be necessary to kill bacterial spores, and even this prolonged time will not kill many viruses. For this reason, boiling water is not recommended for sterilization of tissue penetrating instruments.

Steam Heat

Saturated steam under pressure is the most effective and practical method of sterilization. At a 15 psi pressure, the temperature of steam can reach 121.5° C. Once the objects to be sterilized reach this temperature, only 10 to 12 minutes are needed to kill all living organisms (Fig. 4.5). Higher temperatures at greater pressures can be obtained, and this will shorten the time necessary for sterilization.

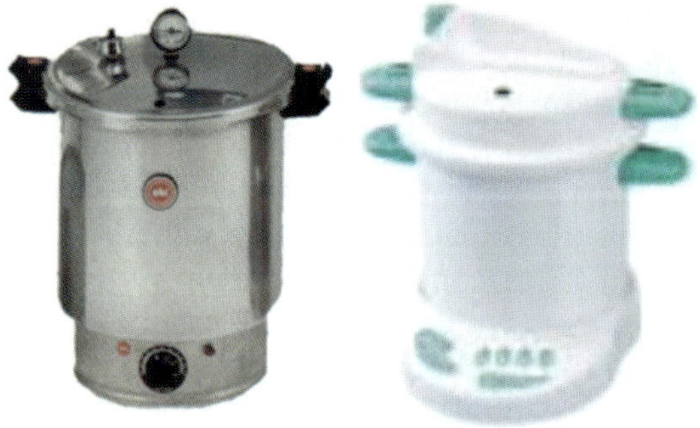

Fig. 4.5: Autoclaves for office to sterilize instruments.

The time needed to sterilize a particular item also varies with the amount of material and thickness of the wrap. Liquids may also be sterilized by autoclave, providing their contents will not be inactivated by the temperatures reached.

Oil

Hot oil baths have been used to sterilize metallic instruments. The oil can reach a temperature of 175° C, and after the instruments reach this temperature, 15 minutes of submersion is necessary for sterilization. To ensure the temperature conversion of the instruments, often 1 hour or more of submersion is used.

Disadvantages of using oil as a means of sterilization

- Oil has poor penetration properties and poor sporicidal activity.
- Presents a fire hazard.
- Difficult to remove from instruments such as handpieces without recontamination.
- It should never be used on hypodermic syringes or needles because of the danger of oil embolization.

Dry Heat

The hot air oven may be used to sterilize items that will not be damaged by the high

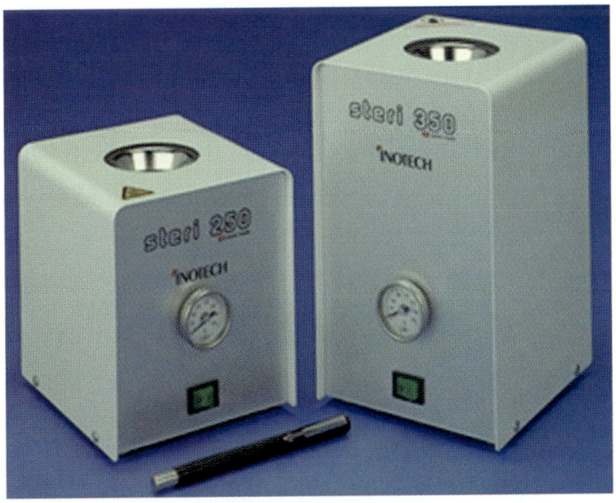

Fig. 4.6: Glass bead steriliser.

temperatures that are generated. Usually 1600° C for 2 hours is necessary to accomplish sterility.

The long time period is necessary, according to Kelsey (1969), because of the poor heat conduction by air and the poor penetration properties of dry heat.

Mechanism of action of dry heat: Dry heat kills by dehydration and oxidation.

It does not penetrate grease, oil, and powders, and equipment containing these substances should be sterilized by other means. One proposed advantage of this method is the maintenance of sharp edges on cutting instruments. Another method of dry heat sterilization employs a heat transfer device. Glass beads (Fig. 4.6), molten metal, and salt are media that are used. Temperatures of 220° C can be reached, and submersion of small instruments such as endodontic files may produce sterility in 10 seconds, provided the instrument is clean. Oliet, Sorin, and Brown (1958) reported that temperatures vary in different areas of the sterilizer.

Gas

Ethylene oxide, a gas at temperatures above 10.80° C, is a highly toxic compound that destroys organisms by alkylation. It is very flammable, but when it is mixed with carbon dioxide or Freon, this danger is minimized. It is an excellent sterilizer of articles that are susceptible to damage by heat, but it is highly toxic and will blister living tissues on contact. The time that the gas must be in contact with the material to be sterilized is dependent on

- temperature
- humidity
- pressure
- the amount of material.

Irradiation

Ionizing radiation, such as x-rays, gamma rays (Fig. 4.7), and high-speed electrons, or nonionizing radiation in the form of ultraviolet light can be used to kill or inactivate microorganisms.

Ionizing radiation has great penetrating properties and is commonly used by industry to sterilize disposable materials such as needles, suture material, cannulas, and pharmaceuticals sensitive to heat (Bellamy, 1959). According to the Radiosterilization of Medical Products and Recommended Code of Practice (1967), much more radiation is necessary to kill microorganisms than that which would be lethal to man. However, no residual radiation remains on materials treated in this manner, and it is very effective for heat labile items.

Nonionizing radiation, such as ultraviolet light, is used most commonly to purify air, such as in the operating room.

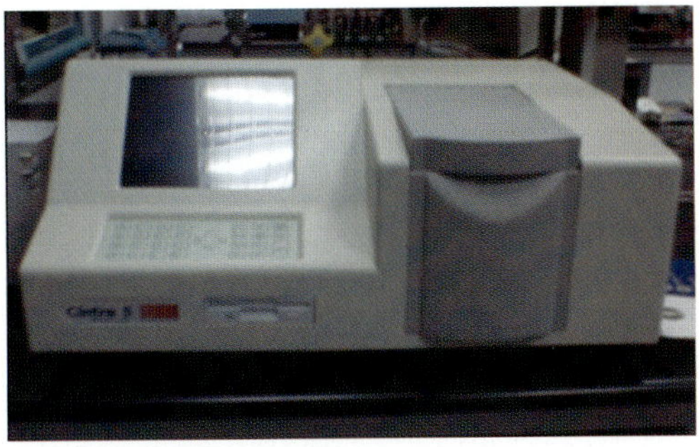

Fig. 4.7: Gamma irradiation unit.

Oliet, Sorin, and Brown (1958) reported that temperatures vary in different areas of the sterilizer.

Nonionizing radiation, such as ultraviolet light, is used most commonly to purify air, such as in the operating room.

ANTISEPTICS

To be tolerated by living tissues, antimicrobial chemicals must be less toxic than the disinfectants or agents used for sterilization and as a result they are generally less effective. However, relatively effective agents with good antibacterial activity, notably the iodophor compounds, have been developed and should be used whenever possible.

Alcohols

Alcohols are frequently used for skin antisepsis prior to needle puncture. They are good organic solvents and their benefit is derived primarily from their cleansing action. To be antibacterial, the alcohol must have prolonged contact with the organisms. Its rapid evaporation prevents this contact and eliminates the possibility of chemical buildup on repeated usage. However, the use of hexachlorophene and iodophor compounds has been shown to be much more effective in reducing the bacterial contamination of skin.

Aqueous Quaternary Ammonium Compounds

Benzalkonium chloride (Zephiran) is the aqueous quaternary ammonium compound most commonly used as an antiseptic. Its antimicrobial activity is primarily against gram-positive bacteria. Reliance on it as a sterilizing medium has resulted in many iatrogenic infections. It is well tolerated by living tissues, but because of the narrowness of its activity spectrum, its use is not widespread.

Hexachlorophene

Hexachlorophene compounds have been used for many years for surgical scrubs and preoperative preparation of the surgical site (Fig. 4.8). They are particularly effective against gram-positive organisms.

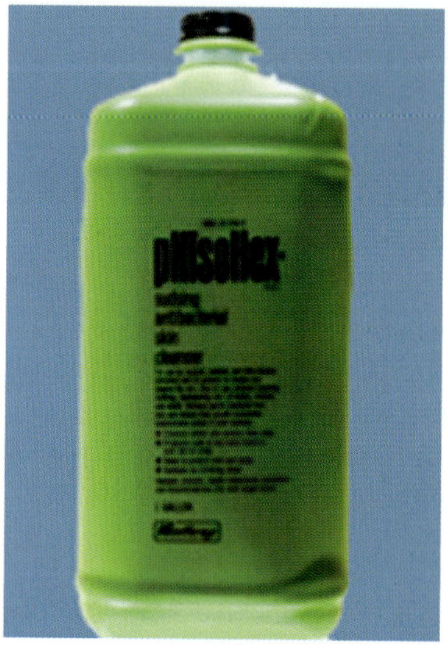

Fig. 4.8: A hexachlorophene compound used as an antiseptic.

They are less effective against gram-negative organisms and fungi and are not effective against viruses, spores, and *Mycobacterium tuberculosis*. Harber, Targovnik, and Baer (1967) reported that hexachlorophene solutions are susceptible to bacterial contamination. Smylie, Webster, and Bruce (1959) have shown that hexachlorophene, to be fully effective, must be applied to dry skin because the com-bination of water and protein will pre-cipitate it.

Iodophor Compounds

According to Joress (1962), Close and co-workers (1964), and Crowder and coworkers (1967), the most effective antiseptics are the iodophor compounds. In them, iodine is

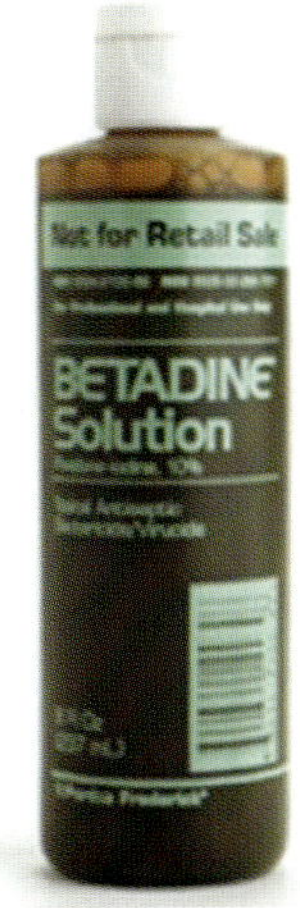

Fig. 4.9: Betadine solution which is used as an effective antiseptic

complexed with organic surface-active agents such as polyvinyl-pyrrolidone (Betadine, Isodine) (Fig. 4.9).

Their activity depends on the release of the iodine from the complex. The surface agent is film forming, which prevents the solution from staining clothes or skin. Because of this complexing action, skin sensitivity to the iodine is not a major problem. These compounds exhibit an effective activity against most bacteria, spores, viruses, and fungi.

PRINCIPLES OF STERILE TECHNIQUE

All materials used as a part of the sterile field for an operation must be sterile. Certain basic items (such as the linen, the instrument set, and the basins) may be obtained from the supply kept in the sterile supply room. Others, such as specialized surgical instruments, may be sterilized the night before or immediately preceding the operation and taken directly from the sterilizer to the sterile operative field. Once an item is removed from a sterile wrapper, it must be used or discarded.

- Linen used in the operating room is usually dyed green. This helps to reduce the glare from lights, thus reducing fatigue and eyestrain.
- Only materials known to be sterile should be used and their sterility should be maintained throughout the operative procedure.
- Sterile areas are set up just prior to use. Scrub attire should not be worn outside the surgical suite. All team members should wash hands before and after the care of each patient.
- Items should be considered unsterile if there is doubt about their sterility.
  If a sterile-appearing package is found in an area not designated for sterile storage, it is considered unsterile and must be reprocessed and resterilized. If there is doubt about the timing of a sterilizer, its contents are considered unsterile. If an "unsterile" person brushes close to a sterile table, the table is considered contaminated. Also, if a "sterile" person brushes close to an unsterile table, the person's sterile gown is considered contaminated. If a sterile table or sterile items are left unmonitored, the table and items are considered unsterile. Do not drop or place clean supplies on the floor. Do not drop or place used supplies or soiled linen on the floor.
- Only the top surface of a draped table is considered sterile. Anything extending over the edge or hanging over the edge is not sterile.
  Linen or sutures falling over the edge of the table should be discarded. The scrub should not touch the part hanging below the table level.
  When the scrub drapes a table with sterile linen, he should see that the part of the linen that drops below the table's surface is not brought up to table level again.
- Once again, neither the circulator nor the scrub may intrude upon the other's area

at any time, although it is very important that they consult with each other and that each is aware of what the other is doing. The duties performed by the scrub and by the circulator are governed by specific procedural rules. Persons who are "sterile" touch only sterile articles; "unsterile" persons touch only unsterile items. All supplies for the "sterile" team members (scrub, surgeon, and assistants) are provided by the circulator ("unsterile" team member) who protects the sterility of items through the use of the wrappers on sterile packages.

- The ***scrub*** is considered a "sterile" person.

  The "sterile" personnel gowns and gloves without touching the outside of the gown or gloves with his bare hands. If a "sterile" team member's glove is punctured during an operation, the glove is to be changed at once. If the glove is pricked by a needle or an instrument, the needle or instrument is discarded from the sterile field. Notify the circulator of the needle's whereabouts.

The ***parts of a surgical gown considered sterile*** are the sleeves (except for the axillary area) and the front of the gown from table level to a few inches below the neck opening.

A "sterile" team member turns away from the sterile field to have perspiration mopped from his brow. The scrub drapes the part of an unsterile table nearest himself first. A "sterile" person should keep his hands in sight and at waist level or above. A "sterile" person should keep his hands away from his face and his elbows close to his sides. He should never fold his arms because his gown may be moist with perspiration in the axillary (under arms) region; thus, his gloves would become contaminated. When a "sterile" person stands on a footstool, the lower part of his gown should not brush the sterile table.

- "Sterile" team members should keep their contact with sterile areas to a minimum. "Sterile" team members should not lean on the sterile tables or on the draped patient. The scrub should keep the large instrument table (back table) and the Mayo stand far enough away that the gowns of other "sterile" team members do not brush them.
- "Sterile" team members keep well within the sterile area. The scrub should allow a wide margin of safety when passing unsterile areas. He and all other "sterile" team members should observe the following practices.

  "Sterile" team members should stand back at a safe distance from the operating table while draping the patient. "Sterile" team members should pass each other back to back. A "sterile" team member should turn his back to an "unsterile" person or area when passing. A "sterile" team member should face a sterile area when passing. "Sterile" team members should stay near the sterile table. They should not wander about the room nor go out into the corridor. When used items or soiled sponges are placed into a basin and maintained on the sterile field, the inside of the basin is contaminated. Handle such a basin by the outside only.
- The circulator is considered the "unsterile" member of the surgical team.

  An "unsterile" team member should never crowd past a "sterile" team member or field. Allow sufficient space between you and the sterile field or between you and gowned individuals when passing them. "Unsterile" team members should keep away from sterile areas. "Unsterile" persons should allow a wide margin of safety when passing sterile areas. "Unsterile" persons should face a sterile area when passing it to be sure you have not touched it. In addition, "unsterile" persons should not go within the sterile "circle" or between two sterile fields. When passing behind a gowned team member, always notify him to avoid possible contamination of his sterile attire if he should turn or move back and brush you.

- The circulator stands at a safe distance from the sterile field when adjusting the light over it.

  Never reach across a sterile field. Stand outside the sterile field and hold the extra supplies needed; allow the scrub to reach for them. Do not enter the sterile field to perform any duties. When moving a sterile table, grasp the table legs well below the tabletop and underneath the sterile drapes. The circulator "flips" the sterile suture material onto back table

- The edge of a cover that encloses sterile contents is not considered sterile. Such covers include the edges of wrappers on sterile packages, the caps on solution bottles, and test tube covers. No definite line separates the sterile from the unsterile area at the edge of the cover; therefore, the edge is considered unsterile.

  The scrub should lift contents from packages by reaching for them with the arm straight out and lifting the items straight up — with the elbow held high throughout the procedure. The circulator lifts the cap from a solution bottle so that the edge of the cap never touches the lip. Caps are not replaced. The entire contents are dispensed and any excess solution is discarded.

- Sterile areas should be protected from moisture because a moist item may become contaminated. When moisture soaks through a sterile area to an unsterile one, or vice versa, a means of transporting infectious organisms to the sterile area is provided.

  Sterile packages should be laid on dry areas. If any portion of a sterile package becomes damp or wet, the entire package should be discarded. If a sterile package falls on the floor, it is considered unsterile.

  Linen packages from the sterilizer should be permitted to cool before being stored on shelves. This procedure prevents their becoming damp from steam condensation when placed on a cool shelf. Sterile drapes should be placed on a dry surface. (Thus, time should be allowed for the prep solution used to paint the patient's skin to dry before draping is begun.)

  During surgery, if a solution soaks through a sterile area from an unsterile one or through an unsterile area from a sterile one, the wet area should be covered with another sterile drape.

- Whenever microorganisms cannot be eliminated from a field, they should be kept to an absolute minimum. Although absolute asepsis in an operative field cannot be reached, every effort is made to control sources of possible contamination. Skin cannot be sterilized. Skin normally harbors staphylococcus and other organisms; however, any agent capable of sterilizing skin will also destroy it. The skin of the patient, as well as that of members of the "sterile" team, is therefore a potential source of contamination in every operation. However, this does not remove the need for strict aseptic technique. Defenses within the patient's body will usually overcome the relatively few organisms left on the skin when the following protective measures are carried out.

The patient's skin is given a shave and scrub just prior to surgery and is again thoroughly cleansed in the operating room just prior to the incision. As much of the operative area is cleansed as is feasible and the surrounding skin is scrubbed. Some areas cannot be scrubbed vigorously. Mucous membranes are gently prepped since scrubbing would damage the tissue. When the site of operation is the mucous membrane of the nose, mouth, throat, or anus, the number of microorganisms present is great. However, these parts of the body do not usually become infected by organisms that normally inhabit them. When scrubbing the patient's skin, a sponge is used only once for prepping an area. Once the sponge is removed from contact with the skin, the sponge is discarded into a kick bucket. All of the patient's skin area except the site of incision is covered with sterile drapes. Sterile towels or other sterile material may be used to cover the skin after the incision is made. The reason for this additional precaution is to protect the surgical wound from the waste products continually excreted by the skin. In addition, airborne organisms continuously pose a threat of contaminating the incision.

When the knife used for the skin incision is no longer needed, the scrub isolates it from other items on the sterile field.

The skin of operating room personnel is another source of contamination. They follow rigid steps in scrubbing their hands and arms using brushes and detergents and adhering to strict technique. This is done to remove the maximum number of organisms. When drying their hands, sterile hand towels should not touch their scrub clothes.

The cap worn on the head of team members should completely cover the hair to prevent particles of dandruff or hair from falling on the sterile field or in the room. Infected areas are grossly contaminated. All team members should avoid scattering the contamination. Team members are required to wear a mask covering the nose and mouth during an operative procedure. The mask must cover the mouth and nose entirely and be tied securely to prevent venting. The strings should not be crossed when tied because the sides of the mask will gap. A pliable metal strip is inserted in the top hem of most masks to provide a firm contour fit over the bridge of the nose. This strip also helps prevent fogging of eyeglasses. Air should pass only through the filtering system of the mask. Masks should be either on or off. They should not be saved from one operation to the next by allowing them to hang around the neck or by tucking them into a pocket. Bacteria that have been filtered by the mask will become dry and airborne if the mask is worn necklace fashion. By touching only the strings when removing the mask, contamination of the hands will be reduced. Masks should be changed between procedures and sometimes during a procedure, depending on the length of the operation and the amount of talking done by the surgical team.

When possible, the respiratory tract of the patient should be isolated from the incision. In some cases, isolation is achieved by using the anesthesia screen. This serves as a barrier between the incision and the respiratory tract. Team members should not talk except when essential. Silence is even better than masking to reduce the number of organisms spread from nose and throat. Team members should avoid sneezing and coughing. Persons who have colds or any active infection should be excluded from the operating room. Main corridors are considered to be contaminated areas; therefore, doors from corridors into the operating rooms should be kept closed. Also, sterile items without wrappers should not be carried through corridors. Walking through and around the operating room should be kept to the necessary minimum. All dusting should be damp-dusting with a germicide solution. Floors should be wet-vacuumed between cases as well as at the end of the day. Dry-dusting and dry-mopping should be avoided in the operating room since the dust created by these methods would continue to settle or float in the room for hours. The bedclothes over the patient should be handled gently when he is being transferred to the operating table in order to avoid throwing lint off into the air. Local policy may require bedclothes to be removed/replaced prior to the entry in the operating room; nevertheless, the patient should be covered with a cover sheet at all times. Dressings removed from a wound should be placed at once in a bag and the bag should be closed and discarded. Drainage that is left exposed to the air may become dried, thus enabling the infectious organisms in it to become airborne and be carried to other parts of the surgical suite and the hospital to infect others.

THE HAND SCRUB

The surgeon begins his efforts at aseptic technique with the hand scrub. Wise and co-workers (1959) have shown that 20—30% of surgeons' gloves are punctured at the end of an average operation. The purposes of the hand scrub are to remove superficial contaminants and loose epithelium and to reduce the bacterial count on the skin.

Many techniques of hand scrub have been suggested, but most are empirically based. Before beginning the hand scrub, the nails should be checked for cleanliness. All gross contamination should be removed with the use of a nail cleaner before the scrub continues. The arms are then wetted to several inches above the elbows. The hands are kept elevated above elbow height so that the direction of water flow will be toward the elbows.

The scrub begins at the tip of one finger of one hand. The long axis of the finger is then divided into four surfaces and 30 scrub strokes are applied to each surface. After this is done, the interfinger webbing is given 30 strokes and the next finger is begun and so on until the fingers of one hand are completed. Then the ventral, dorsal, and lateral surfaces of the hand are cleaned. The length of the forearm is divided into thirds, and each of the four surfaces is scrubbed progressing by thirds toward the elbow. The scrub should extend to 2 inches above the elbow. Once one hand and arm are completed, the surgeon then scrubs the other hand and arm in a like manner, beginning at the fingertips and working toward the elbow. When one area is scrubbed it should not be touched again because of the possibility of contamination from an unscrubbed area. Dunphy and Way (1973) recommend that the scrubbing procedure should take approximately 10 minutes. Successive scrubs that day need last only 5 minutes, if no major contamination has been encountered. After both arms are scrubbed, the brush is discarded and the arms are rinsed of excess soap. Most hospitals have foot or knee pedals for water control, but if the older faucet handles are being used, the surgeon must be careful not to contaminate the scrubbed areas of his arms while turning the water on and off with his elbow. The rinse should be done with elevated arms so that the water will drain from the fingertips progressing down the hands, arms, and finally the elbows.

HAND TOWEL DRYING (Figs 4.10–4.16)

A sterile towel is included within the sterile

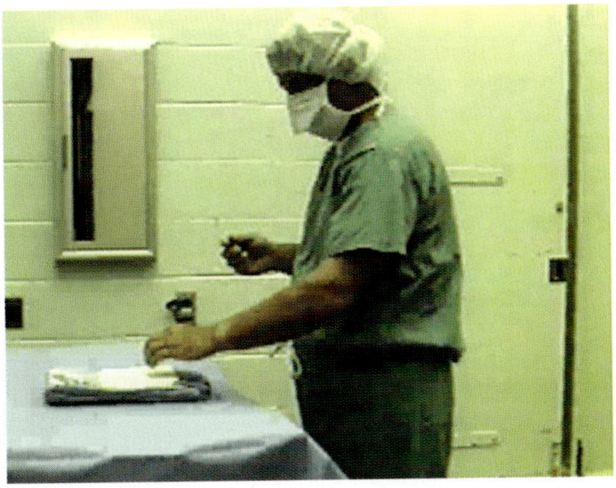

Fig. 4.10

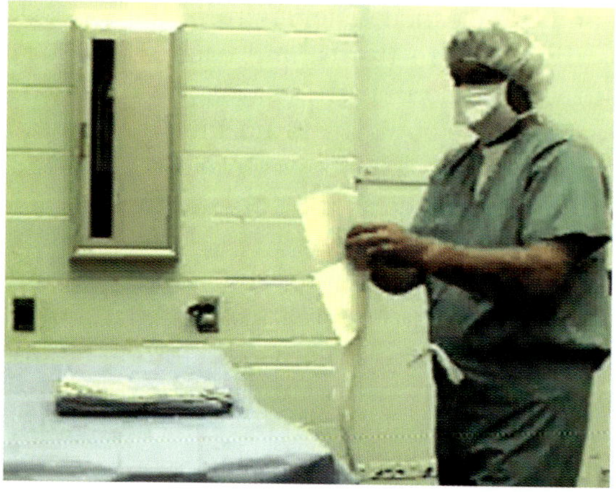

Fig. 4.11

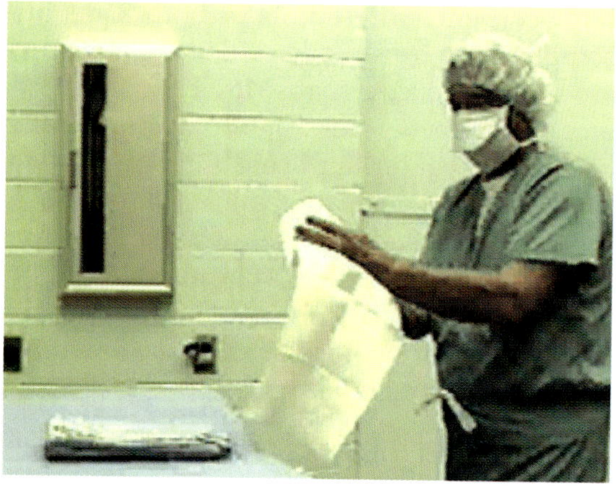

Fig. 4.12

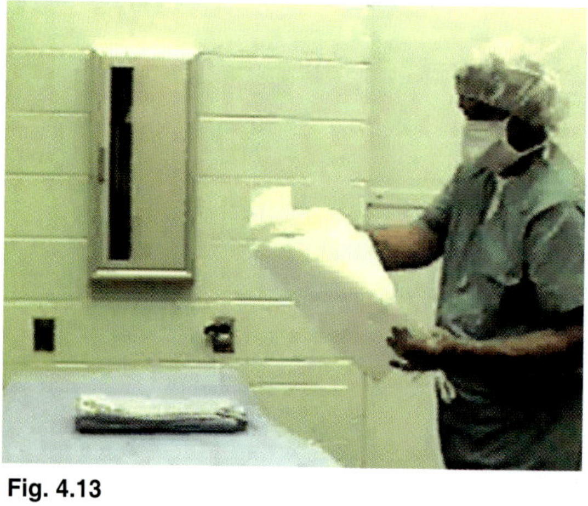

Fig. 4.13

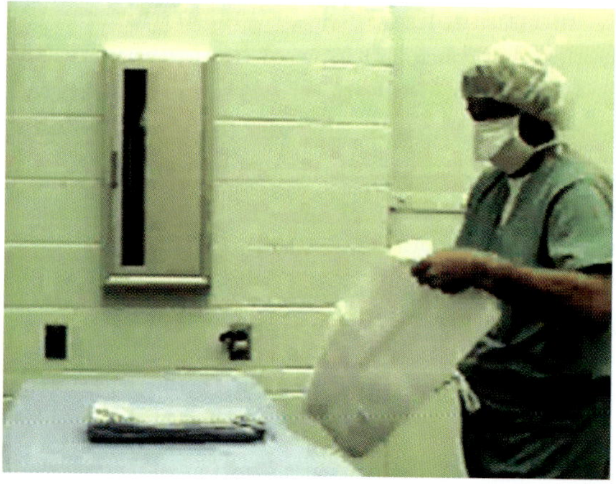

Fig. 4.14

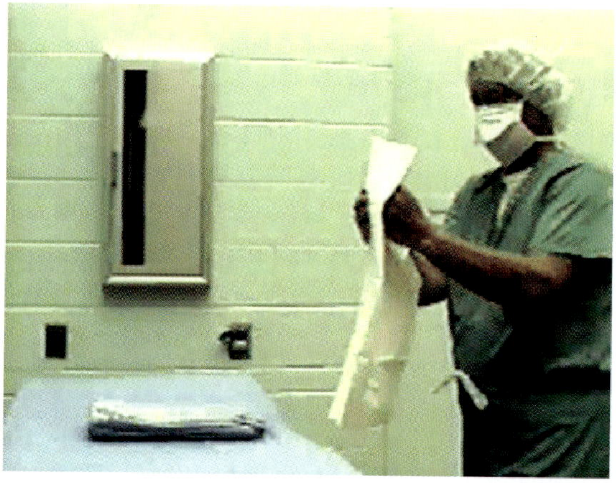

Fig. 4.15

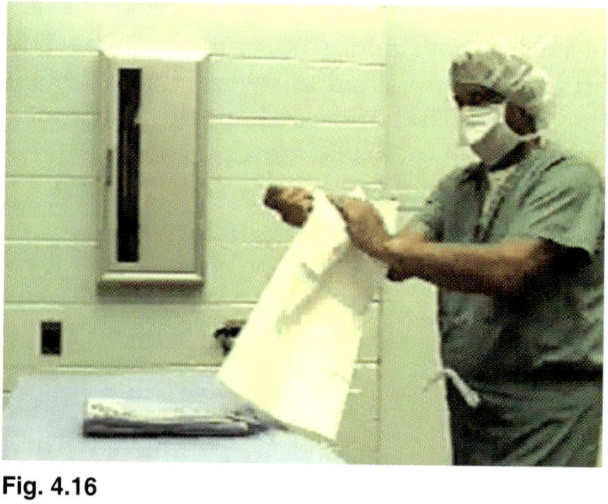

Fig. 4.16

gown pack. The towel is lifted away from the table and folded in half lengthwise. One hand and forearm are dried by one side of the towel. Always dry in the direction of hand to elbow so that contamination of the upper arm is not spread by the towel to the surgeon's hand.

The second hand and forearm are then dried by the other side of the towel in the direction of hand to elbow. The towel is then discarded away from the surgeon, making sure that the towel doesn't contact the sterile gown.

CLOSED GLOVING TECHNIQUE (Figs 4.17–4.31)

Step 1: An assistant opens the sterile pack of gloves and drops them into the sterile field (Figs 4.17 and 4.18).

Step 2: Left hand (within the gown) lifts the right glove by its cuff (Fig. 4.19).

Step 3: Right glove is laid on the palm of the right hand (cuff to cuff with the gown sleeve) with fingers of the glove pointing toward the elbow and the thumb of the glove positioned on top of the surgeon's covered right thumb (Fig. 4.20).

Step 4: The inside of the cuff of the glove is grasped by the right hand (still within the gown) and the left hand folds the cuff of the

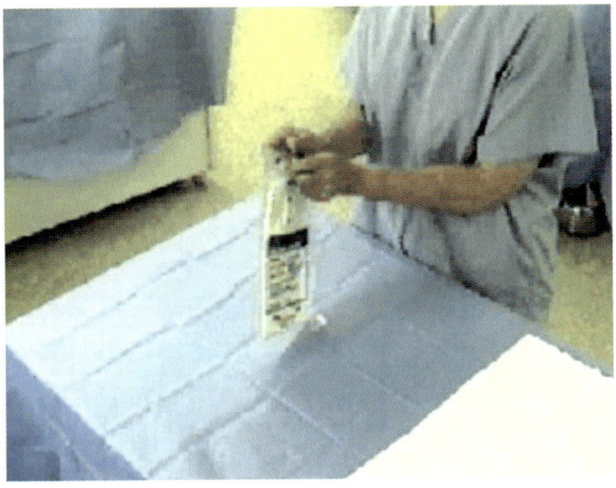

Fig. 4.17

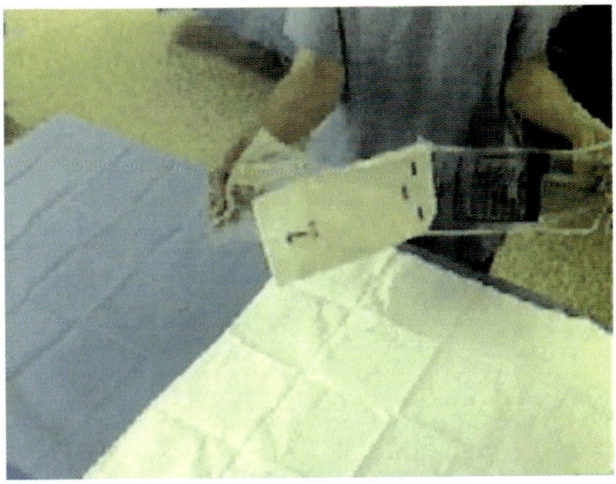

Fig. 4.18

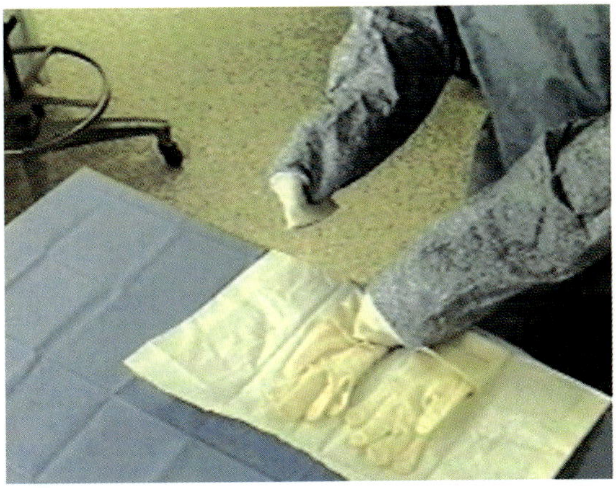

Fig. 4.19

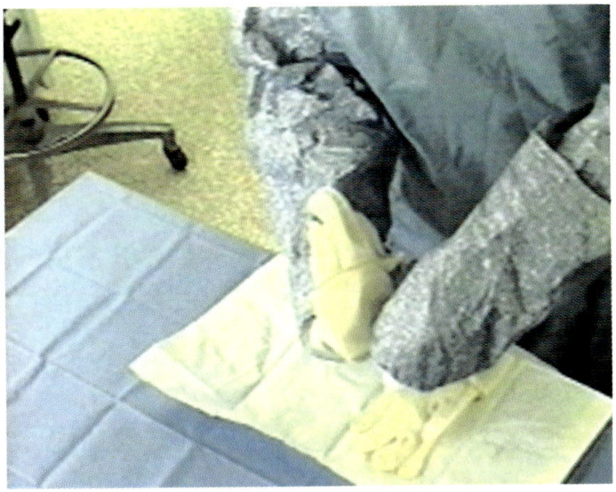

Fig. 4.20

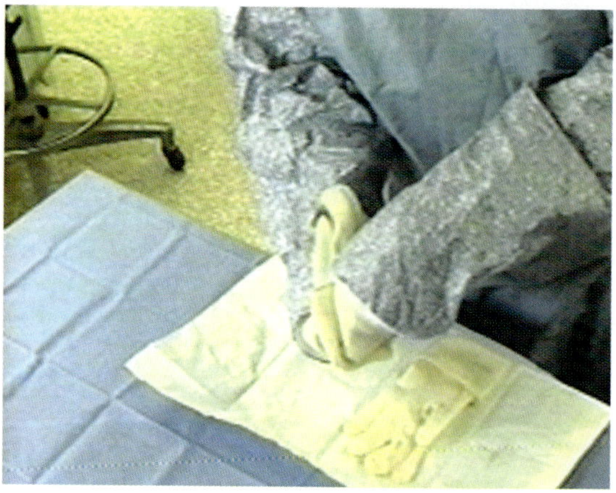

Fig. 4.21

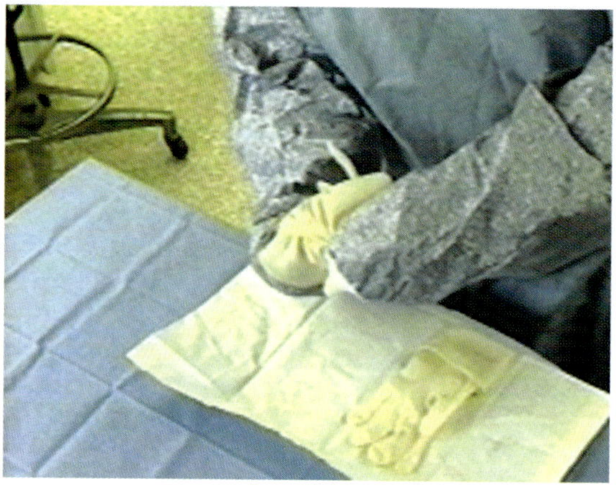

Fig. 4.22

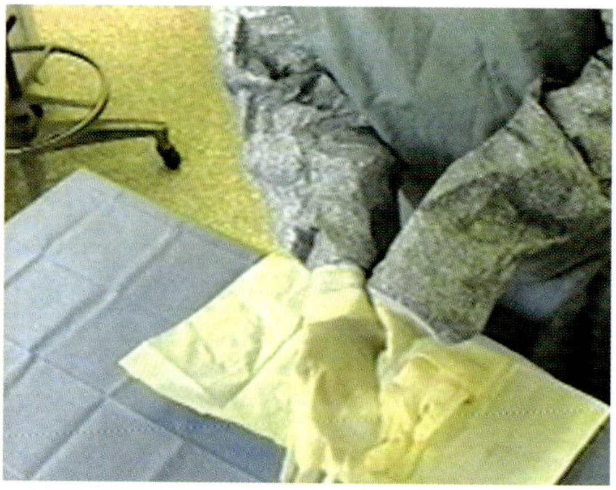

Fig. 4.23

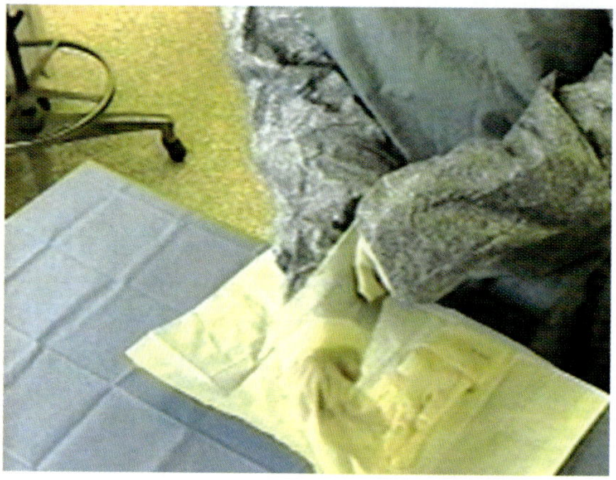

Fig. 4.24

glove over the back of the right hand (Figs 4.21 and 4.22).

Step 5: The left hand then pulls the cuff of the right glove and sleeve of the right gown towards the elbow as the right hand slides into the glove. Wait to adjust the glove until both gloves are on and sterility is ensured (left fingers may slip out of the gown while trying to adjust the right glove prematurely) (Figs 4.23 and 4.24).

Step 6: With the gloved right hand lift left glove by its cuff and place on palm of left hand (aligned with the cuff of the gown), with glove fingers pointing toward the elbow and the left thumb of the glove over the covered left thumb of surgeon (Figs 4.25 and 4.26).

Step 7: Left fingers (still within the gown) grasp the inside of the glove and the right hand pulls left glove cuff over the back of the hand (Figs 4.27 and 4.28).

Step 8: Pull the glove cuff and gown sleeve toward elbow as left hand slides into the glove (Figs 4.29 and 4.30).

Step 9: Now that both gloves are on, pull glove cuffs over gown sleeves and adjust gloves for comfort (Fig. 4.31).

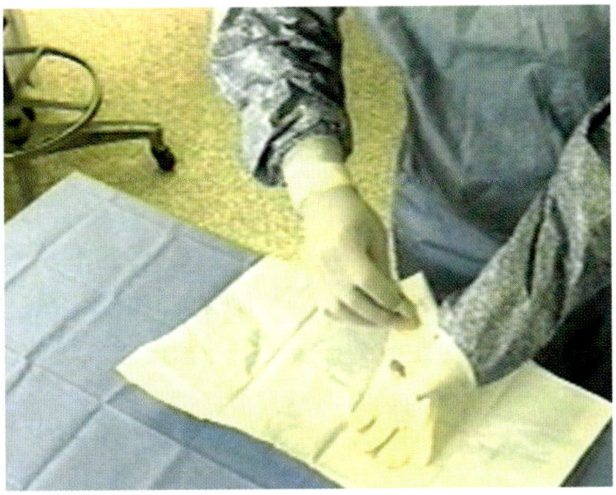

Fig. 4.25

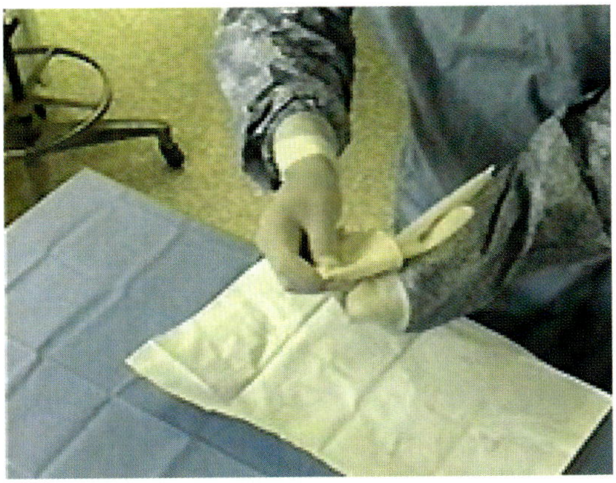

Fig. 4.26

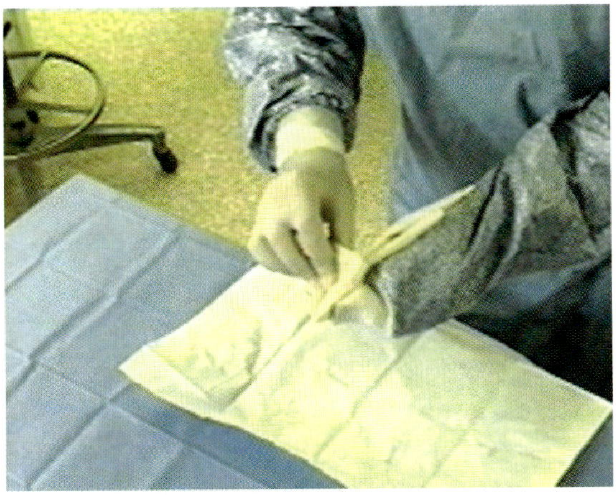

Fig. 4.27

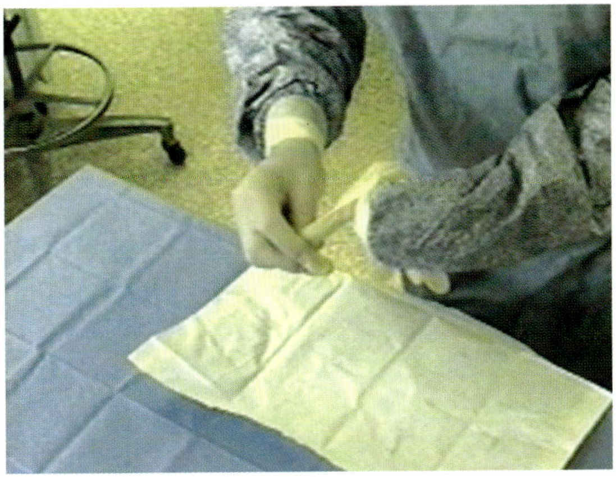

Fig. 4.28

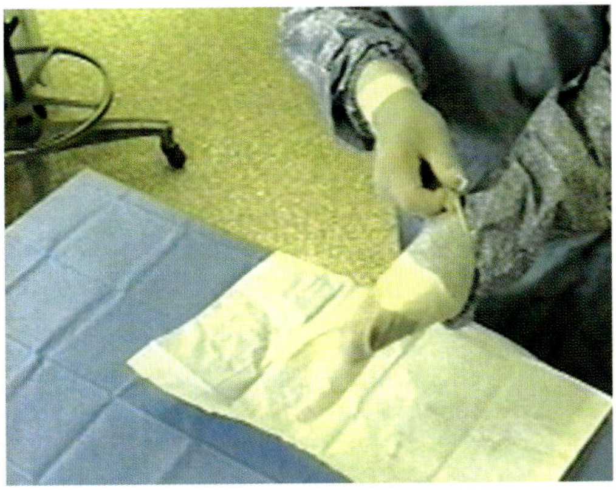

Fig. 4.29

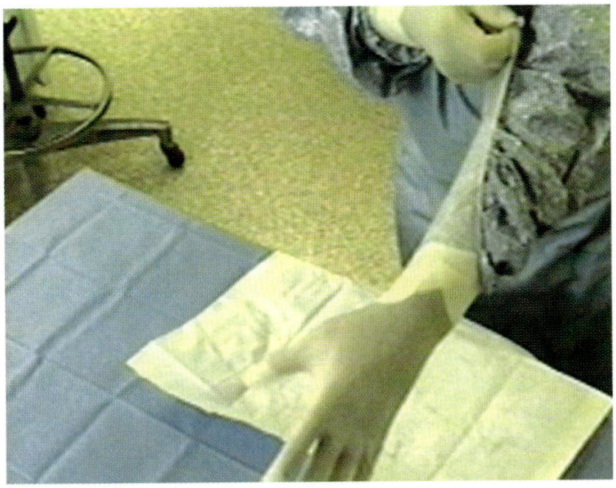

Fig. 4.30

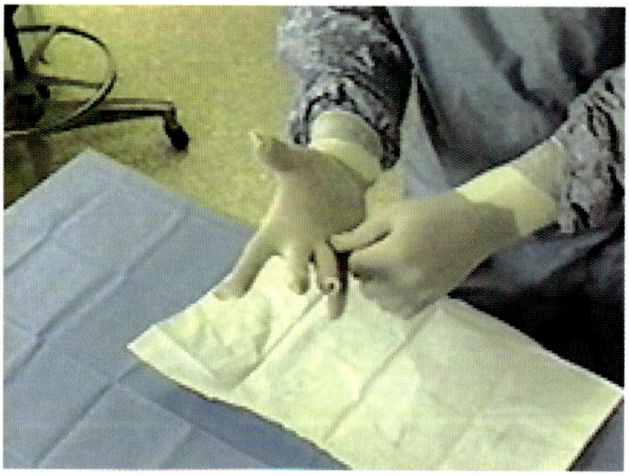

Fig. 4.31

GOWNS FOR SURGERY

Disposable Paper Gown (Fig. 4.32)

Advantages

Paper gowns are resistant to wetting so they are less permeable to bacteria. They are preferred for wet bloody surgery. Donning a new gown for each surgery and disposing of it at the end ensures sterility.

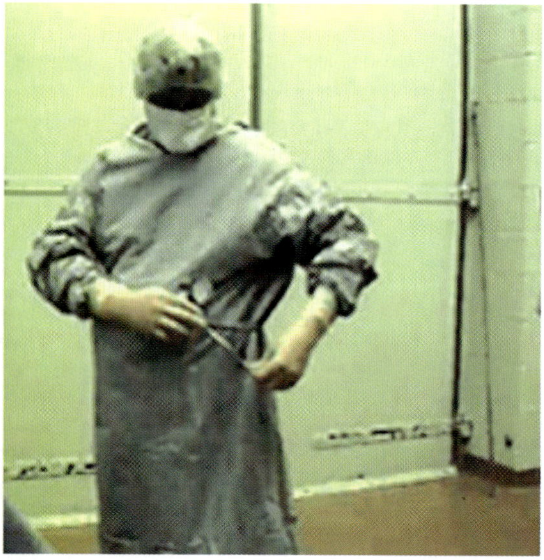

Fig. 4.32

Disadvantages

Paper is less ecologically sound because it is not reusable.

Linen (cloth) Gowns (Fig. 4.33)

Advantages

Linen gowns are both comfortable and reusable. Previously worn gowns can be autoclaved to regain sterility.

Disadvantages

Linen is a woven material so that when it becomes wet, bacteria can permeate through its interstices. Linen is not the gown material of choice for wet, bloody surgical procedures.

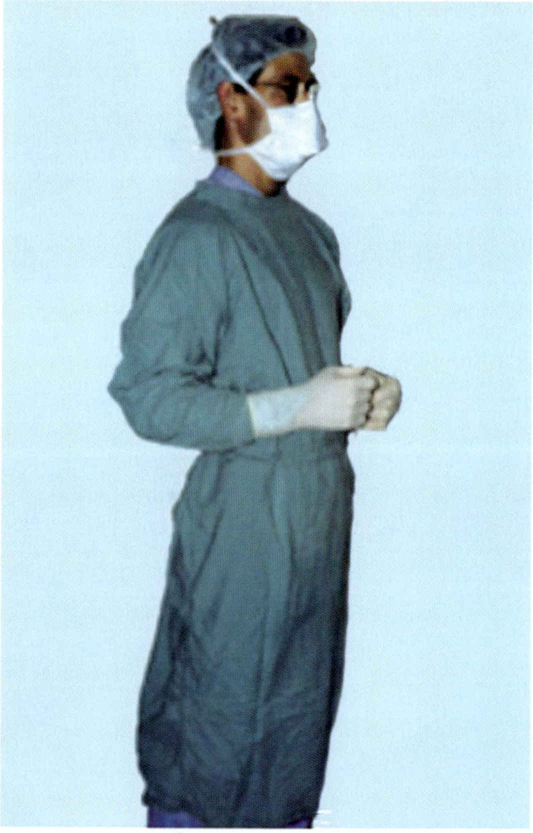

Fig. 4.33

Plastic Gowns (Fig. 4.34)

Advantages

Plastic is superior in its resistance to wetting and bacterial penetration. Plastic can be used to reinforce paper gowns during wet surgery (plastic sleeves for abdominal surgery).

Disadvantages

Plastic is extremely uncomfortable to wear because of the inability to shed heat and perspiration.

FOLDING OF A GOWN FOR STERILIZATION (Figs 4.35 to 4.42)

Hold the gown so that the outside is facing away from you. Place the outside right and left ties into the white tab.

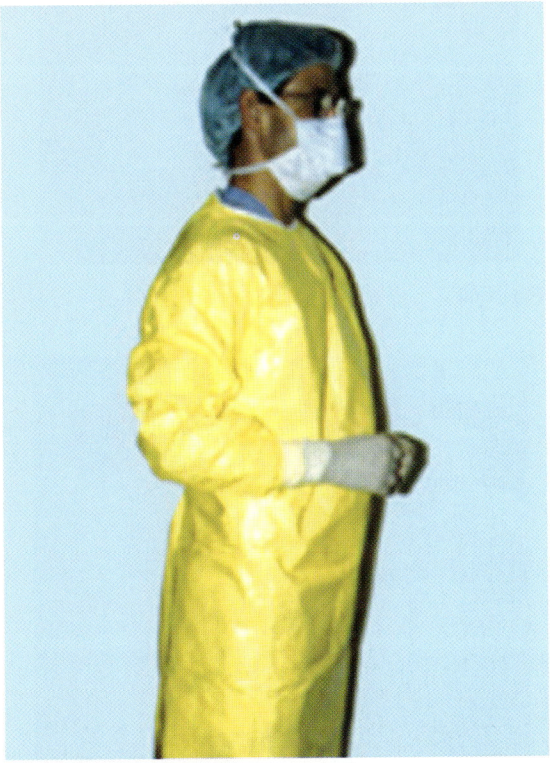

Fig. 4.34

Fold the gown in half lengthwise twice making sure that the inside of the gown is showing.

Lie the gown on a table and fold in half lengthwise again. Then fold end to end twice. The gown is folded in such a way that the top of the inside of the gown is presented when

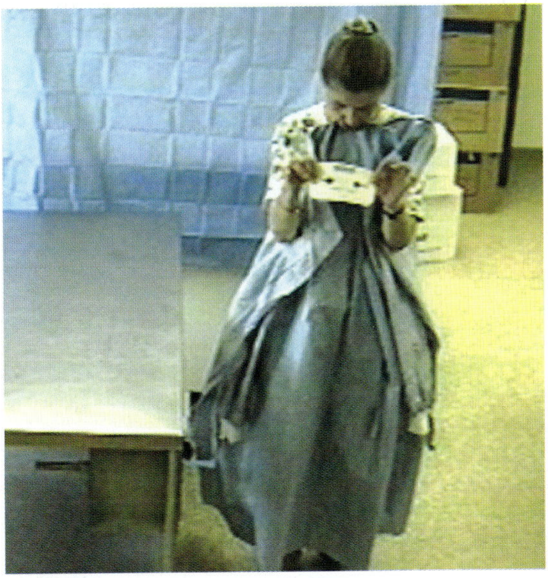

Fig. 4.35

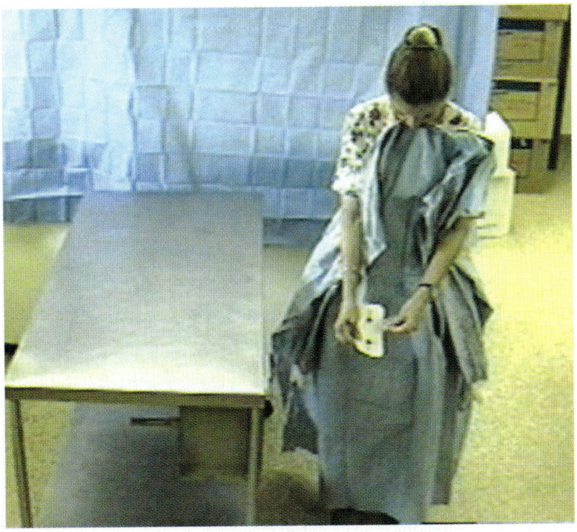

Fig. 4.36

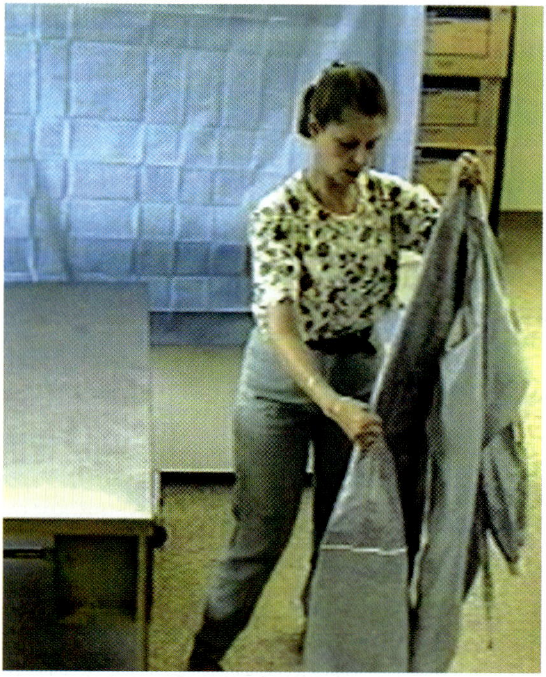

Fig. 4.37

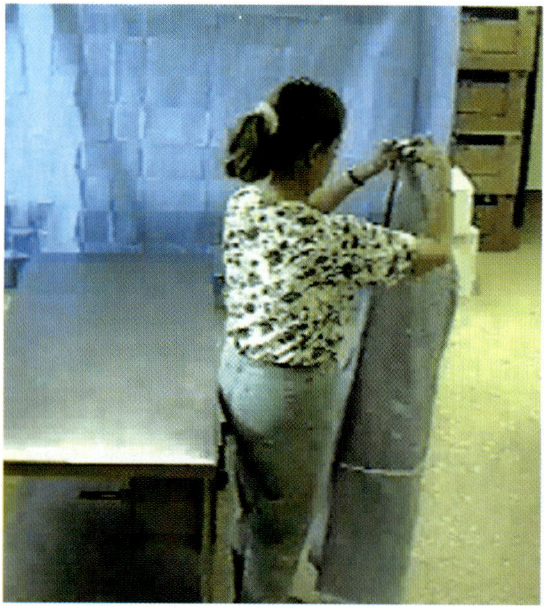

Fig. 4.38

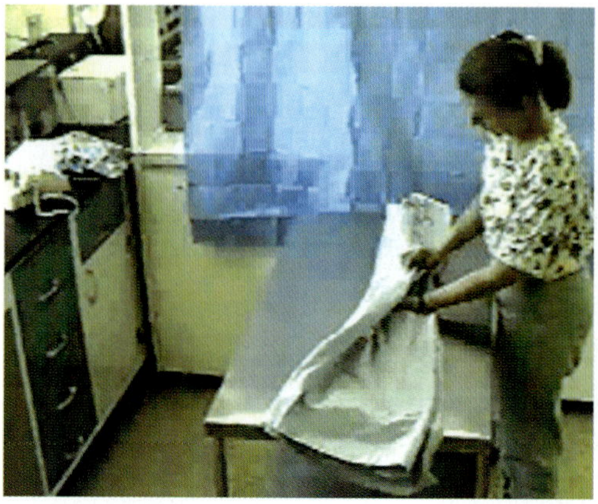

Fig. 4.39

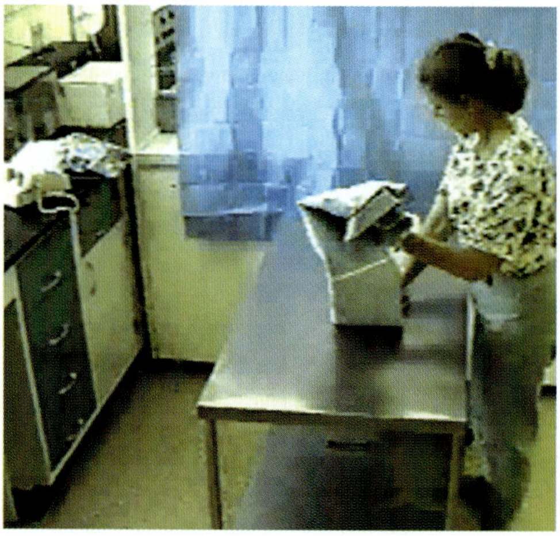

Fig. 4.40

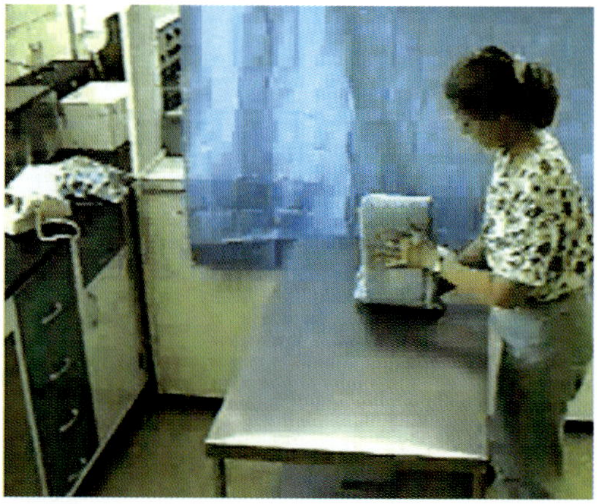

Fig. 4.41

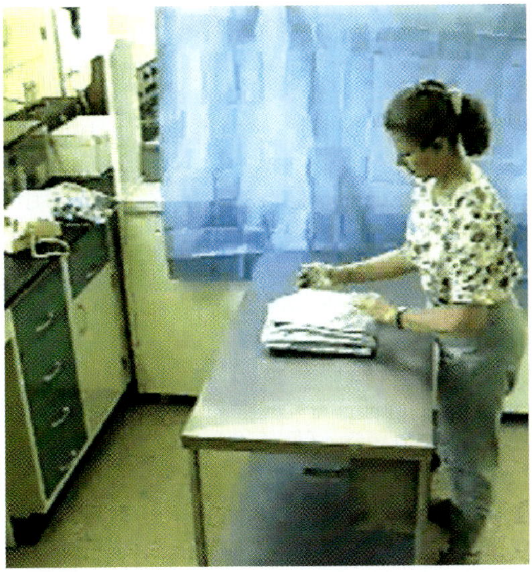

Fig. 4.42

the sterile pack is unwrapped. This is the area grasped by the surgeon to begin donning the gown.

PREPARATION OF THE SURGICAL SITE

Preparation of the surgical site is important to reduce contamination by the patient's own normal flora as well as resistant bacteria acquired from the hospital environment. The operative site cannot be sterilized by current methods, but the gross cleansing action does significantly reduce the incidence of postoperative infections. All extraoral procedures should be accompanied by a presurgical scrub. A circumoral preparation should precede intraoral procedures to prevent transference of the resident skin flora to the intraoral wound.

Before the preparation, a lubricating ointment should be applied to the patient's eyes and the eyes taped shut. Also, if bleeding in proximity to the ear is anticipated, the external auditory meatus should be gently capped with petroleum jelly-impregnated gauze.

If there is hair in the surgical area, it is generally removed just prior to scrubbing the skin. Shaving the area the night before produces small abrasions on the skin and resident bacteria multiply as a result of the injury. This phenomenon is lessened by decreasing the time interval between the shave and the skin preparation. Some surgeons feel the close shave is unnecessary, and indeed in some surgical sites such as the eyebrow the shave is never done routinely.

The scrub should begin in the center of the area to be prepared and then move outward concentrically, if possible. Preparing the central part first and then successive areas away from the operative site will minimize contamination of the already cleansed region from an unscrubbed one. Once the center has been scrubbed it should not be touched again with the same sponge. The surgeon may choose to scrub the area a second time with a new sterile sponge, but this process must again start in the middle and extend toward the periphery. The skin preparation should take about 5 minutes unless the area is grossly contaminated.

Intraoral preparation before surgery traditionally has not been done because of the improbability of significantly reducing the bacterial count of the mouth.

OPERATING ROOM PROCEDURES

The operating room is merely a clean environment in which to do surgery. It is not sterile. The ceiling, walls, and floors are regularly disinfected, especially following a contaminated case. The air may be filtered or flow past an ultraviolet radiation device to reduce bacterial counts. The operating rooms are set away from the hospital by two sets of doors. People are required to remove their street clothes and don scrub suits before entering the operating room area. Masks, gowns, gloves, and special shoes or shoe covers are worn during the operation. The patient and surgical site are draped and isolated. The surgical instruments and related equipment are sterile. All these precautions tend to reduce the chance of wound contamination, but still the operative site is only clean, not sterile.

The scrub suit consists of a pair of pants or skirt and a shirt or blouse, which should be tucked inside. A cap is placed over the hair. If the surgeon has long hair, surgical hoods are available and should be used. A mask is then tied in place over the surgeon's nose and mouth. Conductive shoes should also be worn. These shoes will prevent the buildup of static electricity, which could cause a spark and subsequent explosion involving the volatile inflammable anesthetic gases. The shoes also lessen the chance of patient electrocution. Today the many electrical devices surrounding and attached to the patient in the operating room are potential sources of electrical shock. According to Arbeit, Parker, and Reuben (1972), one tenth of a milliampere of a 60 cycle per second current can produce ventricular fibrillation. By wearing conductive shoes, the surgeon becomes an alternate pathway for aberrant currents. If conductive shoes are not available, the surgeon must use conductive shoe covers.

After entering the operating theater and before gowning, personnel should take precautions to avoid contaminating open packs of draping material or instruments. Once the patient is prepared and draped, only those who are scrubbed, gowned, and gloved may work in the surgical site. The backs of those gowned are considered nonsterile, as are areas below the waist. Therefore one must be careful to keep the arms above the waist when resting and not to back into any sterile areas. Also, one must remember that the mask and surgical cap are not sterile, and these can contaminate any sterile object they touch.

DRAPING THE PATIENT

The purpose of draping a patient is to isolate the surgical area from other parts of the body that have not been prepared for surgery and also from nonsterile operating room equipment and personnel. A double-layered drape is usually considered necessary for effective isolation. To apply this drape without displacing the endotracheal tube, it is suggested that the anesthesiologist temporarily disconnect the tube from the anesthesia machine so that the patient's head may be lifted and the drape placed beneath. An additional two, three, or four towel drape is then placed over the endotracheal tube and adjacent unscrubbed areas to complete the isolation of the surgical site (Fig. 4.43).

An effective way of isolating the mouth from the surgical site is by using a clear plastic drape with an adhesive side (ViDrape).

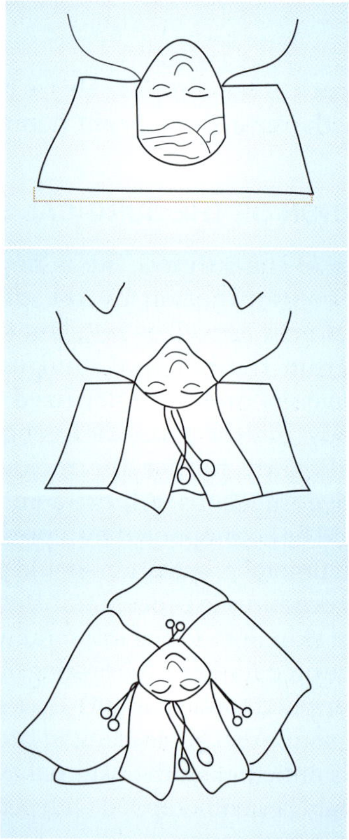

Fig. 4.43: Patient's head is placed on sterile sheet covered by two towels. Towels are used to drape patient's head. Additional towels may then be added to isolate surgical area.

INCISIONS AND SUTURING TECHNIQUES

Knowledge of healthy and diseased actions is not less necessary to be understood than the principles of other sciences. By an acquaintance with principles we learn the cause of disease. Without this knowledge a man cannot be a surgeon .... The last part of surgery, namely operations, is a reflection on the healing art; it is a tacit acknowledgement of the insufficiency of surgery. It is like an armed savage who attempts to get that by force which a civilized man would by stratagem.

(John Hunter, 1728-93, Surgeon, St. George's Hospital, London)

Good surgical care begins with the application and integration of basic sciences—such as anatomy, biochemistry, histology, microbiology, pathology, pharmacology, and physiology to the management of the ill or diseased patient. Clinically, this takes the form of the evaluation process, presurgical preparations, intraoperative management, techniques of asepsis, craft of surgery, and postoperative care.

PRESURGICAL EVALUATION

The first step in presurgical evaluation is the recognition of existing medical conditions. For example, a history of hepatitis B, uncontrolled diabetes mellitus, or sickle cell anemia may alter the usual approach to the patient's surgical problem. The recognition of nutritional deficiency states is also important, and preoperative dietary supplements may be indicated in elective situations. Some patients may also require prophylactic medication before surgery.

Certain disease states such as asthma or epilepsy can be aggravated by psychologic or physical stress.

A consideration of the patient's medical status also helps in the anticipation of complications. For example, individuals with anemia or agammaglobulinemia or those taking immunosuppressive drugs may have increased susceptibility to infection and delayed healing. Patients with a history of alcoholism, recent ingestion of large doses of aspirin, or hypertension may have prolonged bleeding. When complications are anticipated, the proper measures can be taken to prevent them or at least to lessen their severity.

PRESURGICAL PREPARATION

General Considerations

It would be desirable to have every patient who is to undergo a surgical procedure in optimum health. However, this state does not exist in the majority of patients. The tolerance of the surgical procedure, the postoperative course, the incidence of complications, and the quality and rate of healing can all be positively or negatively affected by the health of the patient. Therefore it becomes the goal of the surgeon to maximize the physical condition of the patient prior to surgery. For example, a patient with a history of alcoholism and nutritional deficiency may require vitamin K to prevent bleeding because of a lack of the vitamin K-dependent coagulation factors II, VII, IX, and X. Multiple vitamins including thiamine may also be needed, and, if the patient has a protein deficiency, a high protein diet may be instituted preoperatively to aid wound healing and body defenses.

Prophylactic Medications

Medications are given prophylactically to prevent anticipated complications that arise with some degree of predictability. The two most frequently used drugs for prophylaxis are antibiotics and steroids. Subacute bacterial endocarditis is a serious complication of heart disease carrying a high degree of morbidity and mortality. Antibiotic prophylaxis is recommended for patients with most forms of congenital heart disease, aortic stenosis, pulmonary stenosis, patent ductus arteriosus, mitral valve prolapse syndrome or other acquired valvular heart disease and prosthetic heart valves. Other indications for prophylactic antibiotics include patients with compound fractures, those who are immunologically suppressed or those on long term corticosteroids.

Corticosteroids may have to be administered prophylactically under certain circumstances. A deficiency of corticosteroids in the stressed patient results in a precipitous drop in blood pressure because of pooling of blood in capillary beds and increased vascular permeability. In patients who have adrenal insufficiency, prophylactic use of corticosteroids prior to surgery is important to prevent a possible fatal episode. Patients with adrenal insufficiency include those who have been taking corticosteroids for longer than two weeks or those who have been on long term steroid therapy and have discontinued it within the last year. In these patients, adrenal atrophy attributable to the lack of stimulation by ACTH has started to take place and therefore the adrenal cortex will not respond normally to stress. Corticosteroids are also given prophylactically to limit postoperative oedema.

SURGICAL TECHNIQUE

Skin Incisions

Before the surgeon puts knife to tissue he should plan the incision. On the face it is advisable to map the incision out with pen and Bonney's blue (Fig. 4.44 shows the marking of the submandibular incision). For incisions in the neck it is satisfactory to scratch the line of the cut with the back of the point, provided that the scratch is not carried too deep. Lengthy incisions should be cross-hatched at about three places with Bonney's blue on the face, or with scratches on the neck. Such marks help in the correct approximation of the wound edges at the end of the procedure.

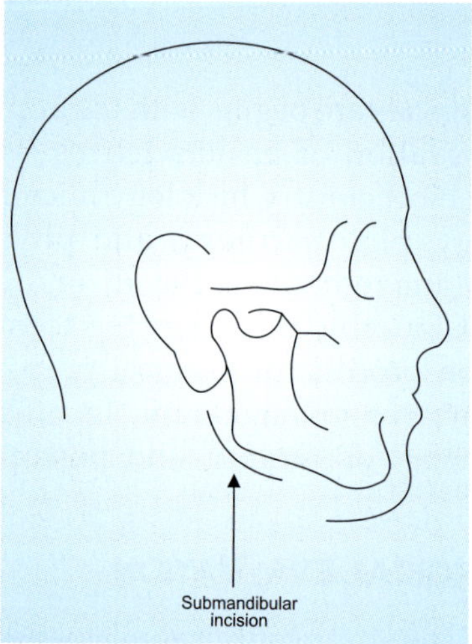

Fig. 4.44: The submandibular incision.

The skin is incised at right angles to the surface except within the eye-brow where the cut should be angled along the line of the eyebrow hairs. Whenever an incision is made, the blade should be held perpendicular to the epithelial surface and not obliquely, which will result in a bias cut. The knife should be passed in one stroke over the predetermined length of the incision to avoid causing irregularities in the wound edges. The skin should be slightly tensed by finger pressure to produce uniform resistance to the passage of the blade and a predictable depth of penetration. When operating in vascular areas, the surgeon may decide to modify the incision technique to reduce bleeding. For example, electrosurgery may be used instead of a scalpel. Another method, used more commonly, is the injection of a vasoconstricting solution into the area prior to making the incision. Because local anesthetic solutions containing a vasoconstrictor such as epinephrine are readily available, these are often used for this purpose. Otherwise, a solution of 1:100,000 epinephrine can be prepared by mixing 0.1 ml of 1:1000 epinephrine with 9.9 ml of sterile isotonic saline solution. The solution should be used that day, as this dilute concentration of epinephrine is very unstable without preservatives.

In patients undergoing general anesthesia with a halogenated hydrocarbon inhalation agent such as halothane or enflurane (Ethrane), the concomitant use of epinephrine can produce ventricular arrhythmias. This complication appears to be dose related (Rosen and Roe, 1963), and therefore it is prudent to use minimum amounts of epinephrine in these patients. A waiting period of at least 5 minutes following the injection is necessary for the epinephrine to act fully. It should be pointed out that with this technique the possibility of postoperative bleeding exists from vessels that did not bleed the time of surgery because of the effect of the vasoconstrictor.

Skin and subcutaneous tissue should be penetrated in one sweep if possible down to the subjacent layer. The tissues should be separated on both sides of the wound over the surface of each succeeding layer and each is opened in turn. In this way, proper layer-by-layer closure is facilitated. Where the subcutaneous fat is thick a subcutaneous suture will be required and the wound edges should be undercut to a depth of about 2 mm about 4 mm deep from the surface. This will permit proper eversion of the wound edges without unnecessarily deep stitches and minor corrections can he made in the lie of the wound margins with the skin sutures. Such undercutting should be done as the wound is established, so that proper haemostasis has been ensured by the time that closure is undertaken. It is particularly important to undercut the opposite edge of a wound where one edge is raised as a skin flap. Unless both margins are equally mobile a nice closure is difficult. Undercutting is also necessary where there is oedema of the skin, as, for example, when osteomyelitis or certain fractures are operated upon. Otherwise the stiff skin is difficult to suture.

The skin edges of neck and facial wounds should not be grasped with dissecting forceps, tissue forceps, or towel clips or they will be crushed and damaged. Where a wound is to be open for some while it must be protected from organisms brought to the surface of the adjacent skin as the patient sweats. Plastic sprays, adhesive drapes, and skin towels should be applied to overcome this problem, particularly where bone surgery is involved. Where skin towels are applied, they should be sewn on with loosely tied horizontal mattress sutures and not clamped on with towel clips. Should a skin flap be everted as the tissues are retracted, a moist pack should be applied to the underside of the subcutaneous fat to prevent drying in the heat of the operating room.

The deep layer should be closed neatly with 3-0 or 4-0 plain catgut. Often a continuous suture is satisfactory, but the stitch should not be drawn up tight like a purse string and the knots should be buried on the deep surface of the layer. Skin hooks and 5–0 or 6–0 nylon on atraumatic curved cutting needles should be used to close the skin. Some surgeons prefer braided silk as it is softer and knots more easily. The stitches should enter not more than 2 mm from the wound edge and pass to a depth of about 4 mm embracing a greater width of subcutaneous tissue. Each edge should be dealt with separately so that accurate passage of the needle through the tissues is ensured. The suture should pass to the same depth through each wound margin to avoid overlapping or stepping of the skin and it must lie at right angles to the wound. When it is closed the wound surfaces should be approximated so that no dead spaces are left and the cut edges at the surface should be slightly raised in order to produce a final scar that is flat and level with the rest of the surface: A spray-on plastic dressing is sufficient since a dry wound stands the best chance of remaining uninfected, unless, of course, a pressure dressing is applied.

Peri-orbital Incisions

Incisions are made in this region to expose the zygomatico-frontal region, the floor of the orbit and infra-orbital margin and the medial wall of the orbit. The zygomatico-frontal region can be exposed by an incision in the lateral end of the eyebrow carried backwards in the line of a crow's foot crease. An alternative is a V-shaped cut made just internal to the lateral margin of the orbit, in the lax tissue lateral to the upper and lower eyelids. Medially an incision can be made medial to the supra-orbital notch and within the eyebrow. If necessary, such an incision can be extended across the root of the nose so as to expose the nasal bones. Inferiorly the incision is usually made in a curve following the line of the infra-orbital margin. It should not encroach on the lateral third of the orbit or the lymphatic drainage from the lower eyelid is affected.

For resections of the maxilla the incision runs through the upper lip, lateral to the philtrum, around the ala of the nose and then up to the margin of the lower lid lateral to the lacrimal canaliculus. It is carried laterally through the lower conjunctival fornix and may be extended further laterally in a crow's foot crease (Crockett, 1963). Incisions involving the free margin of the lip should be broken by lateral cuts and sutured in a Z. Special care should be given to approximating the muscle layer. Both measures are necessary to prevent notching of the lip as the scar contracts. Stepping of eyelid incisions is also necessary to prevent a coloboma of the lid as the wound heals (Kazanjian and Converse, 1959). That is, the conjunctival incision is made a short distance to one side of the skin incision so that a step is created through the muscle layer. Opposite the lower lateral rim of the orbit a radial incision is made. Such cuts not only follow the skin creases, but also do not interfere with the lymphatic drainage of the lower lid.

Pre-auricular Incisions

Pre-auricular incisions are required to approach the zygomatic arch, temporomandibular joint, and parotid salivary gland. Such incisions should start within the hairline, slope backwards to the pinna, and follow the anterior attachment of the auricle on to the free margin of the tragus. From there they may be extended down and then back beneath the cover of the lobe of the ear. If further extension is required, it may be made backwards into the hairline again or downwards and forwards into a submandibular crease.

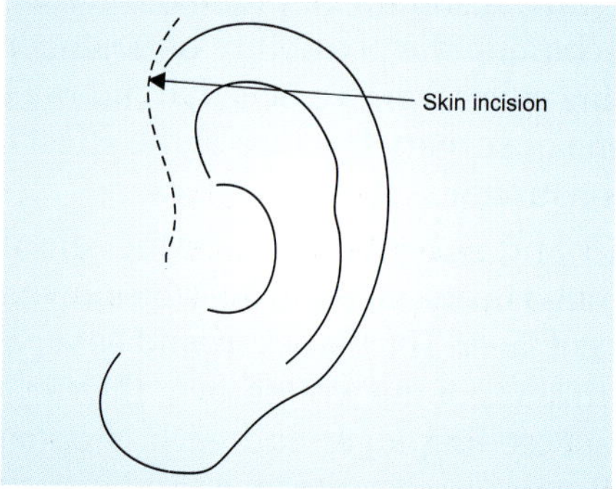

Fig. 4.45: Dingman's approach to TMJ.

INTRAORAL INCISIONS

Many oral and maxillofacial surgical procedures necessitate incisions. A few basic principles are important for performing tissue incisions.

1. A sharp blade of the proper size should be used. In general most oral surgical incisions are made with a No. 15 blade. The only common exception is the use of a No. 11 blade for abscess drainage. A sharp blade

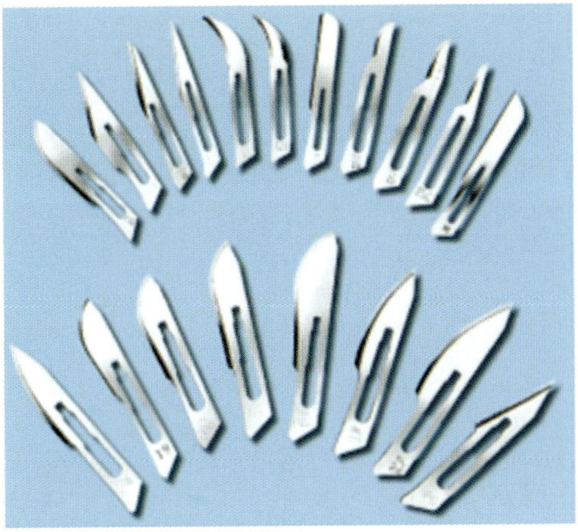

Fig. 4.46: Blades used in surgical practice.

allows incisions to be made cleanly without unnecessary damage caused by repeated strokes.

2. A firm, continuous stroke should be used when incising. Repeated strokes increase both the amount of damaged tissue within a wound and the amount of bleeding thereby impairing wound healing. Long continuous strokes are preferable to short, interrupted ones.
3. The surgeon should carefully avoid cutting vital structures when incising.
4. Incisions through epithelial surfaces should be made with the blade held perpendicular to the epithelial surface. This angle produces wound edges that are squared and therefore both easier to reorient properly during suturing and less susceptible to necrosis of the wound edges.
5. Incisions in the oral cavity should be properly placed. It is more desirable to place incisions over healthy bone than over areas which will not have healthy bone to support the sutured wound.

PRINCIPLES OF FLAP DESIGN

1. The apex of a flap should be never wider than the base. Flaps should have sides that either run parallel or continuously taper from the base to the apex of the flap.
2. In general the length of a flap should be no more than twice the width of the flap (Fig. 4.47).
3. When possible an axial blood supply should be included in the base of the flap.
4. The base of the flaps should not be excessively twisted or stretched because either of these maneuvers may compromise the supplying vessels.

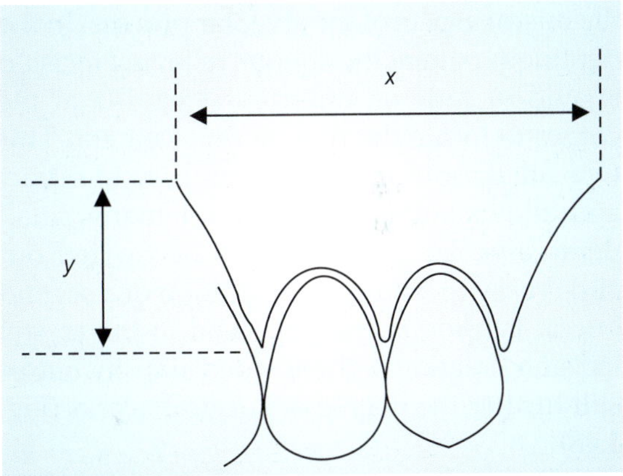

Fig. 4.47: Base (x) must not be less than the height (y) and preferably $x = 2y$

A gingival margin incision which divides the mandibular interdental papillae will permit the insertion of a periosteal elevator and the reflection of either the buccal or lingual mucoperiosteum or both. Similarly, an incision along the crest of the mandibular edentulous ridge will also permit buccal and lingual mucoperiosteal flaps to be raised. Such flaps are described as envelope flaps. If required the incision can be extended backwards into the retromolar region and then distobuccally up the external oblique ridge and anterior border of the coronoid process. No vessel of a size requiring formal ligation will be encountered until this upwards extension of the incision reaches a point just below the level of-the-occlusal surface of the upper 3rd molar. Here, the buccal artery and long buccal nerve lie side by side and cross the anterior border of the coronoid process medial to-lateral on the superficial aspect of the buccinator muscle. The deep facial vein runs either with the artery and nerve or a little higher up.

A second incision can be added which starts at one end of the crestal incision and is carried towards the buccal sulcus. The second incision can be a straight one which leaves the first at an obtuse angle, or with the edentulous ridge the crestal incision can be continued in a curve onto the buccal aspect of the alveolar process. In the dentulous patient the oblique relieving incision should include an interdental papilla at the corner to locate the flap on replacement. This two-sided, or triangular, flap is easy to retract and allows sufficient access for many small dento-alveolar procedures to be carried out and is easy to suture. The addition of a second buccal incision at the other end of the crestal incision creating a three sided flap increases still further the degree of surgical access (Fig. 4.48).

The problem of tension from muscular activity is encountered again when horizontal incisions are made either to deglove the chin or to expose the anterior part of the maxilla during a Le Fort I level osteotomy. Such incisions should be made so that a generous skirt of sulcus mucosa is left on the gingival aspect. In the case of the mandible the incision should be carried out on the labial aspect of the sulcus and then obliquely downwards through the mentalis muscles to provide a sufficient thickness of tissues on the gingival side to hold sutures. A continuous horizontal mattress suture line will bring the deeper tissues together and evert the wound margin, but should not be drawn excessively tight, nor should large bites of tissue be taken at each horizontal step or the wound edge will be strangulated and slough. The epithelial edges are coadapted by oversewing with a continuous plain suture.

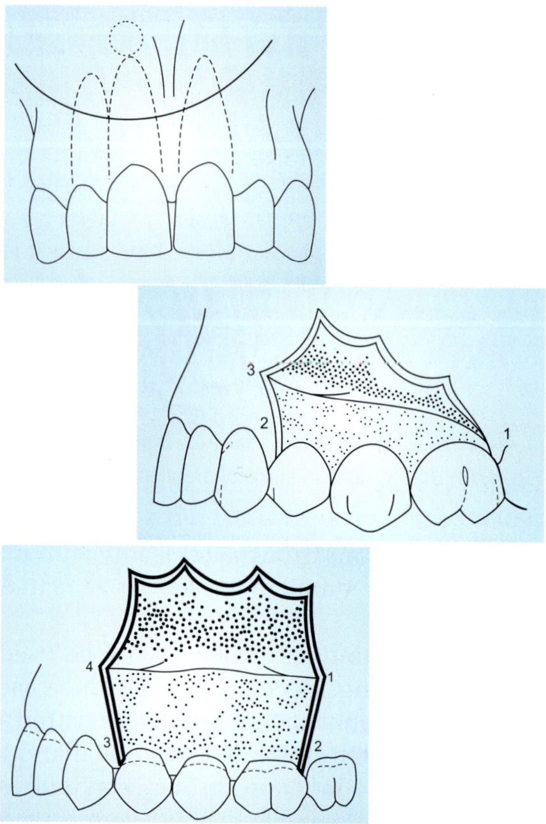

Fig. 4.48: Flap designs used for improved surgical access. (A) Semilunar incision used during apicectomy. (B) Vertical release incision converts envelope flap to 3 cornered flap. (C) Vertical incision on either ends of an envelop flap converts it to a 4 cornered flap.

FLAP REFLECTION

Flaps are raised by dissecting parallel to the surface at the junction of tissue layers. Where these have similar mechanical properties, such as the junction of soft tissue layers, sharp dissection is used. Mostly dental surgeons are intent upon exposing the mandible and maxilla so that flaps are raised subperiosteally. This is done by blunt dissection with a periosteal elevator making use of the well defined plane of mechanical discontinuity between the soft tissues and the hard bone. The attachment of the periosteum to bone varies in strength from place to place. The interdental papillae are firmly attached to the cribriform surface of the tops of the interdental septa. In the edentulous jaw this cribriform bone forms a narrow continuous strip along the crest of the ridge. Connective tissue fibres and vessels which pass from bone to periosteum resist separation by the periosteal elevator and it may be necessary to cut them with a scalpel.

The surface of the bone beyond the alveolar process can be exposed by further elevation of periosteum and overlying soft tissues, but a sufficient mesiodistal length of flap needs to be developed to permit adequate retraction and comfortable access to the bone at the operation site. On the outer aspect of the body of the mandible several structures are encountered which require special attention. Foremost of these is the mental nerve. Gentle use of the periosteal elevator will preserve the mental nerve and vessels inside their conical sleeve of periosteum. Special care should be taken where the patient is edentulous. If the alveolar process is atrophic the mental foramen will be relatively close to the crest of the ridge. Indeed where resorption has been extreme the nerve may emerge on the crest of the residual ridge and can be seen radiating outwards beneath the mucosa.

Anterior to and below the mental foramen there are the origins of the depressor labii and depressor anguli oris muscles and the insertion of the platysma muscle. These add only a marginally stronger attachment of the soft tissues to the mandible. In contrast, the origin of the mentalis muscle below the incisors requires a substantial effort with a rougine to detach it. Indeed the periosteum is firmly attached over the whole mental eminence. The attachment of the buccinator to the mandible is easily disrupted, but it should not be raised unless the additional access is definitely required. Once the edge of the muscle has been separated oedema of the buccal space is facilitated producing a greater degree of facial swelling postoperatively. As the body of the mandible is uncovered buccal to the second molar it should be remembered that the facial artery and vein lie immediately external to the periosteum at this point.

More posteriorly the insertion of the masseter, needs to be separated to expose the outer aspect of the mandibular angle. This requires little effort until the posterior border of the ramus and the lower border of the angle are reached. However the tough, inelastic periosteum may need to be incised by a few gentle strokes across the inner surface to permit adequate retraction of the muscle to allow work on the underlying bone.

The shape of the mandible makes surgical access to its inner aspect awkward and this difficulty is increased by strong muscle origins. The genial muscles can be detached only by cutting through their origin, close to the tubercles and of course if complete detachment is necessary, they should be reattached. The sublingual arteries enter the mandible through a single foramen just above the tubercles and if divided they must be ligated or the bleeding from them arrested with coagulation diathermy. The mylohyoid origin extends from the third molar region to the midline and is not at all easy to separate from the bone, mainly because the muscle slopes downwards and the periosteal elevator more easily perforates the thin lingual periosteum and slips over the surface of the muscle rather than lifting it from the bone.

As the outer surface of the maxilla above the alveolar 'process is uncovered few obstacles are encountered. The buccinator attachment is barely noticed and there is only little resistance from the levator anguli oris. In contrast the depressor septi muscles form a fleshy zone over the central incisors which requires some care during flap reflection. Once the anterior bony aperture of the nose is reached the reflection of the periosteum into the nasal aspect of the maxilla impedes further mobilization of the soft tissues. Caution should be exercised high on the anterolateral aspect of the maxilla to identify and preserve the infraorbital nerve. This is done by elevating the soft tissues with a swab enclosed finger. Behind the zygomatic buttress or zygomatico-alveolar crest on the posterolateral aspect of the maxilla, again the periosteum should be raised gently. It is easily stripped from the bone but care is necessary to avoid unnecessary damage to the posterior superior dental artery as it enters the bone.

The mucoperiosteum of the hard palate is normally raised by incising the interdental papillae or by making an incision around the crest of the edentulous ridge, The palatal mucoperiosteum is tightly attached at the margin of such a flap, so care must be taken not to use a tooth as a fulcrum for the periosteal elevator when it is raised. Initial elevation of the margin may be facilitated by using the spoon-shaped end of a curved Warwick James' elevator. The mucosa is also tightly attached to the median palatal suture and tethered to the contents of the incisive fossa. Normally a generous length of the curvature of the upper dental arch is needed to form a useful flap. However radially placed relieving incisions can be made to limit the amount of mucosa which is raised to gain access to the surgical site. These should be short so as not to cut the greater palatine neurovascular bundle. Division of the palatine artery leads to a brisk haemorrhage which is best controlled by elevation of the posterior margin of the cut, the application of a haemostat and underrunning the vessel with a resorbable stitch which is then tied to form a ligature. In order to raise the full width of the palate elevation is started at a premolar interdental papilla on each side and separation is carried up to and around the incisive fossa structures. The nasopalatine nerves and vessels are divided as they enter the deep surface of the flap and rarely cause trouble either with haemorrhage or postoperative loss of sensation. Posteriorly the greater palatine neurovascular bundles in the adult emerge opposite the second molars and must be preserved with care. Damage to both can result in death of the flap. Damage to one may result in cyanosis of the edge of the flap. If appropriate one-half only of the palatal mucosa may be raised by making an incision along the centre of the palate.

Access just to the centre of the palate can be made by a midline incision. The mucosa is thin, as well as tightly adherent on either side of the midline, but can be raised with care and retracted to expose the underlying bone. A V-shaped extension about the incisive fossa anteriorly increases access if this is necessary, but should not extend so far laterally as to divide the palatine vessels. Further reflection of the mucosa can be achieved by a V-shaped cut at the posterior end but the thickness of the mucosa at this site makes such an extension less helpful. In making a posterior V-shaped cut the incisions should not be carried on to the soft palate nor should they be made so as to endanger the greater palatine vessels.

HEMOSTASIS

Prevention of excessive blood loss during surgery is important for preserving a patient's oxygen-carrying capacity. However, there are other important reasons, to maintain meticulous hemostasis during surgery. One is the decreased visibility that uncontrolled bleeding creates. Even high-volume suctioning cannot keep a surgical field completely dry, particularly in the well-vascularized oral and maxillofacial regions. Another problem bleeding causes is the formation of hematomas. Haematomas place pressure on wounds-decreasing vascularity, increasing wound tension, and acting as culture media potentiating the appearance of a wound infection.

There are five means of obtaining wound hemostasis.

1. Assisting natural hemostatic mechanisms. This is usually accomplished by either using, a cotton sponge to place pressure on bleeding vessels or placing a hemostat on a vessel. Both methods cause stasis of blood in vessels, promoting coagulation. A few small vessels generally require pressure for only 20 to 30 seconds, whereas larger vessels require 5 to 10 minutes of continuous pressure. The surgeon and assistants should dab rather than wipe the wound with sponges to remove extravasated blood. Wiping is more likely to reopen vessels that are already plugged by clotted blood.
2. Thermal coagulation, or the use of heat to cause the ends of cut vessels to fuse closed.

   Three conditions should be created before thermal coagulation can be properly used. First, the patients must be grounded to allow the current to enter their bodies. Second, the cautery tip and any metal instrument the cautery tip comes in contact with cannot be touching the patient at any point other than the site of the bleeding vessel. The third necessity for thermal coagulation is the removal of any blood or fluid that has accumulated around the vessel to be coagulated.
3. Suture ligation. The bleeders are identified, clamped with a haemostat and ligated.
4. Placement of a pressure dressing over the closed wound.
5. Placing vasoconstrictive substances like epinephrine in the wound or by applying procoagulants like commercial thrombin or collagen, on the wound.

A variety of substances have been developed to be applied in the form of a haemostatic dressing that aims to stop bleeding at the entrance or exit point of the injury. All these substances induce coagulation, with different intervention points within the coagulation system.

QuikClot

QuikClot (manufacturer, Z-medica, Newington, CT) consists of a proprietary formula of zeolite volcanic mineral granules, and is marketed as being able to stop high-volume bleeding from open wounds (Fig. 4.49). It has US Food and Drug Administration (FDA) approval. QuikClot sterile granules are poured into a wound, and absorb the water content of blood through microscopic holes in the granules.

This concentrates the clotting factors and blood cells. QuikClot creates a stable clot that can be removed by irrigation and suction. QuikClot has been tested in an experimental animal model. The granules are non-allergenic. Use of QuikClot leads to an exothermic reaction. The temperature rises more sharply when the QuikClot granules encounter water compared with blood. The temperature rises within 30–60 seconds and lasts several minutes, with a peak between 42°C and 44° C for about 30 seconds.

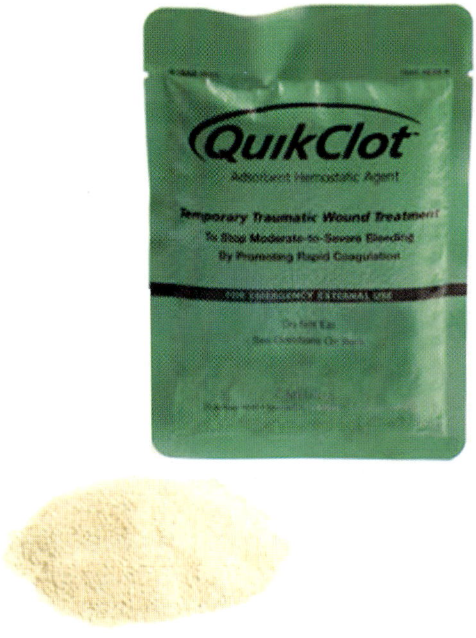

Fig. 4.49

There are inadequate data to support use of QuikClot in body cavities. QuikClot dressings are being trialled by the US Marine Corps in Afghanistan and Iraq, and have already been incorporated in the new Marine Corps individual first aid kit. QuikClot is also being used with a new pressure bandage called CinchTight.

Rapid Deployment Hemostat Bandage

The Rapid Deployment Hemostat (RDH) bandage (manufacturer, Marine Polymer Technologies, Cambridge, MA) consists of fully acetylated poly-N-acetyl glucosamine (p-GlcNAc) applied to a gauze bandage. It has been approved by the US FDA as a dressing for treating bleeding after extremity trauma.

Chitosan Bandage

Chitosan bandage (manufacturer, Hem Con Inc, Tigard, OR) was developed by the Oregon Medical Laser Center through a grant from the US Army Medical Research and Materiel Command. The FDA approved the bandage in November 2002. Chitosan is a biodegradable carbohydrate found in prawns and lobster shells and many other animals. It bonds with blood cells to form a clot, and has some antimicrobial effect. Interestingly, chitosan is not hazardous to those allergic to prawns. Pusateri et al tested the chitosan bandage in a model of severe liver injury in swine, and found it reduced haemorrhage and improved survival.

Recombinant Factor VIIa

Recombinant factor VIIa (rFVIIa, NovoSeven; manufacturer, Novo Nordisk Pharmaceuticals Pty Ltd, Baulkham Hills, NSW) was developed for the treatment of bleeding in haemophiliac patients with inhibitors to factors VIII and IX (Fig. 4.50). It enhances thrombin production on already activated platelets. Its application has been extended to other patients with profuse bleeding who have impaired thrombin production. This includes patients with thrombocytopenia and platelet function deficiencies. rFVIIα seems to enhance haemostasis at the site of injury without systemic activation of the coagulation cascade. rFVIIa can be used for treating uncontrolled massive haemorrhage in the preoperative setting, and it may play a role as an adjunct to surgical haemostasis in trauma patients and in patients with severe postoperative bleeding following general surgery.

Blood Substitutes

Modified haemoglobin solutions, perfluorocarbon emulsions, and liposome-encapsulated haemoglobin are the three types of blood substitutes that have been under development. The first two have reached phase III clinical trials, and the third is in preclinical testing.

Telerobotic Surgery

Robotic surgery provides the potential to undertake more complex and precise tasks with minimal invasion, and is likely to have a major effect on the way surgery is practised. Robot-assisted surgery is already used in cardiac surgery, general surgery, urological surgery, and neurological surgery. The virtual reality systems and telepresence used in the robotic

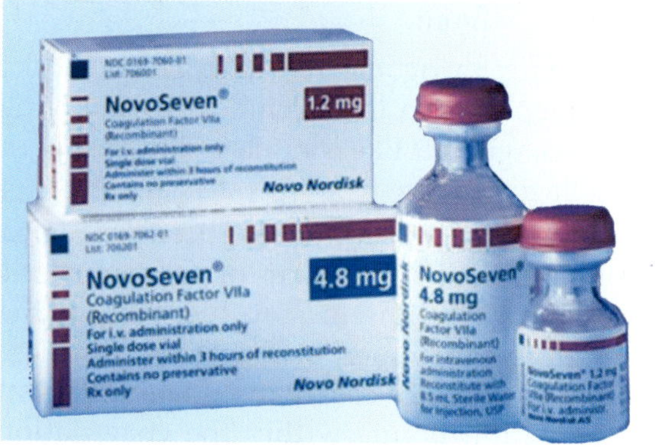

Fig. 4.50

surgery technology could be used for remote surgery, and may therefore have application in military surgery. These systems also have great training potential using virtual reality systems. The sensation of touch, tissue characteristics, and tension are being incorporated into these systems. It is still early days for the evolution of these systems in managing acute patients, and the use of the haemostatic agents will obviate the need for such "immediate" surgery on the battlefield this review.

American Red Cross Haemostatic Dressing

In a model of severe venous and hepatic injury in swine, nine dressing types were trialled, and the American Red Cross haemostatic dressing (Fig. 4.51), which contains microfibrillar collagen, thrombin, oxidised celluloseand poly-N-acetyl-glucosamine (manufacturer, CSL Ltd, Parkville, VIC; distributed by Bioplasma) was effective inreducing post-treatment blood loss and in increasing the proportion of animals in which haemostasis was obtained. Allergic reaction is a potential problem.

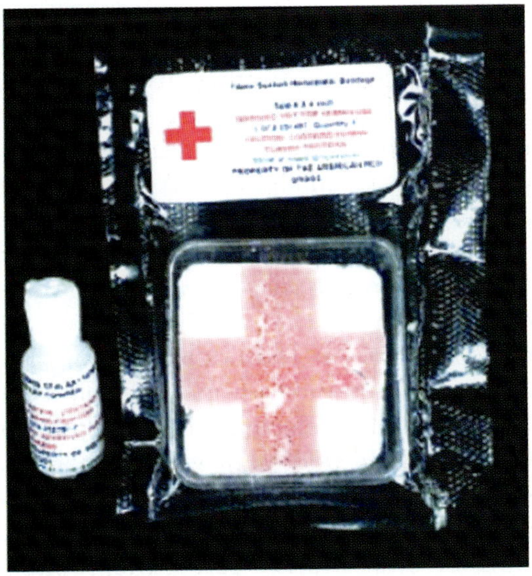

Fig. 4.51

Prostaglandins as Haemostatic Agents

It has been reported that prostaglandin endoperoxides (PGG_2 and PGH_2), possible intermediates in the biosynthesis of PGE_2 and $PGF_{2\alpha}$ from arachidonic acid, may be mediators of platelet aggregation. Kloeze reported that neither PGE_2 nor $PGF_{2\alpha}$ cause platelet aggregation or ADP release, and Willis stated that prostaglandins themselves cannot induce platelet aggregation. But we have found that three synthetic prostaglandins, Wy-16, 991, Wy-17, 185 and Wy-17, 186, induce platelet aggregation in vitro, and two of them, Wy-17, 185 and Wy-17, 186, significantly shorten the Lee White clotting time in rats. The most active of the three, Wy-17, 186, exerts a haemostatic effect on a bleeding wound surface.

NON-TRANSFUSIONAL HAEMOSTATIC AGENTS IN THE MANAGEMENT OF BLEEDING DISORDERS

Desmopressin

Desmopressin, a synthetic analogue of the antidiuretic hormone vasopressin, raises the plasma levels of endogenous factor VIII and von Willebrand factor (vWf). Desmopressin increases about 3–5 fold for a short time after the administration the plasma levels of vWf in patients with a partial deficiency of vWf (von Willebrand disease) or of factor VIII in patients with mild haemophilia A, and also in healthy individuals and in patients with other bleeding disorders; the increase in vWf results in a shortening of the bleeding time and the increase in factor VIII results in a shortening of the activated partial thromboplastin time.

Desmopressin was used for the first time in 1977 by Mannucci et al, to treat patients with mild haemophilia A and von Willebrand disease. After the original clinical study performed in Italy, desmopressin was used in many other countries and the World Health Organization has included it in the list of essential drugs. Desmopressin is the treatment of choice for mild haemophilia A and type 1 von Willebrand disease, inasmuch as it induces a rise in endogenous factor VIII and von Willebrand factor adequate to halt a haemorrhage or to prevent excessive bleeding in surgical procedures; thus desmopressin provides a form of autologous replacement therapy and permits to avoid the use of coagulation factor concentrates. Obviously, patients with unmeasurable levels of factor VIII (severe haemophilia A) or type III von Willebrand disease do not respond at all. Desmopressin is highly cost-effective. The average dose requested to treat a single bleeding episode in mild haemophilia A and von Willebrand disease (20 mg) is at least 10 fold less expensive than the corresponding dose of factor VIII (1000-2000 U).

Pharmacological Profile of Desmopressin

Chemical composition: I-deamino-8-arginine vasopressin

Route of administration and dose: Intravenous infusion: 0.3 mg/kg diluted in 50 ml saline solution over 30 min; Subcutaneous injection: 0.3 mg/kg; Intranasal spray: 300 mg/kg (concentrated solution)

Mean factor increase over baseline: Factor VIII 3-5 times; vWf 3-5 times

Time to peak level: 30-60 min after i.v. infusion; 90-120 min after s.c. injection

Plasma half-life: 6-8 hours for factor VIII; 8-10 hours for vWf

Tachyphylaxis: After repeated administration at 12 or 24 h intervals, the increase in factor VIII and in vWf may be approximately 30% less than that achieved after the first administration.

Desmopressin shortens the bleeding time in a variety of congenital platelet function defects, namely Bernard-Soulier disease, storage-pool deficiency, release defect or abnormal metabolism of arachidonic acid. The ability to shorten the bleeding time in these patients is unpredictable, and must be assessed individually in each patient. In Glanzmann thromboasthenia a positive response is hardly ever seen. The patients taking aspirin or ticlopidine show prolonged bleeding times to antiplatelet pharmacological effect, and desmopressin can promptly normalize primary haemostasis in most of them. Desmopressin may be helpful, in addition to antifibrinolytic lysine analogues, in the management of hemorrhagic teleangectasia (Rendu-Osler disease). Desmopressin significantly shortens the bleeding time in patients with chronic uraemia, despite the fact that von Willebrand factor and factor VIII are normal or even elevated in uraemic patients. Desmopressin is the treatment of choice for uraemic bleeding when only a short-term effect is required; it is indicated to prevent haemorrage after biopsies or minor surgical procedures or to control acute bleeding. A significant reduction in protein C activity after desmopressin administration in uraemic patients has been reported. Desmopressin lacks the pressor effect of vasopressin, but exerts a much stronger antidiuretiuc effect. Desmopressin must be used with caution during pregnancy, as it may cause hyponatremia or induce premature labour. In chronic uremia, liver cirrhosis, congenital or acquired platelet dysfunctions, hereditary haemorrhagic teleangectasia, no quantitative or qualitative vWf abnormality has been demonstrated; the favourable effect of desmopressin may be mediated by the fresh appearance in plasma of ultralarge vWf multimers, that are haemostatically very effective. An additional mechanism of action of desmopressin may be related to the release of P-selectin, which is stored in Weibel-Palade bodies of endothelial cells beside vWf: P-selectin mediates leukocyte-endothelial cell interaction and improves platelet-endothelial cell adhesiveness. Desmopressin also promotes the release into plasma of tissue-type plasminogen activator, resulting in a short-lived generation of plasmin, which is promptly neutralised by circulating antiplasmin; no fibrinolytic activation occurs in vivo. Accordingly, inhibiting fibrinolysis when desmopressin is administered is not usually needed.

DEAD SPACE MANAGEMENT

Dead space in a wound is any space that remains devoid of tissue after closure of the wound. Dead space is created by removing tissue in depths of a wound or by not reapproximating tissue planes during closure. Dead space in a wound usually fills with blood creating a haematoma with a high infection potential. There are 4 means of eliminating dead space.

1. Loosely suturing tissue planes together to minimize the postoperative void.
2. Place a pressure dressing over the repaired wound.
3. Place a packing into the void until bleeding has stopped and then to remove the packing.
4. Use of drains, either by themselves or in addition to pressure dressings.

Suturing

Principles of suturing

1. The needle holder should grasp the needle at approximately ¾ of the distance from the point. The suture end of the needle is the weakest area because either it is hollow, as in the case of a swaged needle, or it contains the eye. Grasping the suture end will result in at least a bent needle, if not a broken one.
2. The needle should enter the tissue perpendicular to the surface. If the needle pierces the tissue obliquely, a tear may develop.
3. The needle should be passed through the tissue following the curve of the needle.
4. The suture should be placed at equal distance (2 to 3 mm) from the incision both sides and at an equal depth. This principle can be modified in cases where the tissue edges to be sutured are at different levels: then passage of the suture closer to the edge of the lower side and farther from the edge of the higher side will tend to approximate the levels. Another method involves passage of the suture at an equal distance from the wound margins on both sides but deeper into the tissue on the lower side and more superficially on the higher side.
5. If one tissue side is free (as with a flap) and the other fixed, the needle should be passed from the free to the fixed end.
6. If one tissue side is thinner than the other, then the needle should be passed from the thinner to the thicker side.
7. If one tissue plane is deeper than the other, then the needle should be passed from the deeper to the superficial side.
8. The distance that the needle is passed into the tissue should be greater than the distance from the tissue edge. This will ensure a degree of tissue eversion. Some degree of tissue eversion is desirable in anticipation of scar contracture.
9. The tissues should not be closed under tension, since they will either tear or necrose around the suture. If tension is present, the tissue layer should be undermined to relieve it
10. The suture should be tied so the tissue is merely approximated, not blanched.
11. The knot should not be placed over the incision line.
12. Sutures should be placed approximately 3 to 4 mm apart. The closeness of the sutures depends on the anticipated tension across the suture line. Closer spaced sutures are indicated in areas of underlying muscular activity such as the tongue or in other areas of increased tension.

13. Occasionally extra tissue may be present on one side of the incision and cause a 'dog-ear' to be formed in the final phase of wound closure. Simply extending the length of the incision to hide the excess will provide an unsatisfactory result.

KNOT TYING

The surgeon may use either the instrument tie or the one-or two hand tie The instrument tie is more convenient in closed areas such as the mouth but can be used in open areas as well.

Square Knot

The basic knot is the square knot. It is prudent to provide at least three ties for surface knots (Fig. 4.52).

Certain types of suture material such as nylon, polypropylene, polyglycolic acid and gut may require more ties.

Surgeon's Knot

Because of the double throw, the surgeon's knot offers the advantage of reducing slippage of the first tie, while the second tie is put in place. This is particularly useful in confined or difficult to reach places where the first tie would ordinarily be loosened in the process of producing the second tie. A third tie squared on the surgeon's knot is usually made for security (Fig. 4.53).

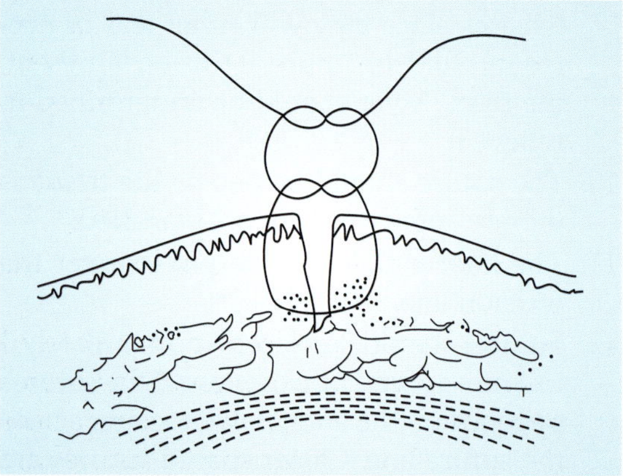

Fig. 4.52: The square knot is formed by wrapping suture around needle holder once in opposite directions between ties

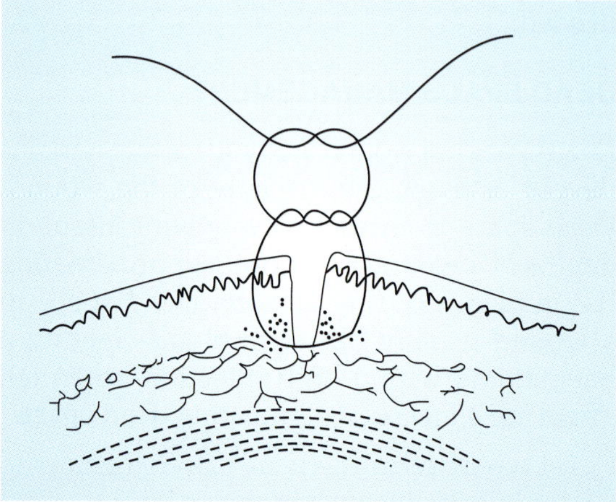

Fig. 4.53: Surgeon's knot is formed by two throws of suture around needle holder on first tie and then one throw in opposite direction on second tie.

Granny Knot

This knot involves a tie in one direction followed by a single tie in the same direction as the first. This will allow the knot to be slipped to place and provide initial holding similar to the surgeon's knot. However, a third tie squared on the second must be made to hold the knot permanently (Fig. 4.54).

SUTURE METHODS

Interrupted Suture

The interrupted suture is the most commonly used. Its advantages are that it is strong and that successive sutures can be placed in a manner to fit the individual requirements of the situation. Each suture is independent of the next, and the distance between each suture and between the sutures and the incision line can be easily varied (Fig. 4.55).

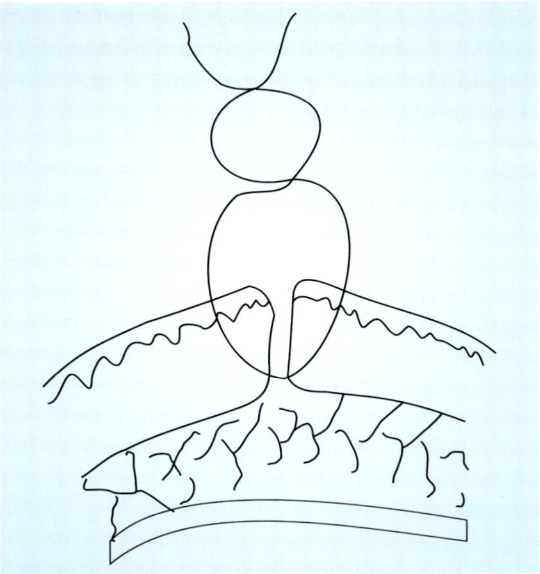

Fig. 4.54: Granny knot

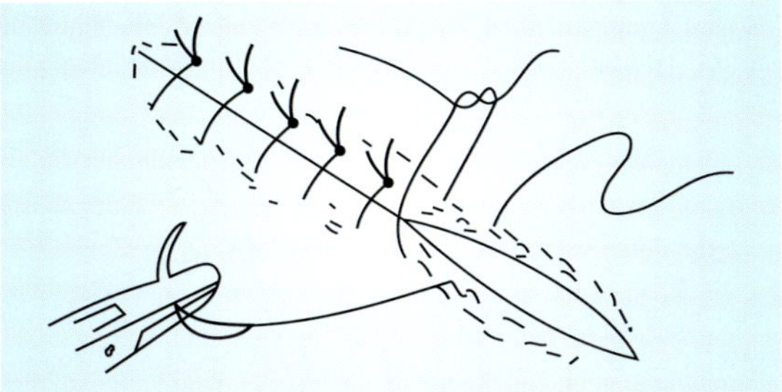

Fig. 4.55: Simple interrupted suture.

The loosening of one suture will not produce loosening of any of the other sutures. A degree of eversion of the incision can be produced by ensuring that the depth of the bite is greater than the distance from the suture to the wound edge. Should the wound become infected, removal of a few selected sutures may be satisfactory treatment. For a strong closure or in areas of tension, this technique is preferred over the continuous suture.

Continuous Suture (Figs 4.56–4.58)

The continuous suture provides a rapid technique for closure. Another advantage of the

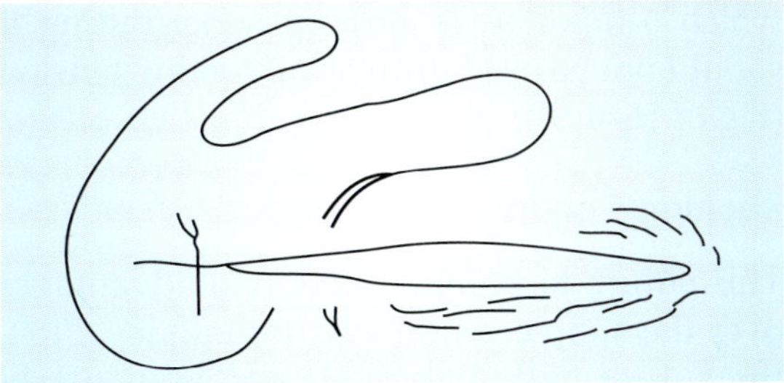

Fig. 4.56: Simple interrupted suture is placed and needle is then reinserted in continuous fashion.

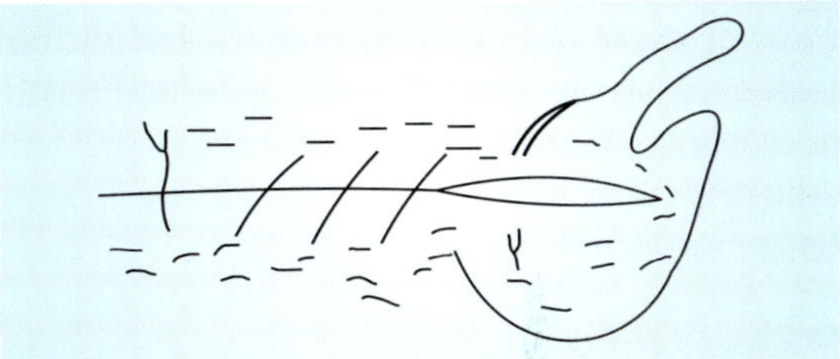

Fig. 4.57: Suture passes perpendicular to incision line underneath tissue and diagnoally on surface.

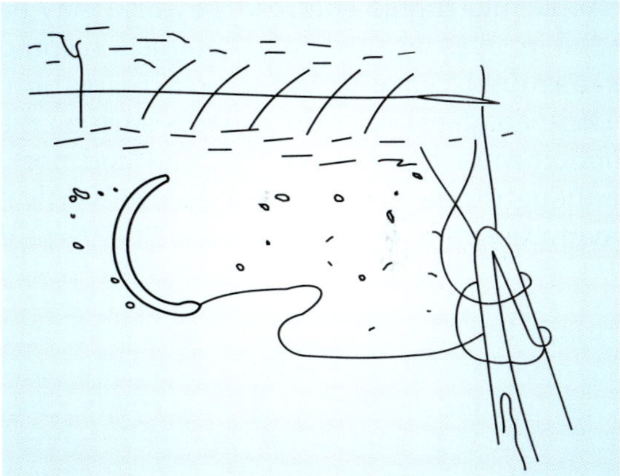

Fig. 4.58: Suture is ended by tying to last untightended loop on suture.

continuous suture is the even distribution of tension over the entire suture line. If the tissues should swell in one area, as for example with the formation of a hematoma, the remaining sutured area can provide a degree of slack that will help relieve the pressure. The continuous suture also provides a more watertight closure which is important in intraoral bone grafting. It should not be used in areas of existing tension (Figs 4.56–4.58).

Locking Continuous Suture

This suture technique offers two advantages over the simple continuous technique First, the suture will align itself perpendicularly to the incision. Second, the locking feature prevents continuous tightening of the suture as wound closure progresses. However, care must be exercised not to tighten the individual lock excessively, since this can produce tissue necrosis. Also, the locking feature may prevent adjustment of tension over the suture line as tissue swelling occurs (Fig. 4.59).

Mattress Suture

The main purpose of mattress sutures is to provide more tissue eversion than occurs with simple interrupted sutures. They also may be used in areas where wound contraction could cause dehiscence or broad scar formation. These are generally skin surfaces such as the abdomen or hip and not the head and neck, although some surgeons do use the vertical mattress suture in neck closures. The vertical mattress suture offers the advantage of running parallel to the blood supply to the edge of the flap and therefore not interfering with healing (Fig. 4.60).

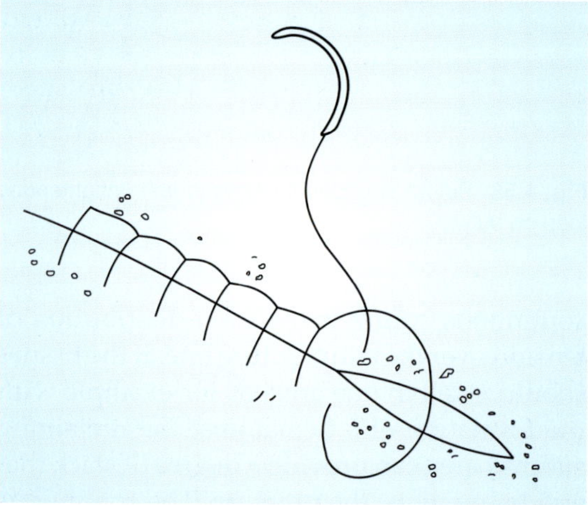

Fig. 4.59: Continuous locking technique

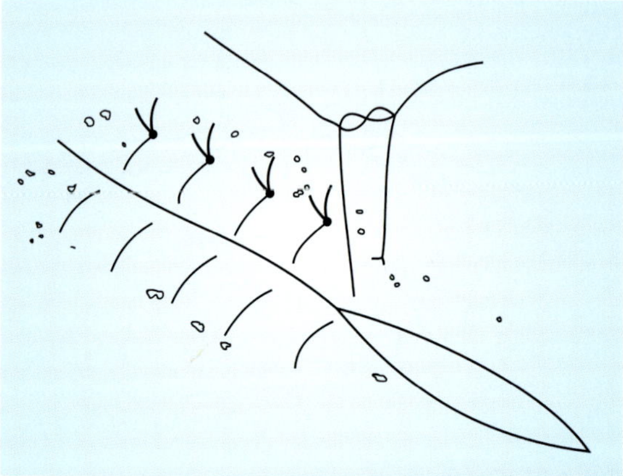

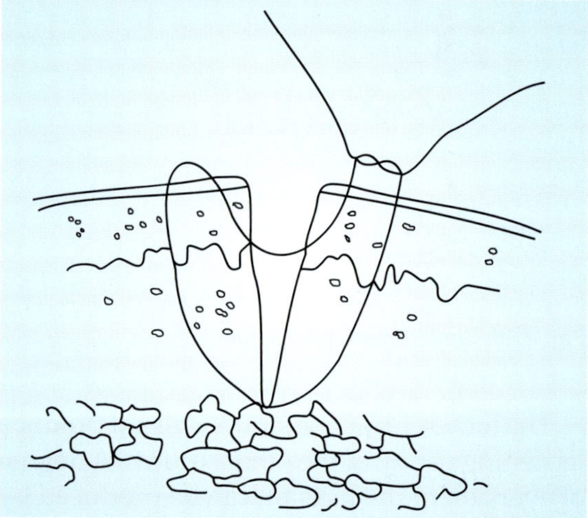

Fig. 4.60: Vertical mattress technique.

The interrupted horizontal mattress suture produces broad contact of the wound margins and is useful where such a condition is needed. However, it suffers from the disadvantage of constricting the blood supply to the edges of the incision. If improperly used, this can cause necrosis and dehiscence. The continuous horizontal mattress suture does limit the blood supply to the flap edge but only minimally and does not interfere with wound healing (Figs 4.61, 4.62).

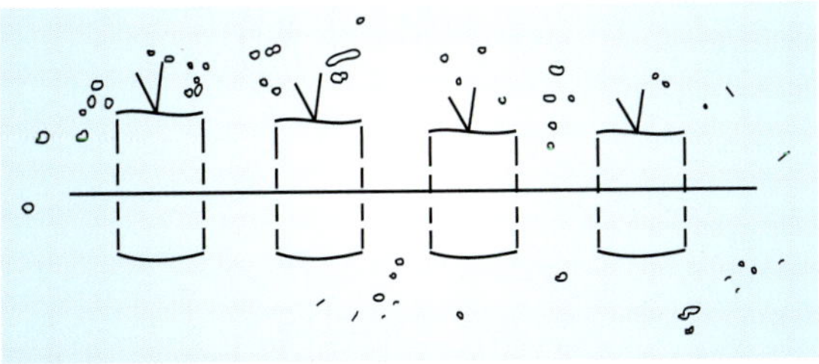

Fig. 4.61: Horizontal mattress technique

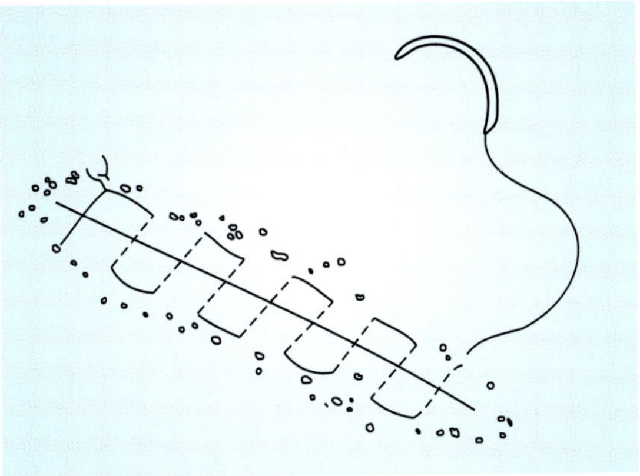

Fig. 4.62: Continuous horizontal mattress sutures.

Figure-of-8 Suture

The figure-of-8 suture is used over extraction sites, where it provides some protection to the surgical area as well as adaptation of the gingival papillae around the adjacent teeth (Fig. 4.63).

Subcuticular Suture

An absorbable 4– 0 suture material is generally used for closure of the subcuticular layer. If individual subcuticular sutures are placed, they should be buried with the knot inverted. A continuous subcuticular suture,may be used with no knots by having the ends exit a short

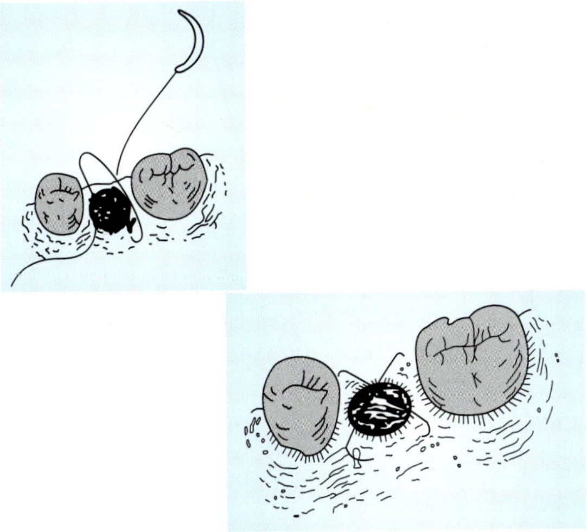

Fig. 4.63: Figure-of-8 stitch

distance from the wound and taping them to the skin (Fig. 4.64). A continuous subcuticular suture may be left for 7 to 10 days and removed by untaping both ends.

SUTURE REMOVAL

The removal of sutures should be performed with care. They should be swabbed gently with chlorhexidine, then each knot gripped in turn with non-toothed forceps. The external part of the suture is raised and the thread cut below the knot and flush with its point of emergence. In order to avoid a strain upon the healing wound the sutures drawn out across the wound. This draws the deep part of the suture out of the opposite puncture creating tension towards the wound rather than away from it. This prevents dehiscence of the healing wound and also draws only the previously buried part of the stitch through the wound. Never cut through a stitch in such a way that part of the contaminated external loop is drawn through the wound. Above all, avoid cutting the suture in two places so that part of the suture is left in the tissues. As the suture is divided some compression of the tissues is released and the

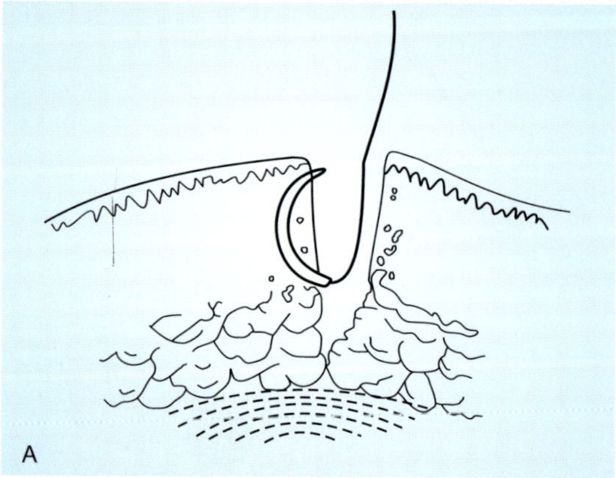

Needle is inserted in deeper tissue first and directed towards the surface

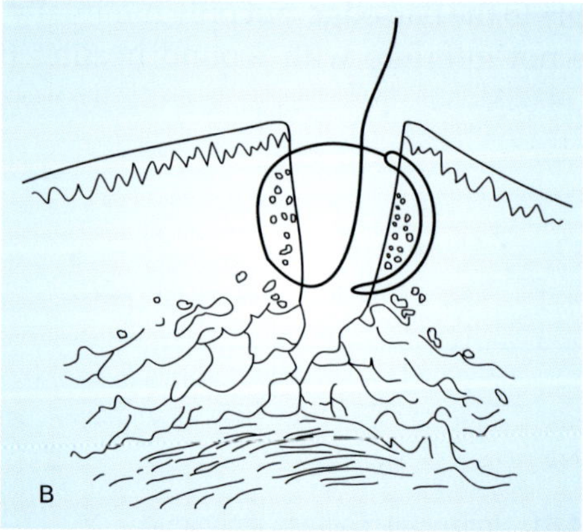

Needle is inserted in opposite side going from superficial to deep tissue.

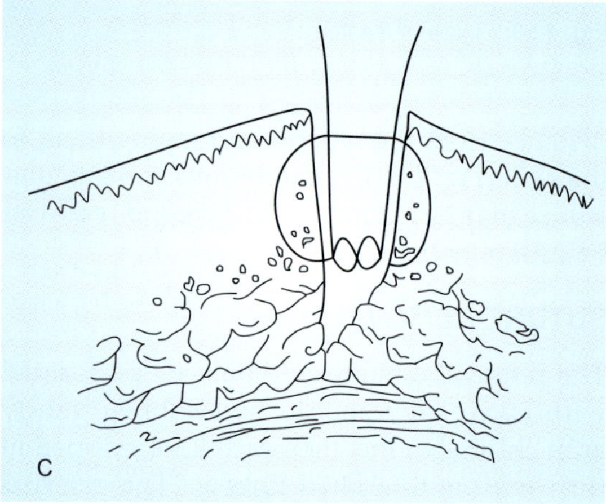

Square knot is tied in usual manner

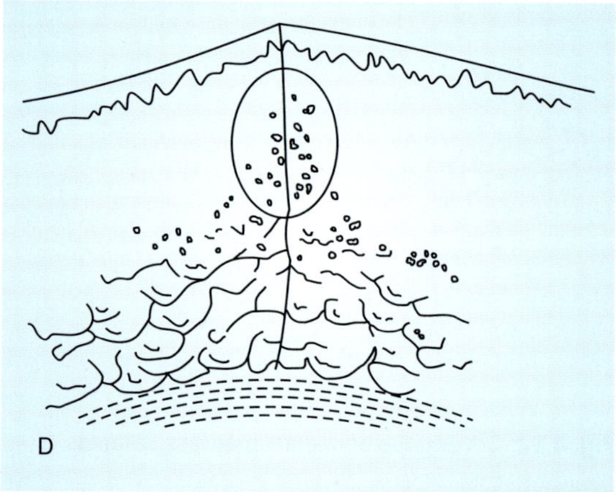

Suture ends are cut short to minimize amount of material that is buried. Knot will be inverted within the tissue.

Fig. 4.64: Steps in subcuticular suturing techniques.

retained segment retreats into the depth of the tissues. Even if some micro-organisms have travelled along the suture material they do not produce a clinical infection in the ordinary way because a suture creates a wound which is drained at both ends.

Sutures are normally left for 5–7 days where closure is completely without tension. Where tissues have been displaced and some degree of tension created, as in the rotation or advancement of a flap to close an oro-antral fistula, it is better to leave them for 10–14 days. Preferably sutures should be left until local tissue oedema has subsided at which time the loop will probably lie loosely over the wound and can be removed easily and without causing the patient discomfort.

Suture Material

Sutures are made of a variety of material and come in several sizes, each designed for a particular purpose. The two basic types of suture material are resorbable and non-resorbable. In general resorbable sutures do not require removal whereas non-resorbable sutures do.

Resorbable Sutures

Three types of resorbable sutures are commonly used for oral and maxillofacial surgery: gut, polyglycolic acidpolyglactin 910. Gut is fabricated from the submucosa of sheep intestines or the serosa of beef intestines. Plain gut is susceptible to rapid digestion by proteolytic enzymes produced by inflammatory cells. For procedures requiring more prolonged suture strength, some gut is treated with basic chromium salts (chromic catgut) to provide more resistance to proteolytic enzymes. Plain gut sutures retain their strength for 5–7 days whereas chromic sutures retain strength for 9–14 days. Plain and chromic guts are supplied in foil packages that prevent desiccation and the suture should be kept moist during suturing with water or saline. Polyglycolic acid and polyglactin 910 do not enzymatically break down. Rather they undergo slow hydrolysis, eventually being resorbed by macrophages. Resorbable sutures are highly reactive compared to non-resorbable sutures.

Non-resorbable Sutures

The most commonly used non-resorbable sutures in oral and maxillofacial surgery are silk, nylon, polyester, and polypropylene. Although silk is classified as a nonresorbable suture material, it loses its tensile strength and disappears in about 2 years if not removed.

Non-resorbable sutures are either monofilamcntous, multifilamentous, or both. The multifilamentous form increases its strength, but also increases suture abrasivencss and is more likely to convert contamination into infection. Silk and polyester sutures are available only in a multifilamentous form; polypropylene is produced only in a monofilamentous form; and nylon comes in both monofilamentous and multililamentous forms.

All nonresorbable Sutures have sonic reactivity.

Suture Sizes

Sutures are available in various sizes that range from the largest size, 7, down to the extremely fine 11–0 suture. The increasing number of zeros correlates with a decreasing suture diameter and strength. For example, size 1–0 suture is larger in diameter than size 2–0, size 3–0 is larger than size 7–0, and so forth Because suture material is foreign to the human body, the smallest diameter suture sufficient to keep a wound closed properly should be employed. Most oral and maxillofacial surgical procedures the use of 3–0 or 4–0 suture.

Needles

Sutures are manufactured with and without needles attached. A wide variety of needles are available on those sutures with pre-attached needles. Sutures without attached needle are used to ligate blood vessels or to thread closed or French-eyed needles. Most sutures used for oral and maxillofacial surgery are swagged on needle: that is during manufacture the suture has been placed into a hallow end of a needle and the end then slightly crimped to retain the suture. Swagging sutures onto needles simplifies handling and causes less tissue damage during suturing than is caused by closed or French-eyed needle.

Needle points also vary (Fig. 4.65). The basic point types are cutting and tapered. Cutting needles have sharp edges that allow the needle to penetrate tough tissues such as gingival and skin. The tapered point is round and without cutting edges. It causes less tissue damage during penetration but cannot easily go through relatively firm tissue. Most oral and maxillofacial surgery is performed with a cutting needle. Different curvatures for the

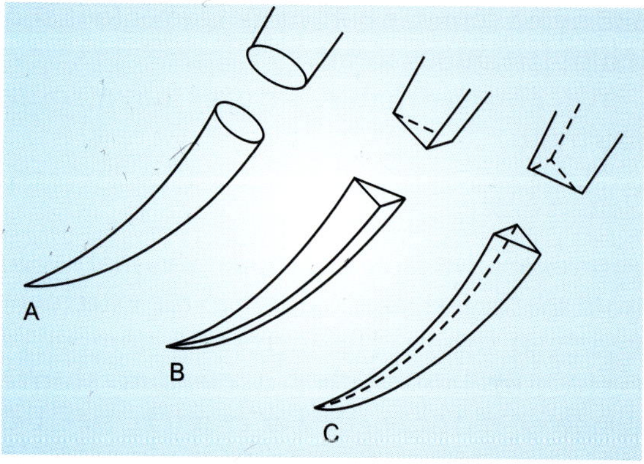

Fig. 4.65: Needles in cross-section. (A) Tapered, (B) Cutting, (C) Reverse

needles are available such as 1/4 circle, 3/8 circle, 1/2 circle, 3/4 circle curved ended straight and straight needles (Fig. 4.66).

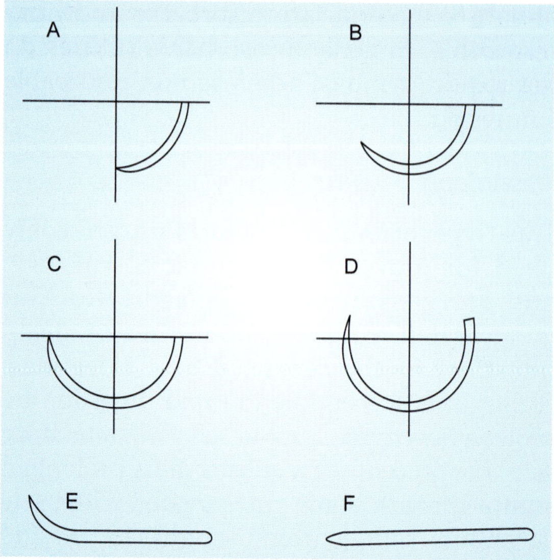

Fig. 4.66: Needles (A) ¼ circle, (B) 3/8 circle, (C) ½ circle, (D) ¾ circles, (E) Straight with curved end, (F) Straight

ARMAMENTARIUM

SPONGE HOLDING FORCEPS

Sponge holding forceps is a long and straight instrument with round fenestrated ends that have transverse serrations on the inner surface (Fig. 4.67).

Indications

1. Preparation of the part for an operation by application of a detergent, ether and povidone-iodine in that order.
2. Blunt dissection by pressure of a folded piece of gauze.
3. Hemostasis by pressure of a swab.
4. To dry operative field by application of a dry swab.
5. To hold tongue during operations on the tongue.
6 To retract bowel by the pressure of a moist gauze during an abdominal operation.

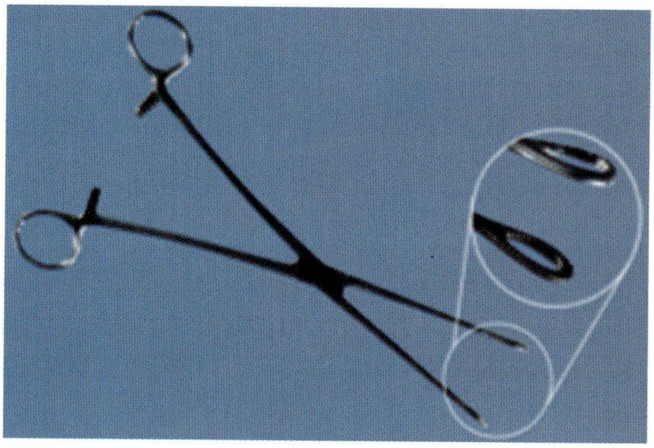

Fig. 4.67: Sponge holding forceps.

7. To hold bowel or stomach during operations involving these organs.

TOWEL CLIP

Doyen's towel clip is a short instrument with curved ends that end in sharp points. The handles are joined at the proximal ends so that when pressed, the tips open and when released the tips close (Fig. 4.68).

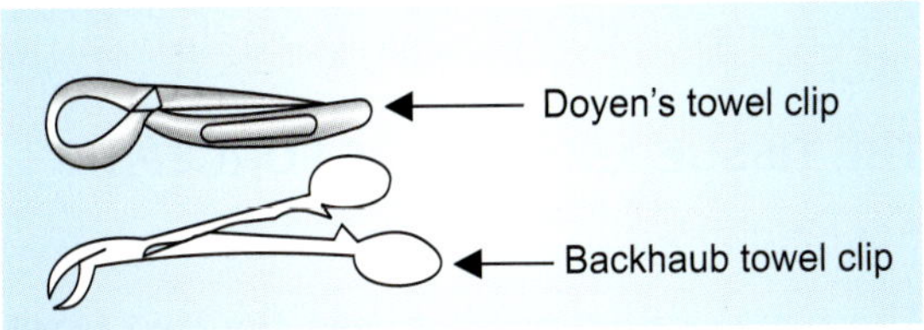

Fig. 4.68: Towel clip

Indication

1. To fix the draping towels in position.
2. To fix suction tube to draping towel.
3. To hold the tongue during operations on the tongue: it is less traumatic than tongue forceps, and the injury caused by it tends to heal quickly.
4. To fix faciomaxillary fractures.

MOYNIHAN'S TETRA FORCEPS

This instrument is somewhat like Mayo's towel clip. It differs in that it is longer, has a curvature in the shaft and has two teeth in each blade. A ratchet catch secures a firm grip on the towels held (Fig. 4.69).

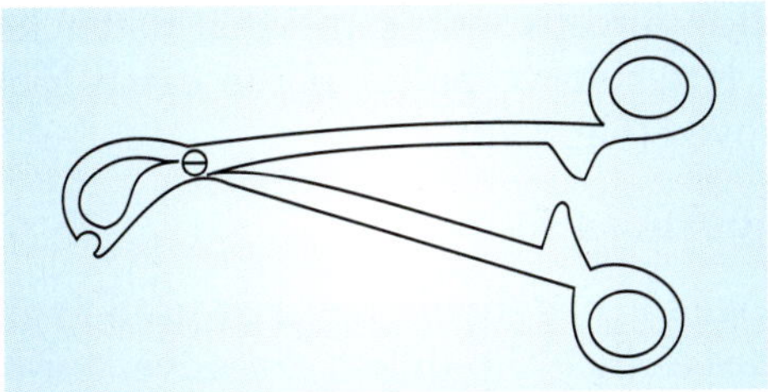

Fig. 4.69: Moynihan's tetra forceps.

Indications

This instrument is used to fix four-cornered or tetra-towels to the cut edges of skin during an operation for isolation of the operative field. Such isolation prevents migration of bacteria from skin into the operative field during prolonged operations.

THE SCALPEL

For Incising Marginal Gingiva

1. The number 15 Bard Parker blade, or equal, is used.
2. The fourth and fifth finger tips are rested on a solid base. The instrument is held like a fountain pen (Fig. 4.70).
3. The curved portion of the blade is placed on the tissue surface, firm pressure made downward, and the blade drawn with a steady stroke for the desired distance.
4. Even pressure is made throughout the entire incision; at the end of the stroke the handle is raised, finishing with the tip of the blade.
5. The beginner tends to use the scalpel and periosteal elevator alternately for a total of five or six exchanges. This results in more trauma and lost time. It must be determined that the incision is down to bone before the scalpel is laid down.

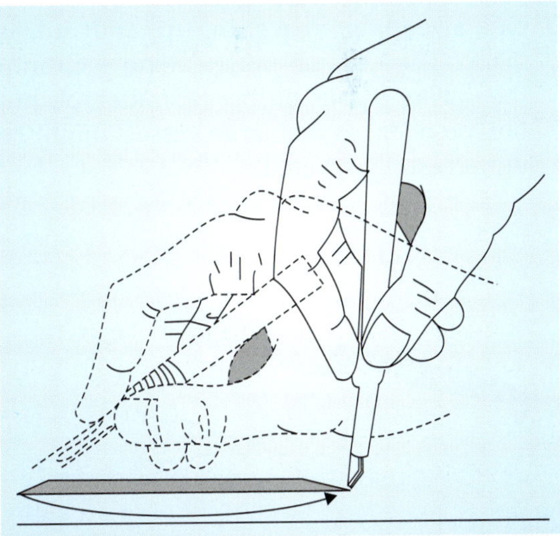

Fig. 4.70: Demonstrating how the scalpel is to be held in a pen grasp and the incision completed in one smooth stroke without lifting the blade and with only movement at the wrist joint without moving the hand.

For Incising Loose Tissues, such as Mucosa of Cheek

1. The number 15 Bard Parker blade, or equal, is used.
2. The tissue is placed on a definite stretch by the retractor in the left hand, or with a gauze square to aid the intra-oral finger to grasp the cheek or lip without slipping.
3. The line of the incision is visualized mentally.
4. The complete incision is made boldly, with firm, steady pressure, finishing up with the point of the blade. The cut should extend into the submucosa.
5. There should be no stopping midway through the incision to clamp bleeders. They are controlled after the scalpel has performed its function.

To Incise Well-Localized Abscess

1. The number 11 Bard Parker blade, or equal, is used.
2. The point of the blade is placed at the edge of the swelling, directed at the center, with the cutting edge up (Fig. 4.71).
3. One sweeping stroke, in, up, and out, is made. The incision must extend well into the pocket of pus on the first attempt, but not too deep, so that large vessels might be unnecessarily severed.
4. If performed in the manner described, incision of pointing gingival abscesses may be done without anesthesia, for the pain, which is of very brief duration, is not perceived until the act is accomplished.

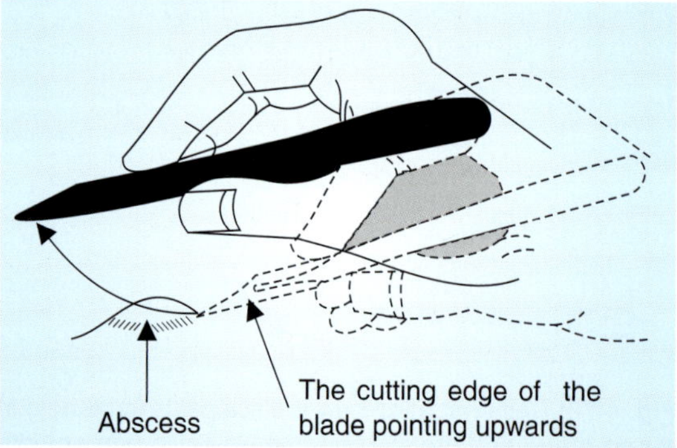

Fig. 4.71: Demonstrating the manner in which the scalpel is to be used for incising a well localised abscess

THE TISSUE AND SPONGE FORCEPS

Specifications

The prime difference between the two types of instruments is that those used for grasping tissue have sharp teeth, while those employed in manipulating gauze, cotton, or suture material have only a moderate roughness on the inner surfaces of their beaks to prevent slipping. The familiar foil carrier or cotton plier is classified with the sponge forceps, even though the beaks are smooth.

Examples of the general group of sponge forceps which are commonly used in oral surgery are: the foil carrier, the common hospital straight sponge forceps, and the nasal dressing forceps. The latter has a bayonet handle and long slender beaks well-suited for carrying gauze into the depth of a cavity such as the antrum or large cyst.

Examples of the general group of tissue forceps are the common hospital straight tissue forceps with sharp teeth, and the O'Brian fixation forceps with somewhat flatter teeth. The latter serve better if the catch lock is removed (Fig. 4.72).

Suggestions for Use

Sponge forceps should never be used to grasp tissues as they slip unless excessive, crushing pressure is applied. Tissues should never be handled with anything except sharp traction hooks, sharp toothed forceps, or properly designed retractors. In working upon the skin of the face, where minimal edema, fibrosis, and scarring are imperative, plastic surgeons now use traction hooks for virtually all immobilization or manipulation purposes.

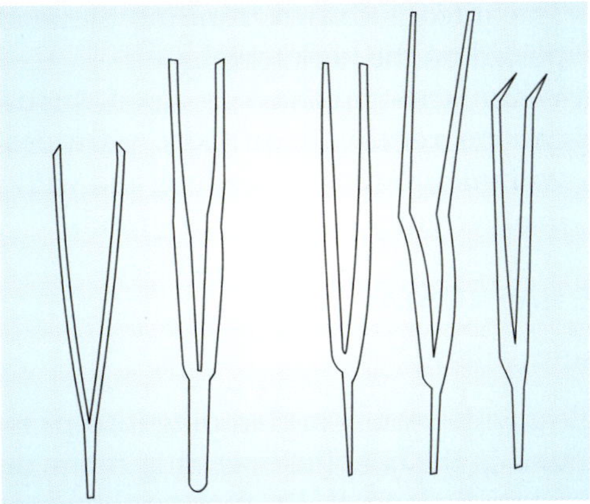

Fig. 4.72: Tissue and sponge forceps (from left to right) (1) O'Brian tissue fixation forceps, (2) Hospital type tissue forceps, (3) Hospital type sponge forceps, (4) Nasal dressing forceps, (5) Foil carrier

The foil carrier is well suited for postoperative dressings in oral surgery. It may be used to carry a cotton pledget into a tooth socket or bony cavity to dry it prior to placement of a dressing, or to carry the dressing to place.

For suture removal the O'Brian fixation forceps, straight sponge forceps, or nasal dressing forceps are somewhat better than the foil carrier as their broad beaks make it easier to grasp the small thread on the first attempt.

THE SCISSORS

Specifications

The straight Stille or Mayo 6 inch instrument with two slender blunt tips will serve well for dissection as well as for cutting sutures or trimming wound margins.

Additional convenience may be derived from the acquisition of scissors of two other designs: a serrated blade type for trimming gingival flaps and a one-sharp-one-blunt blade type for suture removal (Fig. 4.73).

Method of Use

1. *For Trimming Wound Margins*
   a. The tissue is immobilized by use of the traction hook or tissue forceps, or by resting the scissors against the tissue, with the redundant portion extruding through the open blades.
   b. The cut should be made at right angles to the tissue surface.

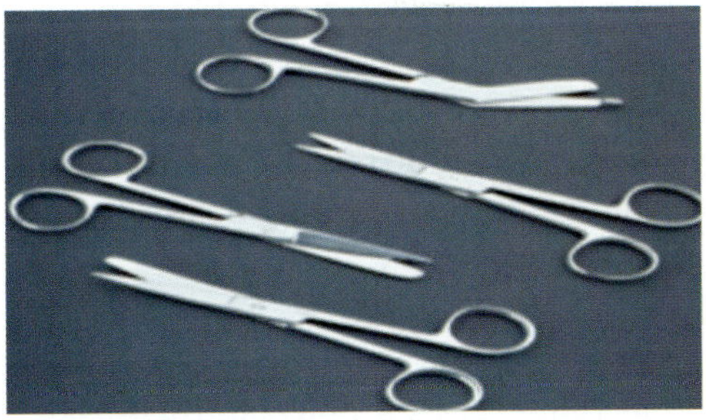

Fig. 4.73: Surgical scissors

2. *For Blunt Dissection or Undermining*
   a. The wound margin is immobilized with the traction hook or tissue forceps.
   b. The blades of the scissors are thrust into the tissue closed, and forcibly spread apart. The intent is to open up the tissues with minimal risk of severing nerves or blood vessels.
   c. The above method may also be used to enter a deep abscess, though the hemostat is generally employed for that purpose.
   d. An important use of the scissors is that of undermining wound margins to prepare them for advancement to a new location, there to be sutured with less tension than would be the case if they had not been freed up.
   e. The tissue margin is immobilized with the traction hook or tissue forceps. The scissors may be used in the manner described above for blunt dissection, but the operator will find that eventually he will have to sever the restraining bands of tissue by boldly cutting them with the scissors to achieve the desired relaxation.
   f. The bed thus created will present bleeding vessels which must be dealt with by direct

clamping or firm, sustained pressure. However, adequate undermining is the prerequisite for success in any plastic procedure in the mouth which contemplates moving tissue to a new location.

3. *For Cutting Sutures*
   a. As the strands of suture material are held on a slight stretch, one blade of the opened scissors is rested against them and made to slide down to within 1/4 inch of the knot (1/8 inch for buried sutures).
   b. The blades are closed together smartly. An effort should be made to achieve a rhythm or tempo for this oft-repeated act.
   c. In all techniques described in this book, the operator always cuts his own intra-oral sutures, using the right hand, and the scissors are returned to the same location at the right rear of the tray after each use. This prevents operator and assistant from always being uncertain who is going to cut the knots. This is one of many decisions made in advance for all cases. The operator is selected for this function because the assistant is retracting with one hand and aspirating with the other. Further, there are many inaccessible spots in the mouth where the operator alone has clear vision.
4. *For Removing Sutures*
   a. This action requires three hands.
   b. The assistant retracts the lip or cheek with a retractor, mouth mirror, or tongue blade.
   c. The operator holds in his left hand the foil carrier, sponge forceps, or tissue forceps.
   d. He holds the scissors in his right hand.
   e. The operator secures a hand rest for the grasping instrument, and then lightly picks up the free end of the suture, placing it on a slight tension. With the scissors lightly rested on lip or cheek he snips one of the taut strands.
   f. The stitch is drawn from the tissue and placed on the neck towel.
   g. When this method is used sutures can be removed quickly, painlessly, without producing bleeding, and without inadvertently cutting both strands.

THE HAEMOSTAT

Specifications

While a wide variety of clamping forceps may be found in the hospital operating room, only the mosquito and Kelly type are generally used for intra-oral work. These are available in both straight and curved design. Variations such as the Kochers, Allis, and Carmault will be occasionally needed in the more major procedures in the hospital (Fig. 4.74).

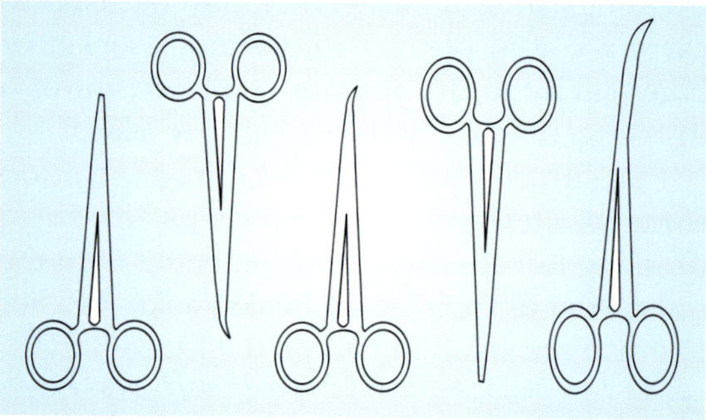

Fig. 4.74: Artery forceps. (A) Straight mosquito, (B) Curved mosquito, (C) Curved Kelly and (D) Alli, (E) Carmault.

Mode of Use

1. *For Clamping Bleeders*
   a. The bleeding site should be well exposed by good retraction and illumination.
   b. The area is compressed with a gauze sponge and as the latter is quickly removed the beaks of the hemostat grasp the bit of tissue which appears to contain the bleeding vessel. Some degree of skill is required to unerringly clamp the bleeder without including an excessive amount of extraneous tissue.

c. Careful reflection on the anatomy of the region and the probable origin of the vessel will help the surgeon to know where to clamp proximal to the bleeding point.
d. The bleeding vessel is often more superficial than would be expected. The actual white-walled vessel can frequently be seen.
e. A vessel only partially severed, and thus unable to retract, constitutes one of the most dangerous types of bleeders.

2. *For Blunt Dissection*
   a. For the second step in incision and drainage, the closed beaks of the hemostat may be used forcibly to enter the abscess without undue hazard of injuring vessels and nerves. When the deepest point is reached the beaks are forcibly spread apart to permit the pus to escape and enlarge the passage for future drainage.
   b. For undermining a flap preparatory to advancement the instrument is used in the same manner, but the scissors will often serve to better advantage.
3. *For Removal of Tooth Fragments or Root Tips*
   Due to its slender beaks and the firm control provided by the long handles, a hemostat will often succeed in lifting out a stubborn, movable fragment due to the traction and rotation effect provided by a grasping instrument.
4. *For Grasping and Holding Tissue such as Cyst Membranes*
   Where an indefinite plane of cleavage exists, separation can often be accomplished by steady traction in one or more directions after the tissue has been firmly grasped with the hemostat. However, the portion which is crushed becomes unsuitable for pathological study.
5. *For Grasping Traction Sutures*

BABCOCK'S FORCEPS

Babcock's forceps is a non-traumatic instrument. It has two ring shaped finger grips, a ratchet catch and fenestrated curved blades. Each blade has a transverse bar which has a fine transverse serrations (Fig. 4.75).

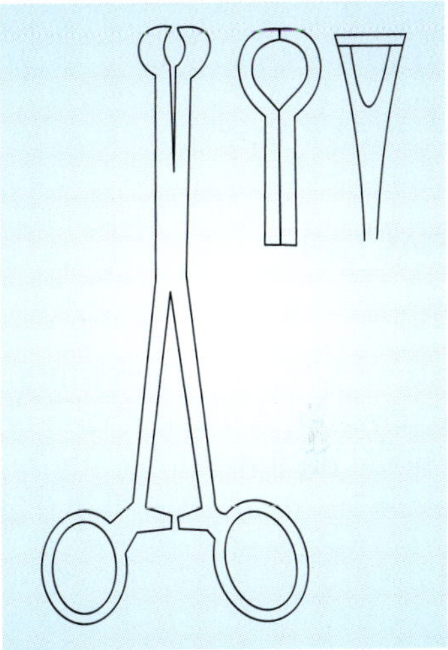

Fig. 4.75: Babcock's forceps.

Indications

To hold the lymph nodes during lymph node biopsy.

ALLIS' FORCEPS

Allis' forceps have two finger grips, a ratchet catch and tips which are flattened, curved inwards a little, and with fine teeth on the distal edges for a secure grip on the structure held (Fig. 4.76).

Indications

1. To hold fascia and apponeurosis.
2. To hold fibrous capsule of different structures.
3. To hold the subcutaneous tissues under the skin at the two extremes of a skin incision.

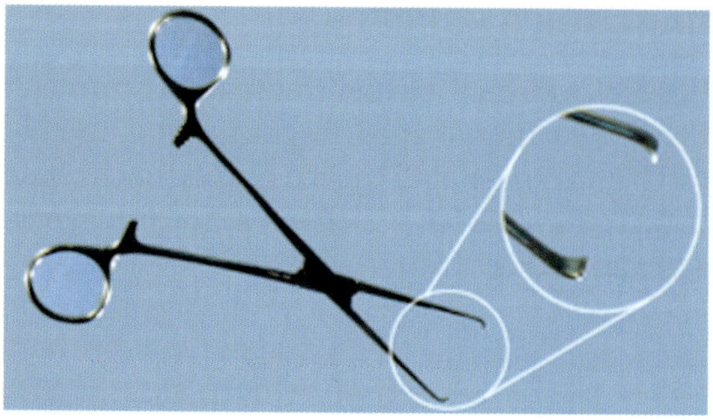

Fig. 4.76: Retractors for surgery

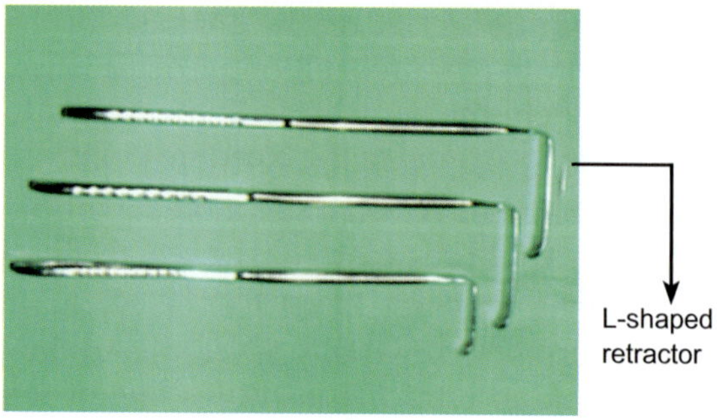

Fig. 4.78: L-shaped retractor

THE RETRACTOR

Specifications

1. University of Minnesota hand-fitting cheek and flap retractor. A metal ribbon type with smooth blade designed to gently hold back the cheek or mucoperiosteal flap (Fig. 4.77).

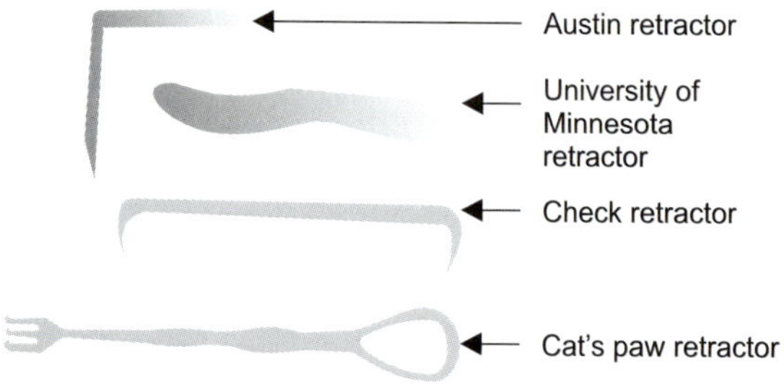

Fig. 4.77: Allis' forceps.

2. Alternate choice: Austin right angle flap retractor with two semi-sharp teeth at the end (Fig. 4.78).

Advantages of Retractor over Finger, for Flap Retraction

1. The retractor can be boiled and is thus more sterile than the finger.
2. The retractor is safer. Fingers are kept away from the bur, chisel, or sharp-pointed elevator.
3. The retractor is less bulky, provides more room in the small operative field.
4. The retractor is more efficient, holds the flap back better, results in less slipping (which produces trauma) of the flap.

Retracting Lip or Cheek for Examination or Postoperative Treatment

1. The retractor is held in the operator's left hand. For use on the left side of the mouth the operator's arm encircles the patient's head.
2. The blade of the retractor draws the cheek or lip away from the alveolar ridge, putting the former on a stretch.
3. Resting the end of the retractor on the gingiva pinches, hurts, and traumatizes the tissue.

For Retracting the Mucoperiosteal Flap

1. The retractor is held in the operator's left hand (except at the time of tying knots in suture, when the assistant automatically takes it).
2. The operator's left wrist or forearm rests lightly on the patient's head or forehead, to steady the instrument and prevent undue arm fatigue.
3. The retractor is placed in position in three steps:
   a. The cheek or lip is raised with the retractor.
   b. The flap is gently raised with whatever instrument is in the right hand.

c. Then the tip of the retractor is put to place and pressed firmly against bone, to prevent slipping. The retractor is never rested on the reflected base of the flap, as this would thrombose nutrient vessels to the flap.

4. The retractor performs two important functions: it draws the soft tissues aside, permitting an unobstructed view of the hard tissues beneath, and it holds the delicate soft tissues out of the way, protecting them from trauma from the bur, chisel, or elevator.

SINUS FORCEPS

Sinus forceps are slender, long, straight with slightly expanded tips but no ratchet catch on the handles. The blades have transverse serrations on the inside of the tips (Fig. 4.79).

Indications

1. Incision and drainage of an abscess, to explore the abscess cavity and break all the septa within by Hilton's method, to drain all the pus inside.
2. To remove foreign bodies from sinuses or wounds.

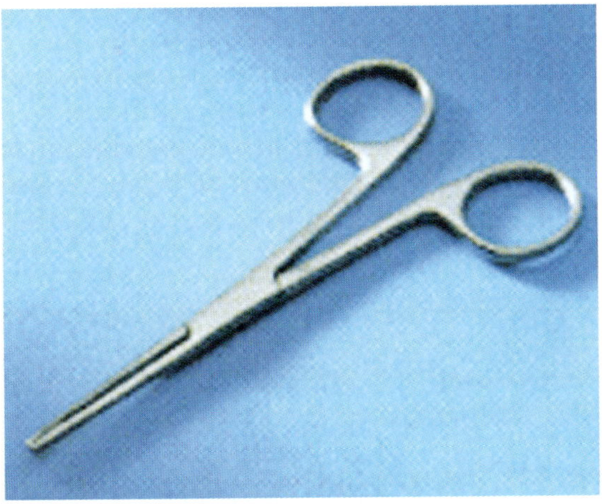

Fig. 4.79: Sinus forceps

3. To place a drain in an abscess or a sinus.
4. To pack an abscess cavity.
5. To drain a hematoma.
6. To place nasal or oral dressing.

THE SUCTION ASPIRATOR HANDLE AND TIP

Specification

The Hu-Friedy Coupland item is used. Four tips of various sizes are supplied, of which the three smallest will be most useful. An iron wire pick may be made in the dental laboratory to be used as a ramrod to dislodge particles of bone which may become caught inside the lumen during use. A large ramrod of coat hanger wire is needed to thoroughly clean the inside of the handle prior to sterilization (Fig. 4.80).

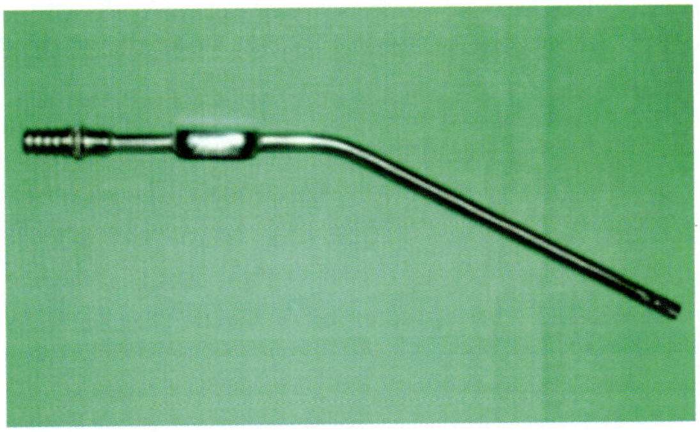

Fig. 4.80: Suction aspiratory tip.

Use of the Aspirator

The assistant must be trained to methodically keep four areas free of blood, saliva, and debris. They are:

a. The floor of the mouth,
b. The right and left retromolar triangles,
c. The junction of the tongue with the soft palate, and
d. The operative field.

In policing the operative field the assistant must strive to provide excellent visibility for the operator. This requires a certain amount of judgment for if the aspirator is providing a dry field but is blocking the view of the operator; no useful purpose will be served. Also as far as possible the assistant must try to avoid excessive movement with the suction when not required which would distract the surgeon. The aspirator tip and all instruments should be slanted away from the center of the field like petals of a flower, so that the headlight beam and line of vision may be directed at the center of interest. When not needed the aspirator should be held 6 to 12 inches from the field, to give the operator all possible room. When it is indicated, the assistant should lightly flood the operative field with intermittent streams of saline delivered from the irrigating syringe. Simultaneously the aspirator tip should be applied nearby, as close to the field as possible but at the lowest point. Care should be taken not to flood the patient's throat with irrigating fluid.

Whenever the operator reaches for the dental handpiece the assistant automatically reaches for the irrigating syringe to provide the action described above, without verbal request of the operator.

The assistant must be prepared instantly to give up the aspirator to the operator without verbal request, and instantly to accept it from him in the same way, for the operator occasionally has to police a small recess that is not visible to the assistant. The operator may thus keep his vision uninterruptedly on the operative field throughout this exchange.

Whenever the assistant's trained ear detects that the aspirator is partially plugged, she must immediately free the obstruction. This is done by thrusting into the orifice the iron wire pick or one beak of the foil carrier. A finger rest should be secured to make this action successful on the first try, so that the aspirator will not be out of function for more than two or three seconds.

Effective use of the aspirator will make it unnecessary for the patient to use the cuspidor at any time during the operation, and this should be explained to the patient as surgery begins. If the patient makes an effort to reach the basin the assistant should gently push the head back into the headrest, then immediately remove the previously overlooked fluid or debris.

CHEATLE FORCEPS

They are available in two sizes, large and small. It is a long instrument; the blades are flat and angled away from the handles for ease of handling. The blades have a wavy shape, so that instruments can be held with a secured grip. There is no ratchet catch. The forceps are used to pick up instruments from a sterilizer or an arranged trolley, to be transferred for use to another trolley. The forceps are kept vertically with the blades immersed in a antiseptic solution when not in use. Thus the blades are kept sterile.

THE PERIOSTEAL ELEVATOR

Anatomical Considerations

The labial and buccal mucoperiosteum is tightly attached to alveolar bone at the gingival margin; but it is more loosely attached as we move apically and a plane of cleavage exists.

The palatal mucoperiosteum is tightly bound down.

The mandibular lingual mucoperiosteum is thin and extreme care must be taken to raise the mucoperiosteum to avoid tearing of the flap (Fig. 4.81).

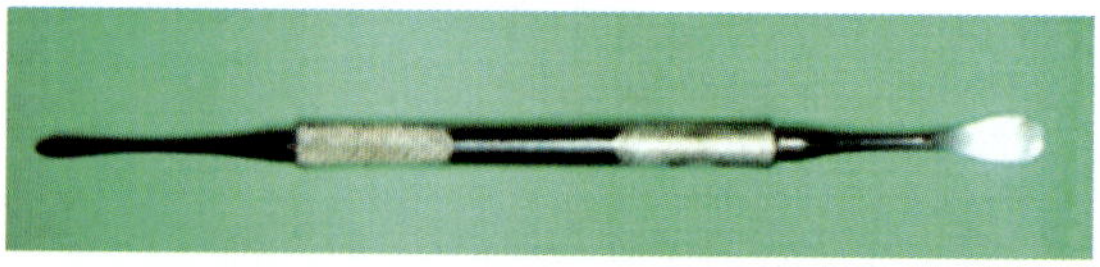

Fig. 4.81: The mucoperiosteal elevator (the most commonly used instrument for raising flaps during a surgical procedure).

Pathological Considerations

Previous or chronic inflammation (draining sinus tracts and periodontal pockets) produce heavy fibrosis and the soft tissues become tightly bound to the underlying bone.

Methods Used for Raising a Labial or a Buccal Mucoperiosteal Flap

i. The 'push stroke'.
ii. The 'pull stroke'.
iii. The 'pry stroke'.

The Push Stroke

1. The wide end of the instrument is kept at a 45 degree angle to the surface of the bone. Repeated shovelling thrusts are made.
2. The fibers that would bind the flap to bone must be severed, by sliding the instrument on bare bone.
3. The flap will split and tear if excessive, bursting force is applied to a tightly bound down edge of mucoperiosteum. Advantage should be taken of the less tightly attached portion, away from the free gum margin, in getting the flap started. It is usually well to do easy things first, when raising flaps, so that the plane of cleavage will be readily established.
4. The retractor, in the operator's left hand, raises the edge of the flap as soon as possible, so that the uncut fibers may be seen and severed under direct vision. By putting fibers on a stretch it makes them easier to sever from bone.

The Pull Stroke

1. Often the flap can be peeled from the bone somewhat as the skin of a tangerine is removed from the fruit.
2. The wide blade of the spatula is used to draw the flap toward the operator.
3. This technique is often useful in raising flaps when alveolectomy is being performed after the teeth have been extracted, either at the same sitting or a week or two afterward.

The Pry Stroke

1. The interdental papillae are tightly bound down but are also thick and strong. The small end of the spatula is used to detach them from bone.
2. The point of the instrument is inserted firmly under the triangular mass of tissue and, by using the adjacent tooth as a fulcrum, the tissue is pried away from its bed. The interdental septum will usually break away readily.
3. Since this pad of tissue is thick, it will not split. Raising one or more papillae will reveal the bony plateau beneath so that further raising of the flap may be accomplished easily, without laceration of the thinner mucosa lying over the center of the tooth.

With effective use of the periosteal elevator, retractor, light and aspirator, no more than twenty seconds should be required to raise a flap.

NEEDLE HOLDER

A needle holder is available in different sizes, small, medium or large. It has two finger grips, a ratchet lock and small blades. The ratio of the lengths of the handles to blades is 4:1 thus the grip on the needle is quite strong. The inner surface of the blades has criss cross serrations for a secure grip on the needle held each blade has a longitudinal groove on its inner surface which makes the grip on the needle strong and prevents wobbling of the needle during use. For intraoral placement of sutures a 6 inch (15 cm) needle holder is usually recommended (Fig. 4.82).

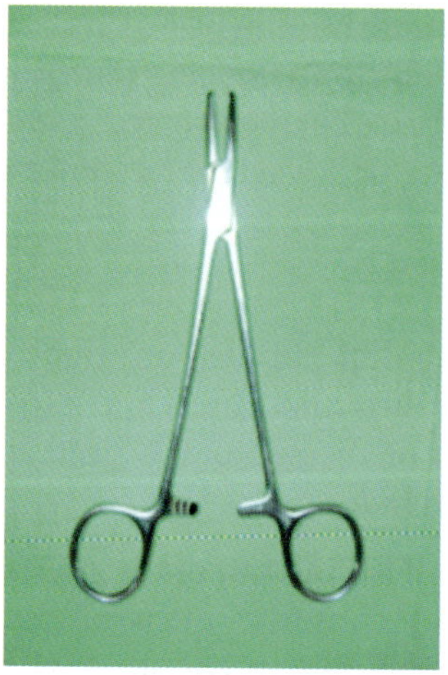

Fig. 4.82: The 6-inches needle holder used most commonly in oral and maxillofacial surgery.

THE SURGICAL BUR

Specifications

A bur is always discarded after use on one operation. Sharp instruments are always safest, can be used with a lighter touch. The straight handpiece is used whenever possible, so as to have minimal bulk of instrument in the operative field.

General Principles

- The revolving bur is never used free-handed. The tips of the fourth and fifth fingers are rested very heavily on nearby teeth or alveolus. If the teeth are sharp the fingers are protected with folded gauze square.
- The revolving bur is never used without an intermittent stream of water or saline being played upon it by the assistant. At the same time, the suction aspirator tip must be held at a low point nearby, to pick up waste water and debris.
- Periosteum and other soft tissues must be firmly held away from the revolving bur or they will catch and wrap around it with mutilating effect.

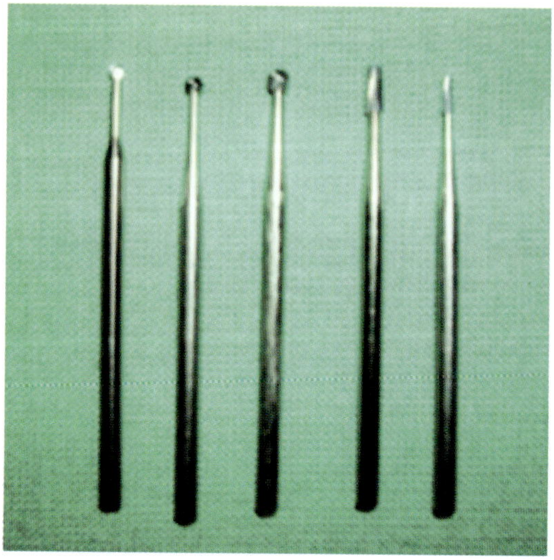

Fig. 4.83: Surgical burs (from left to right). (1) E 0123 (Maillefer), (2) SSWhite HP-6, (3) SSWhite HP-8, (4) SSWhite HP-703, (5) SSWhite HP-560),

- It is often best to run the bur at a constant, high speed, with a pumping action to permit the coolant to reach frequently the cutting end of the bur.

Indications for Use

- To remove bone.
- To cut into and divide tooth substance for ease in removal.

To Remove Bone

1. ***To expose an unerupted tooth or retained root fragment.***
   a. An estimation is made of the location with regard to nearby landmarks visible on the radiograph and in the mouth.
   b. A circle of drill holes is made over this area, even larger than would be thought necessary. The bur should cut just through the cortical plate.
   c. The drill holes are connected by inserting the tip of the bur and pulling outward through each bridge separately. When this method of trephining is used, there will

be little excuse for the bur to "travel" into soft tissue, producing mutilation.

d. The disc of bone is pried out as one piece.

e. Further entry into the bone is done with the hand chisel, used in a scooping manner, when a small root tip is being sought. If an entire tooth is being exposed, the bur may be used to "clean" it with light brushing strokes.

2. *To release hypercementosed, curved, or fractured root*

   a. If adjacent teeth are not to be saved, a series of drill holes in the shape of a U is made on the buccal, the holes are connected, and the plate of bone thus outlined is pried off with a chisel. Bone is then cleaned from the mesial and distal surfaces of the root, with the bur resting lightly on the root surface for guidance. This method not only provides wide access promptly but also affords an excellent opportunity for application of the inclined plane elevator at the mesial or distal aspect of the root.

   b. When adjacent teeth are to be retained, or when working near the mental foramen, the bony wound is opened up more cautiously by drilling a single hole in a spot known to be over the tooth to be removed, then the exposure extended occlusally, mesially, and distally, until the excavation reveals the exact location of the root. Undercuts or areas of ankylosis which have prevented removal are cut away.

To Section Teeth for Ease in Removal

1. The rotating bur is passed straight into the center of the crown or root, cutting approximately four-fifths of the way through. The handpiece is used with a pumping action to permit the water to cool and clean the bur. *It is advised by senior surgeon's to begin sectioning at the neck of the teeth because this is the portion of the tooth which is covered with a thin layer of dentin and also the pulp chamber is widest in this region (Fig. 4.84).*
2. Lateral pressure is then made toward the mesial, cutting nearly through.
3. Lateral pressure is then made toward the distal, cutting nearly through.
4. Into this slot a screwdriver-shaped instrument is inserted and turned, breaking off the fragment.

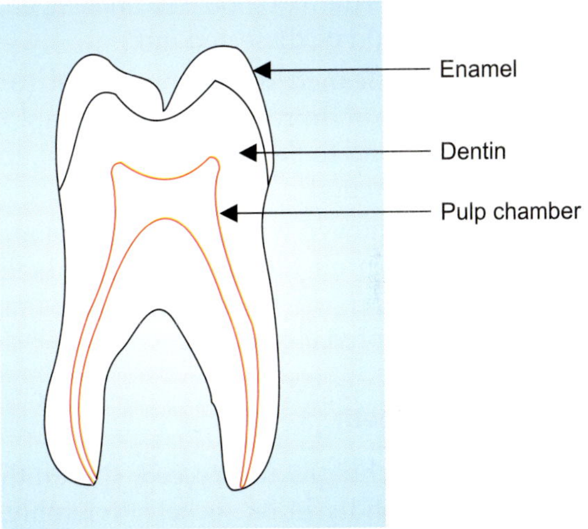

Fig. 4.84

THE MALLET AND CHISEL

General Principles

1. Chisels must always be razor sharp, with an acute bevel.
2. The single bevel type is used for cutting bone.
3. The bi-bevel type is used for splitting teeth.
4. Any heavy headed small surgical mallet that can be readily sterilized is satisfactory.

For Removal of Bone

1. It must be made certain that the flap is reflected back well beyond the point to which bone is to be removed.
2. The chisel is placed nearly in line with the long axis of the tooth. (To pound at right

angles is disagreeable to the patient and chips into the tooth.) The bevel may be either up or down, at the discretion of the operator, but the chisel should not be allowed to bind.

3. With either hand pressure or by use of the mallet, bone is shaved off. The mallet blows should be continuous: tat-tat-tat-tat, in fairly rapid sequence, and hard enough to effect rapid bone removal.
4. The anatomy of the root should be unchanged. The root should be dissected out.
5. All bone is cleaned off of the buccal (or labial) surface of the root way up to the apex and also around to the mesial and distal, to remove undercuts.
6. The root is removed with the inclined plane or sharp-pointed elevator. (The chisel, already in hand, can frequently be used as the sharp-pointed elevator.)

For Splitting Teeth

1. For this technique to succeed, the tooth must be solidly in its socket. Preferably, there should be some preliminary bone removal so that the sections can fall apart when the split is made.
2. When a lower third molar is to be split and the patient is under local anesthesia, it is a good plan to have him bring up his hand, beneath the drapes, and support the angle of the mandible with the heel of the hand.
3. The cutting edge of the chisel is placed in a well-developed groove or fissure and held firmly in place.
4. A single strong, sharp blow is made with the mallet. The handle should be held at the end for best results.
5. The chisel is placed in the crevice thus created and, with caution, slowly but resolutely forced deeper and deeper, so that the free fragment is pried loose and extruded.
6. If the tooth does not split after one or two tries it is well to abandon this method in favor of the bur technique, for the enamel may be gnarled and further efforts would involve unwarranted trauma.

THE RONGEUR FORCEPS

Specifications

Any of several forceps-like instruments designed to cut bone by their nipping, biting, or shearing action. Two types are used, the round-nosed rongeur and the side cutting bone forceps.

Round-Nosed Rongeur-Indications for Use

1. To open up the side of a socket to expose a fractured root tip.
2. To enlarge a window into a cyst or the antrum, by bone biting action.
3. To remove or smooth bone in alveolectomy (not as effective for this purpose as the side cutting bone forceps. When a point of bone is nipped off with the tips of the beaks, two small points are left. The resulting surface has a nutmeg-grater feel).
4. To grasp and securely hold tough, fibrous tissues that are to be drawn away from bone (pericoronal sac, cystic membranes, or scar tissue masses). The foil carrier or frail tissue forceps are not suitable for this purpose.
5. To extract a portion of a tooth from a deep bony wound when a rotation and lifting movement is required.

Side Cutting Bone Forceps-Indications for Use

1. To remove bone or smooth bone in alveolectomy. It is excellent for this purpose, surpassing the round-nosed rongeur due to its planing action, the ease with which it cuts through bone, and the ease with which it is cleaned of debris after each cutting stroke.

2. To open up the side of a socket to expose a fractured root tip.
3. To enlarge a window into a cyst or the antrum, by scissors action.
4. Occasionally to trim soft tissue such as fibrous tuberosities or interdental papilla prior to wound closure.

Method of Bone Removal in Alveolectomy

1. The flap is held well back by the retractor in the operator's left hand.
2. The assistant has open 3 × 3 inch gauze square in her left hand.
3. With the rongeur in the right hand, the operator takes bites of bone and after each fragment has been detached points the opened beaks toward the assistant without taking his eyes or light from the operative field. The assistant wipes the beaks clean, using the gauze square, with a single milking action.
4. This procedure is repeated in rhythmic fashion so that successive bites are removed, steadily contouring the bone to the desired shape. All action is automatic except for the sculpturing of the alveolar ridge which receives the full attention of the operator. The bone fragments quickly pass from the ridge, to the rongeur, then to the gauze square, in systematic fashion.
5. Particularly with the side cutting bone forceps, when the cutting strokes are all made tangent to the desired convex ridge form, a curved surface will result, even though each cut has been on a straight line.

Caution

Both of these instruments can cause brutal crushing injuries of the lips, cheeks, tongue, or flap. All soft tissues should be drawn well away from the working parts of the rongeurs.

THE RASP OR BONE FILE

Indications for Use

1. For final smoothing of bone in ridge trimming procedures, after gross removal has been accomplished with the rongeur or side cutting bone forceps. Its use may be compared to that of sandpaper in carpentry.
2. For bone smoothing in sites that cannot be conveniently reached with the rongeur.

Mode of Use

1. Long, sweeping strokes are used, with a carry through, ending out in a safe area. The instrument cuts on the pull stroke.
2. Cleaning is accomplished by laying the blade on the assistant's sponge, then making one lateral motion. Bone dust will be left on the sponge.

COMPARISON OF BONE CUTTING INSTRUMENTS FOR RIDGE TRIMMING (ALVEOLECTOMY)

Rongeur

When cutting is done with the side of the beaks it acts like a plane and will not cut too deeply. The resulting surface is virtually finished and needs little or no smoothing with the rasp. The action is simple and rapid. The instrument is readily wiped clean in one motion by the gauze square in the assistant's hand.

Chisel

Two instruments are required-the mallet and the chisel.

The chisel has poor control of depth of penetration. When indicated, it can remove a large mass of bone quickly.

Rasp

This instrument will not cut too deeply by accident, but is slow, and difficult to clean after it becomes filled with bony debris.

THE GILMORE PROBE

Specifications

A slender, stiff, tempered instrument with a slightly curved point, somewhat heavier than a dental explorer (Fig. 4.85).

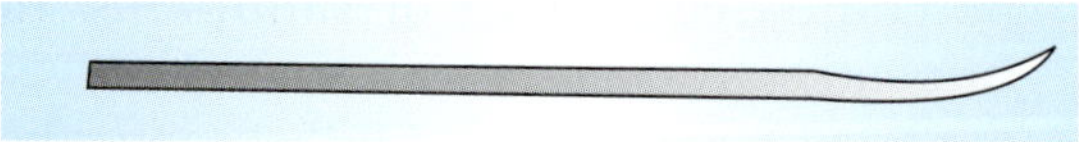

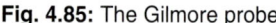

Fig. 4.85: The Gilmore probe

Indications for Use

1. For teasing out small root tips, or wiggling them to visually outline their size, shape, and position (Fig. 4.86).
2. For exploring structures in the depth of a wound such as the inferior alveolar nerve or the lining membrane of the antrum. It is delicate and may be used without producing trauma, when held in the fountain pen grasp.
3. For blunt dissection, to separate the capsule of a cyst or benign tumor from the surrounding normal tissue, when the two are intimately fused. The probe is used in a lateral, scratching manner, thus separating a few fibers at a time. Figure 4.87 shows the incorrect and the correct method for separating the cystic lining.

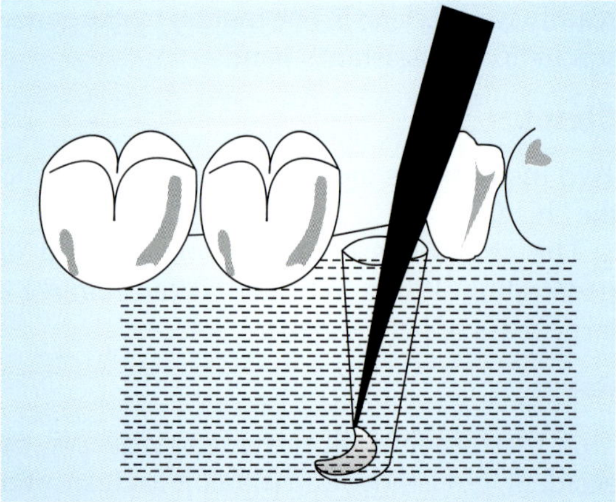

Fig. 4.86: Using Gilmore probe

The probe should never be forced against the cystic lining but should be rested against the bony surface gently lifting up the lining. This practice is very important, especially in cases of keratocysts where the lining is extremely thin and friable. A roller gauze may be useful for separation of the cyst lining from the underlying bony cavity.

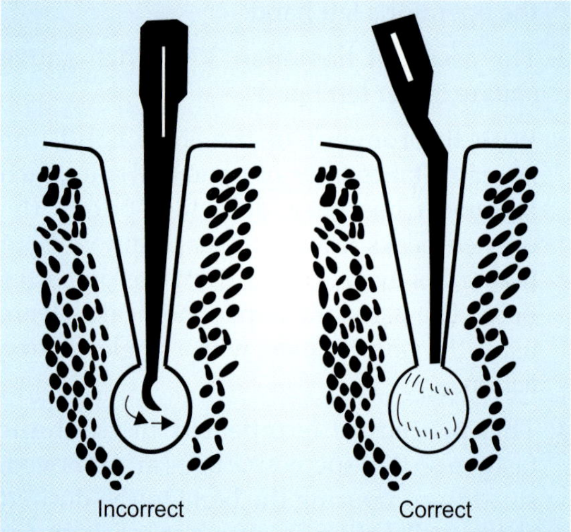

Fig. 4.87: Incorrect and correct method for separating cystic lining

Contraindications for Use

1. It is not used for heavy elevation of root fragments, as it will break. Elevators should be used for large roots.
2. It should not be used for cleaning the suction aspirator tip as it may break. The beak of the foil carrier or an iron wire pick will serve better.

THE DOUBLE-ENDED CURET

Indications for Use

1. For enucleating granulomas, soft tissue tumors lying within bone, cysts, or other membranes.

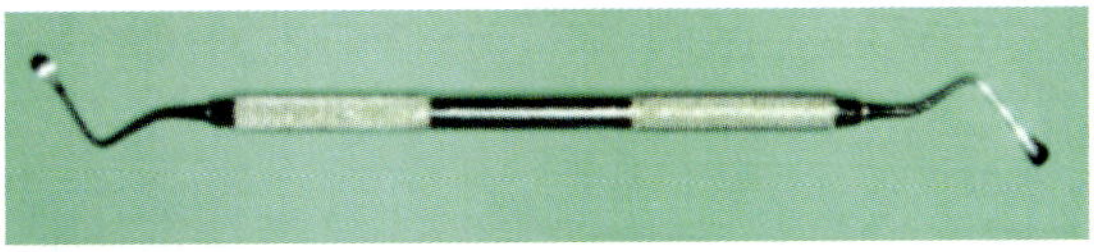

Fig. 4.88: Double-ended curet

2. For removal of bone chips from sockets and alveolectomy wounds (Fig. 4.88).

To Enucleate Granulomas or Cysts

1. By push strokes the mass is peeled from each of the four walls of its bony bed. Each end of the curet will clean two walls. The blade should be inserted so that the concave side faces the outside wall, so that it will curve under the overhanging margin of bone.
2. Lastly, the blade is placed beneath the mass and the tissue lifted out from the bony cavity as with a spoon.

THE DENTAL MIRROR

Specifications

The boilable, plane dental mirror is used.

Indications for Use

1. For preoperative examination, either as a mirror or as a retractor. The glass face of the mirror is held against the cheek to permit inspection of buccal and labial aspects of ridges by direct vision.
2. For cheek retraction in postoperative treatment, such as changing of gauze dressings or suture removal.
3. Rarely, for examining the depth of a socket during tooth removal procedures. Every effort is made to work by direct vision, which is usually possible with the aid of the headlight.
4. Occasionally for retraction of the tongue, when the retractor is already in use, during surgical procedures.

ARMAMENTARIUM FOR EXODONTIA

The more experience the exodontist acquires and the greater volume of work he or she sees, the simpler and more standardized the armamentarium becomes. Wide variation is found in individual likes and dislikes as well as in various techniques that call for specialized instruments.

Forceps

The most widely used instruments employed in the extraction of teeth are the dental forceps. The use of this instrument makes it possible for the operator to grasp the root portion of a tooth and dislocate the latter from it's socket by exerting pressure upon it.

Basic components of extraction forceps (Fig. 4.89).

1. Handle.
2. Hinge.
3. Beaks.

The *handles* of the forceps are usually straight but may be curved. This helps the operator to have better control over the instrument. Maxillary forceps are held with the palm underneath the forceps so that the beak is directed in the superior direction. The forceps used for removal of mandibular teeth are held with the palm on top of the forceps so that the beak is pointed down toward the teeth.

The *hinge* of the forceps, like the shank of the elevator, is merely a mechanism for connecting the handle to the beak. The hinge transfers and

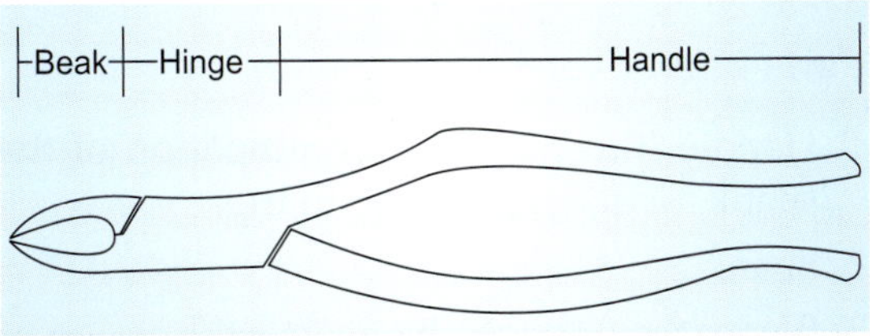

Fig. 4.89: Extraction forceps

concentrates the force applied to the handles to the beak.

The *beaks* of the extraction forceps are the source of the greatest variation among forceps. The beak is designed to adapt to the tooth root at the junction of the" crown and root. It is important to remember that the beaks of the forceps are designed to be adapted to the root structure of the tooth and not to the crown of the tooth. The beak is designed to adapt to the tooth root at the junction of the crown and root.

A final design variation is in the width of the beak. Some forceps are narrow, because their primary use is to remove narrow teeth, such as incisor teeth. Other forceps are somewhat broader, because the teeth they are designed to remove are substantially wider, such as lower molar teeth. Ideally the whole of the inner surface of the forceps blades should fit the root surface. In practice the size and shape of the roots vary so greatly that it is not possible to achieve this aim and the root is gripped by the edges of the blades, 'two-point' contact. If there is only a single linear contact, 'one-point' contact between roots and forceps blade, the tooth will probably be crushed when it is gripped.

Narrow blades are described as being "fine" and wide blades are called "heavy".

ELEVATORS

"Luxate a tooth (to be extracted) with an elevator and deliver it with a forceps."

These are the words of experienced surgeons and highlight the importance of the knowledge of the use of elevators.

Parts of an Elevator (Fig. 4.90)

1. Handle (this may be a continuation of the shank, or at a right angle to it).
2. Shank
3. Blade (the part which engages the crown or root).

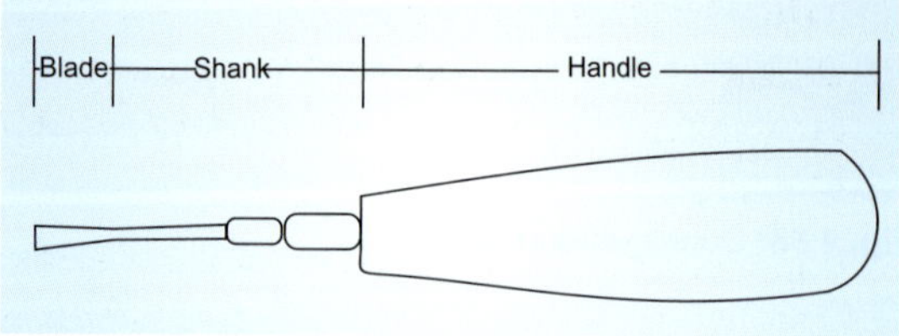

Fig. 4.90: Elevator

Indications for the use of Elevators

1. To reflect mucoperiosteal membranes.
2. To luxate and remove teeth which cannot be engaged by the beaks of the forceps such as impactions and malposed teeth.
3. To remove roots (fractured or carious).
4. To loosen teeth prior to the application of forceps.
5. To split teeth which have had grooves cut in them.
6. To remove intraradicular bone.

Rules when using Elevators

1. Never use an adjacent tooth as a fulcrum unless that tooth is to be extracted also.
2. Never use the buccal plate at the gingival line as a fulcrum except where odontectomy is performed or in the third molar areas.
3. Never use the lingual plate at the gingival line as a fulcrum.
4. Always use finger guards to protect the patient in case the elevator slips.
5. The elevator should be grasped in the fingers and forced down the periodontal membrane at an angle of 45° to the long axis of the root. The tip of the index finger rests against the alveolar bone and enables the operator to have complete control over the instrument.

"The point of application of an elevator, that is the site on the root at which force must be applied to effect delivery, is determined by the line of withdrawal of the tooth or root".

"The line of withdrawal is the path along which the tooth or root will move out of it's socket with the least application of force to it".

6. When cutting through interseptal bone, take care not to engage the root of an adjacent tooth, thus inadvertently forcing it from it's alveolus.

Classification of Elevators

Elevators are classified according to their use or according to form.

1. *According to use*
   - Elevators designed to remove the entire tooth.
   - Elevators designed to remove the roots broken off at the gingival line.
   - Elevators designed to remove roots broken off halfway to the apex.
   - Elevators designed to remove the apical third of the root (apical fragment ejectors).
   - Elevators designed to reflect the muco-periosteum (periosteal elevators) before forceps or extracting elevators are used.
2. *According to form*
   - Straight: wedge type (straight apex).
   - Angular: right and left.
   - Cross bar: handle at right angle to the shank.

Work Principles in the use of Elevators

1. Lever principle.
2. Wedge principle.
3. Wheel-and-axle principle.

Protection of the Patient During the use of Elevators

Two principles apply in protection of the patient

1. The patient's jaws must be supported to prevent dislocation of the mandible.
2. Other tissues in the oral cavity must be protected from potential damage, i.e., the accidental slipping and plunging of the point of the elevator into adjacent or distal soft and hard tissues.

Protection is best accomplished by:

1. Careful and continuous control of the direction of force so that it is directed into the bone surrounding the tooth or against the tooth being luxated.
2. Surrounding the immediate operative area with the fingers.

THE SHARP-POINTED ELEVATOR

Specifications

Any of several stone-sharpened, pointed, single-bladed instruments designed to remove a root by biting into the cementum and dragging it from its socket (Figs 4.91, 4.92).

To Remove Root Fragment Adjacent to an Empty Socket

1. The handle of the instrument is grasped firmly in the palm.
2. The fulcrum, rest, or axis for turning is secured on the alveolar process, usually on the edge of an already empty socket.
3. The point of the elevator is brought to bear on the cementum, by biting through a bony septum if necessary, to reach the root.
4. The root is lifted or dragged from its socket as the non-slipping point retains its bite in the cementum. The point engages the tooth in the same manner as an ice tongs bites into a cake of ice.

The point of the elevator should be sunk into the root as near the apex as possible, for best results. The path of force should be in line with the long axis of the tooth. If the first application of force does not succeed, a slightly different path should be tried. The point of the instrument must be razor-sharp, able to raise shaving from the thumb nail when drawn across it.

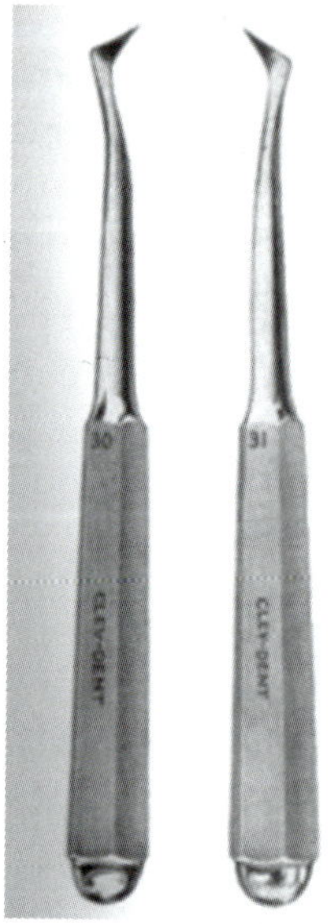

Fig. 4.91: Sharp-pointed elevators

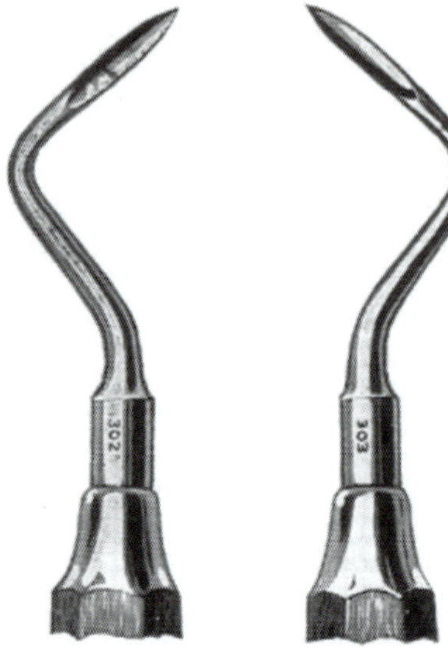

Fig. 4.92: Sharp-pointed elevators

THE INCLINED PLANE ELEVATOR (Fig. 4.93)

Specifications

Any of several unsharpened, single bladed instruments with wedge-shaped working end. The end may be in line with the shaft (straight elevator), at a slight angle (LeCluse), or at nearly a right angle (upper third molar elevator) (Fig. 4.93).

Principles of Physics Involved

Displacement effect

Two objects cannot occupy the same place at the same time. The intent is to cause the metal point of the instrument to occupy the socket instead of the tooth.

Lever effect

When the end of the elevator has entered well into the socket a slight lever action will have extreme expulsive effect. It lifts the root out of its bed (Fig. 4.94).

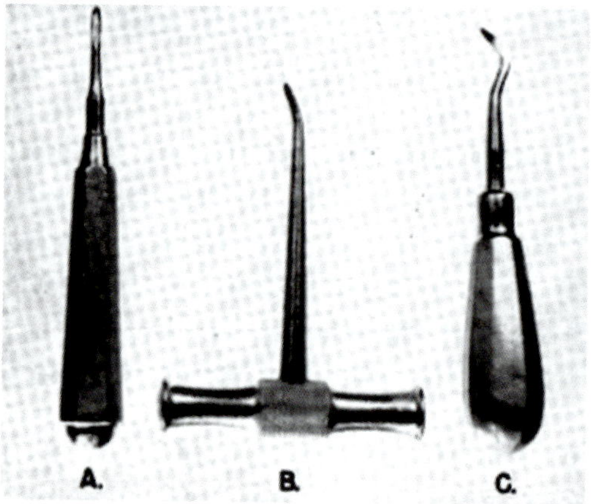

Fig. 4.93: Types of inclined planes elecators: (A) Straight type, (B) LeCluse type with crossbar handle, (C) Upper third molar type

To Remove Root Where There is no Adjacent Empty Socket

1. The tip of the elevator is placed against the neck of the tooth or root, in line with its long axis.
2. With firmly applied pressure an attempt is made to slide the blade up alongside the

root to the apex. Worming, slightly prying, but always intruding forces should be employed.

3. If no seat for entrance of the elevator can be found, the surgical bur may be used to provide a point of entrance.
4. The end of the instrument must be carried to the apex of the socket so the root will not fall back into its bed. The operation must follow through (Fig. 4.94).
5. Without delay, the root should be recovered with the index finger, removed from the mouth, and placed on the table.

Proper understanding of the use of instruments helps the surgeon to use them with less force and gives maximum results. It is rightfully said

"It takes a lot of effort to appear effortless."

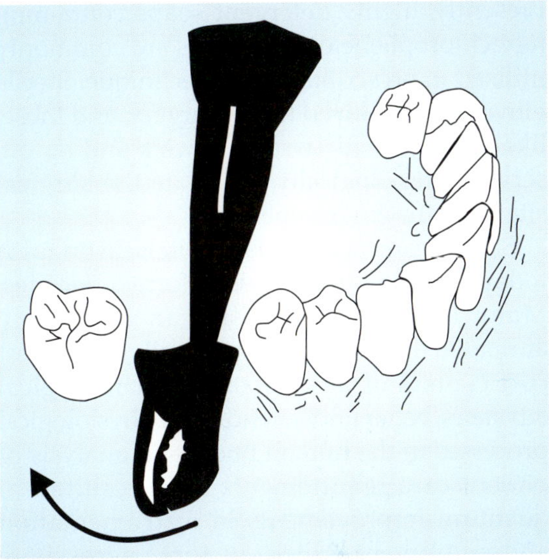

Fig. 4.94: Use of sharp pointed elevators to remove lower molar root

OPERATING ROOM DECORUM

The work of Lister has proved conclusively the role played by bacteria in wound infection. It is now mandatory in all surgery, including oral surgery, that all intelligent, precautionary measures be taken to avoid the contamination of wounds.

Although the means for providing strictly aseptic mouth surgeries are still unavailable, this is no reason for completely abandoning an aseptic technique. At the very least an aseptic routine for mouth surgery markedly eliminates some of the pathways of cross infection: the infection of the doctor from the patient, the infection of the patient from the doctor, or the infection of the patient from another patient through the doctor or through the contaminated armamentarium employed be the doctor. It has long been established that surgical wounds are contaminated chiefly from microorganisms harboured in the skin or mucous membranes that have been incised. Furthermore the oral cavity is normal breeding ground for wide variety of organisms. The nose throat and hands of the operating team are the next most common source of wound infection unsterile instruments and supplies follow in the order of frequency. Complete asepsis in surgery may well be an ideal that is never fully attained. There may always be some doubt regarding sterility of the skin or the mucous membranes to be incised. The air contamination of wounds is an omnipresent problem, but if wound infection in surgery is to be minimized, all logical precautions and preparations must be instituted. This should include the proper preparation of the operating team as well as the patient. Whenever surgery is done, in the hospital operating room or in the clinic, the surgeon wears a face mask. The surgeon's hands are adequately scrubbed.

Presently, highly detergent soaps containing hexachlorophene or iodophors are commonly utilized in prescribing scrub technique. Sterile gloves are employed for all surgery, and these, like sterile sheets, wraps, towels and so on, serve bacteriologically to isolate the surgical site from the environment.

Special care facilities in hospitals distinguish today's hospital from those of former decades. Many hospital care costs can be largely attributed to such facilities, generally the highest cost centers of any hospital. Technological advances, better understanding of physiological processes in the human body, and analysis of patient care requirements have resulted in quantum improvements in instrumentation and equipment which, in turn, necessitate special facilities.

The operating room system complex consists of four main systems:

- Surgical support system (the environment)
- Traffic and commerce (the activities)
- Communication and information (the record)
- Administration (the management).

By appropriate meshing and balance of these systems, the surgery is performed on the patients.

BASIC REQUIREMENT FOR DESIGN

- The design and performance criteria of the suite must be determined and defined for a given institution.
- The objectives of the surgical discipline of the institution must be kept in mind.
- A sensible traffic pattern should be provided.
- Specific requests of individual specialties should be given every consideration.
- Decisions must be made regarding location of the surgical suite in relation to other services (laboratories, surgical in patient areas, imaging department, etc.).
- Caution should be exercised in design planning to accommodate fixed equipment. It is desirable that the design provide for ease of installing and changing fixed equipment.
- Scope for further expansion and flexibility.

Figure 4.95 shows the diagrammatic representation of an ideal operating department showing breakup of each functional zone into facilities.

PLANNING CRITERIA

Functional Criteria

The design of the operating suites must follow the functional requirement of the operating department.

Ergonomic or Workflow Criteria

The flow of the patients, supplies and staff in an operating department is to be conceived and preplanned. This will ensure optimization of relationship between various functional areas of the operating departments.

Figure 4.96 in the form of a diagrammatic sketch shows the traffic flow in and around an operating room.

Environmental Criteria

The environmental aspects should also be considered for the safety and comfort of the patient and staff.

PLANNING CONSIDERATIONS

The essential planning considerations while designing an operating department are as follows.

Zoning

It is universally agreed that surgery is to be performed under the most aseptic conditions. To ensure this aseptic condition, the operating department is divided into four distinct

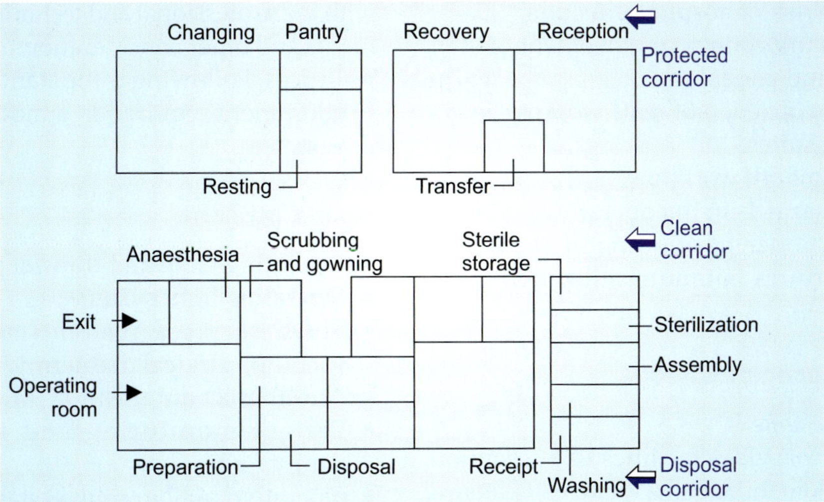

Fig. 4.95: Functional zones

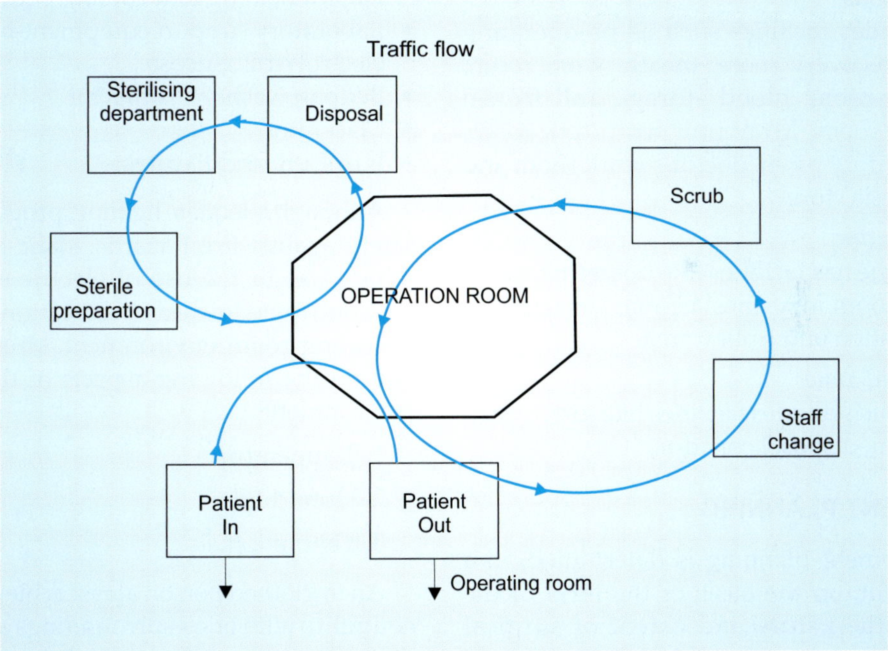

Fig. 4.96: Traffic flow

zones: protective zone, clean zone, sterile zone and disposal zone (Fig. 4.95). These zones are bacteriological zones of varying degrees of cleanliness. The bacteriological count diminishes from the outer to the inner zones. Hundred percent sterility must be ensured in the sterile zone. The zoning of the operating department has the following advantages.

- Minimise risk of hospital infection.
- Minimise unproductive movement of staff, supplies and patients.
- Increases efficiency of staff working in the operating suites.
- Ensures smooth workflow.
- Reduces hazards in the operating suites.
- Ensures proper positioning of the equipments. Ensures optimum utilization of the operating.

Scales of Accommodations

- *Protective zone*
  It usually provides facilities like reception, waiting room for patients relatives, changing rooms, autoclave, trolley bay, control area of electricity
- *Clean zone*
  It provides facilities such as preoperating room, recovery room, theatre work room, plaster room, blood storage and frozen section room, X-ray unit with dark room, nurse's duty room, doctor's work room and anesthesia store.
- *Sterile zone*
  This zone has facilities like operating room, scrub room, anesthesia room, instrument sterilization and trolley area.
- *Disposal zone*
  This zone provides facilities like dirty wash-up room, disposal corridor.

EQUIPMENT PLANNING

The equipment planning is determined, to a large extent, on the basis of the level of the hospital, the nature and extent of surgical procedures are contemplated, and extent of and the constraints of financial, physical and human resources in their acquisition, installation and use.

While planning the equipment mix for an operating department therefore, it is necessary to match their characteristics and specification with the professional and technological requirements and other considerations of logistics and resources. Following is the standard inventory of equipment required in a modern operating department.

Operating Zone

- Operating table and transfer trolley system
- Operating light system
- Fixed services system (medical gases, vacuum, surgical diathermy, cold light)
- Anesthesia equipment
- Patient monitoring and resuscitation equipment
- Operative radiography system
- Operating microscopy equipment
- Extra-corporeal circulation equipment
- Patient heating and cooling equipment
- Laboratory support equipment-blood gases, electrolytes, glucose.
- Bedpan washer/disinfector
- Macerator
- Furniture and fixtures.

Although adequate lighting, proper acoustics, safety against fire hazards, static charge and other risks in the use of electric equipment, etc, contribute towards the creation of an ideal operating room environment, stress must be laid on the following aspects of the physical environment:

1. Temperature
2. Humidity
3. Ventilation.

An unclothed person at rest achieves thermal neutrality with one's surroundings at 24°–27° C at a relative humidity of 50°. When conditions vary the body's own temperature regulating mechanisms come into play.

During anesthesia patients lose body heat. This heat loss is due to the following factors, which are related to the surgical intervention as well as operating room environment:

- Low ambient temperature and high humidity
- Infusion with cold fluids
- Ventilation with cold anesthetics
- Exposure of body cavities
- Absence of muscular movement
- Subcutaneous vasodilatation

Under normal circumstances a relative humidity of 45° to 60° C is recommended for operating rooms. When flammable anesthetic agents are not in use, a relative humidity of 40° is considered adequate. Further when young children and infants are involved, a higher range of 55° to 65° is recommended.

AIR CHANGES

Ventilation at the rate of one change per hour will reduce the level of air contamination by 63 percent, two air changes per hour by 86 percent and ten air changes by about 99 percent.

AIR DISTRIBUTION

Room air distribution systems used in operating room ventilation have many configurations and variations in air handling equipment and patterns of air flow. Some of the prevalent systems are as follows.

- Turbulent or mixing air distribution system promotes uniform mixing of air including the airborne contaminants throughout the entire room (Fig. 4.97).
- Downward displacement piston system, which takes air in the top of the operating room and exhausts at the lower levels, is highly effective and economical system and transports contaminants arising below the operating table out of the operating room environment (Fig. 4.98).
- Unidirectional air flow system, sometimes popularly known as laminar flow ventilation system, is observed in literature with many modifications such as downflow, tunnel, horizontal, and crossflow patterns (Fig. 4.99).

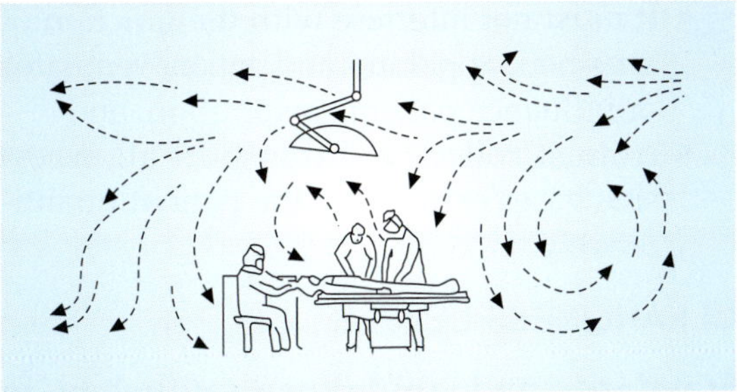

Fig. 4.97

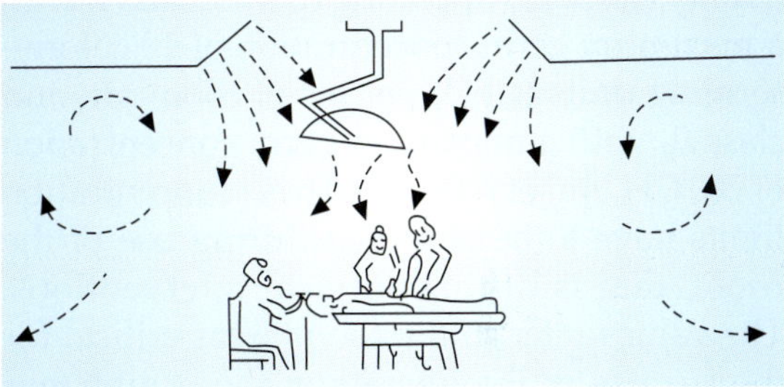

Fig. 4.98

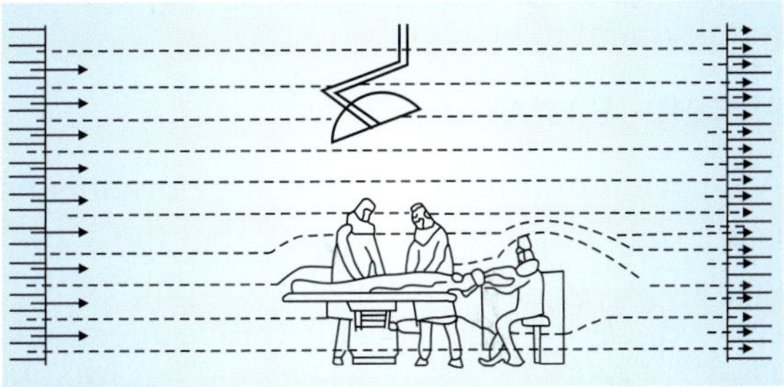

Fig. 4.99

SCAVENGING

Scavenging system essentially is a piped vacuum system which can be hooked onto the patient ventilators used in anesthesia practice so that the expired gases are sucked out of the operating room environment.

Although standards for scavenging system have not been formulated, the following guidelines have been offered.

- The system must not require the attention of the anesthetists during the course of anesthesia,

- It must not interfere with the function of anesthetic apparatus and patient ventilator or influence patients respiration, and
- It must collect and transport all excessive gases expired by the patient quantitatively.

CLEANLINESS LEVELS

Standards and guidelines published in Switzerland and Austria distinguish two quality classes of operating rooms: class I, with a maximum germ concentration of 10 colony-forming units (CFU) per m^3 of room air, and class II, with a maximum germ concentration of 200 CFU/m^3 of room air. These concentration limits have to be observed during use of the room, that is during surgical interventions. The values refer to the room areas critical for the success of the operation: the compliance with an adequate level of discipline during the course of the operation is a complementary requirement to be met.

FILTER CEILING

A clean environment without microorganisms is not only important to ensure that the actual operation is performed without complications; it also reduces the risk of postoperative infections. The filter ceiling consists of 600 mm^2 modules to simplify installation. To prevent contaminated air from flowing into the operating zone, the ceiling is divided into two separate, perforated zones in which air is supplied in a vertical flow at different velocities. Each ceiling consists of three frames: a top frame, a centre frame with 60 mm^2 filter modules, and a third frame. Perforated stainless steel screens (550 mm^2) are attached to the frame, to determine the velocity of the supply air flow. To prevent contaminated air from entering the operating area, the perforated screen ceiling is divided into an outer zone, in which air is supplied vertically at a higher velocity in the inner zone and at a lower velocity in the outer zone. The perforated screens are made of stainless steel and can be easily disassembled for cleaning by hospital personnel. The air is changed 60–70 times an hour in the operating theater. Efficient and cost-effective concepts are now available for meeting the air cleanliness requirements in operating rooms, and to provide the desirable environmental conditions for the surgery.

REFERENCES AND BIBLIOGRAPHY

1. Primary Content Providers: The U. S. Army, The U.S. Navy Ancillary Content and Online Version: David L. Heiserman Publisher: SweetHaven Publishing Services.
2. Oral and Maxillofacial Surgery; Daniel M.Laskin
3. General Haemostatic Agents –Fact or Fiction?; Ulla Hedner; Pathophysiol Haemost Thromb 2002; 32(suppl 1):33–36.
4. Prostaglandins as haemostatic agents; Richard L. Fenichel, David D. Stokes & Harvey E. Alburn; Nature 253, 537–538 (13 February 1975); doi:10.1038/253537a0
5. Contemporary Oral and Maxillofacial Surgery; Fourth edition; Larry J.Peterson, Edward Ellis, James R.Hupp, Myron R.Tucker.
6. Killey and Kay's Outline of Oral Surgery; Second edition. Gordon R.Seward, Malcolm Harris, David A.McGowan.
7. The Extraction of Teeth; Geoffrey L.Howe; Second edition.
8. Oral and Maxillofacial Surgery; Volume One; Harry Archer; Fifth Edition.
9. Practical Oral Surgery; Henry B.Clark; Third edition.

Chapter 5

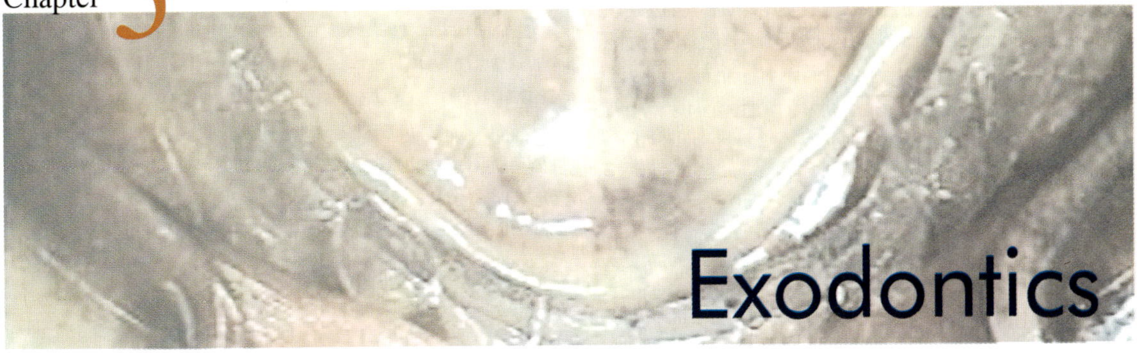

Exodontics

UNCOMPLICATED EXODONTIA

Extraction of teeth is a procedure that incorporates the principles of surgery and many principles from physics and mechanics. When these principles are applied correctly, a tooth can probably be removed intact from the alveolar process without untoward sequelae. Removal of a tooth does not require a large amount of force but rather it can be done well with controlled force in such a manner that the tooth is not pulled from the bone but instead is gently lifted from the alveolar process.

Ideal Tooth Extraction

The ideal tooth extraction is the painless removal of the whole tooth, or tooth-root, with minimal trauma to the investing tissues, that the wound heals uneventfully and no postoperative prosthetic problem is created.

INDICATIONS FOR TOOTH EXTRACTION

1. Severe caries.
2. Pulpal necrosis.
3. Severe periodontal disease.
4. Orthodontic reasons.
5. Malopposed teeth.
6. Cracked teeth.
7. Preprosthetic extractions.
8. Impacted teeth.
9. Supernumerary teeth.
10. Teeth associated with pathologic lesions.
11. Pre-radiation therapy.
12. Teeth involved in jaw fractures.
13. Esthetics.
14. Economics.

CONTRAINDICATIONS FOR REMOVAL OF TEETH

Systemic Contraindications

Severe Uncontrolled Metabolic Diseases

Brittle diabetes and end-stage renal disease with severe uremia are part of this group. Patients with mild diabetes or well-controlled severe diabetes can be treated as reasonably normal patients. It is only when the disease process becomes uncontrolled that the patient should not have a tooth removed.

Uncontrolled Leukemias and Lymphomas

Patients who have uncontrolled leukemias and lymphomas should not have teeth removed until the leukemias can be brought under control. The potential complications are infection as a result of nonfunctioning white cells and excessive bleeding as a result of an inadequate number of platelets.

Cardiovascular Conditions

Patients with any of a variety of severe uncontrolled cardiac diseases should also have their extractions deferred until the disease can be brought under control. Patients with severe myocardial ischemia, such as unstable angina pectoris, and patients who have had a recent myocardial infarction (MI) should not have a tooth extracted. Patients who have severe uncontrolled hypertension should also have extractions deferred, because persistent bleeding, acute myocardial insufficiency, and cerebrovascular accidents are more likely to occur as a result of stress caused by the extraction. Patients who have severe, uncontrolled cardiac dysrhythmias should have their extraction procedures deferred as well.

Pregnancy

Pregnancy is a relative contraindication; patients who are in the first or last trimester should have their extractions deferred if possible. The latter part of the first trimester and the first month of the last trimester may be as safe as the middle trimester for a routine uncomplicated extraction, but more extensive surgical procedures should be deferred until after the child has been delivered.

Bleeding Disorders

Patients who have a severe bleeding diathesis, such as hemophilia, or severe platelet disorders should not have teeth extracted until the coagulopathies have been corrected. Most severe bleeding disorders can be controlled by the administration of coagulation factors or platelet transfusions. Close coordination with the patient's hematologist can result in an uncomplicated recovery from the extraction procedure in most situations. Similarly, patients who take anticoagulants can have routine extractions performed when care is taken to manage the patient appropriately.

Medications

Finally, patients who take or have taken a variety of medications should have surgery performed with caution. Drugs to watch for include corticosteroids, immunosuppressives, and cancer chemotherapeutic agents.

Local Contraindications

Therapeutic Radiation for Cancer

Extractions performed in an area of radiation may result in osteoradionecrosis and, therefore, must be done with extreme caution.

Teeth in an Area of Neoplasm

Teeth that are located within an area of tumor, especially a malignant tumor, should not be extracted. The surgical procedure for extraction could disseminate cells and thereby hasten the metastatic process.

Pericoronitis

Patients who have severe pericoronitis around impacted mandibular third molar should not have tooth extracted until the pericoronitis has been treated. Nonsurgical treatment should include irrigations, antibiotics, and removal of the maxillary third molar to relieve impingement on the edematous soft tissue overlying mandibular impaction. If the mandibular third molar is removed in the face of severe pericoronitis, the incidence of complications increases.

Acute Dentoalveolar Abscess

Most rapid resolution of an infection secondary to pulpal necrosis is obtained when the tooth is removed as early as possible. Therefore acute infection is not a contraindication to extraction. However, it may be difficult to extract such a tooth because the patient may not be able to open the mouth sufficiently wide, or it may be difficult to reach a state of adequate local anesthesia.

If access and anesthesia considerations can be met tooth should be removed as early as possible.

CLINICAL EXAMINATION OF TEETH TO BE EXTRACTED

Access to Tooth

Any limitation of opening may compromise the ability of the surgeon to do a routine uncomplicated extraction. The surgeon should look for the reasons for the reduction of opening. The most likely causes are trismus associated with infection, temporomandibular joint (TMJ) dysfunction (especially internal joint derangement with displacement of the disk without reduction), muscle fibrosis.

Mobility of Tooth

The mobility of the tooth to be extracted should be assessed preoperatively. Greater-than-normal mobility is frequently seen with severe periodontal disease. Teeth that have less-than-normal mobility should be examined to rule out hypercementosis and ankylosis of the tooth. Ankylosis should mostly be expected be deciduous teeth that have been retained and are submerged.

Condition of Crown

The assessment of the crown of the tooth before the extraction should be related to the presence of large caries or restorations in the crown. It large portions of the crown have been destroyed by caries, the likelihood of crushing the crown during the extraction is increased: thus causing more difficulty in removing the tooth. Similarly, the presence of large amalgam restorations will produce a weakness in the crown, and the restoration will probably fracture during the extraction process.

INDICATIONS FOR A PREOPERATIVE RADIOGRAPH

1. A story of difficult or attempted extractions.
2. A tooth which is abnormally resistant to forceps extraction.
3. If, after clinical examination, it has been decided to remove the tooth by dissection.
4. Any teeth or roots in close relationship to either the maxillary antrum or the inferior dental and mental nerves.
5. All mandibular third molars, and misplaced canines. The root pattern of such teeth is often abnormal.
6. Heavily restored or pulpless teeth. These teeth are normally very brittle.
7. Any tooth affected by periodontal disease accompanied by some sclerosis of the supporting bone. Such teeth are often hypercementosed and brittle.
8. Any tooth which has been subjected to trauma. Fractures of the roots and/or alveolar bone may be present.
9. An isolated maxillary molar, especially if it is unopposed and over erupted. The bony support of such a tooth is often weakened by the presence of a large maxillary antrum. This may predispose to either creation of an oroantral communication or fracture of the maxillary tuberosity.
10. Any partially erupted or unerupted tooth or retained root.
11. Any tooth whose abnormal crown or delayed eruption might indicate the

possibility of dilacerations, germination or a dilated odontome.

12. Any condition which predisposes to dental or alveolar abnormality, for example:
    a. Osteitis deformans in which the roots are hypercementosed and there is a predisposition to chronic osteomyelitis.
    b. Cleidocranial dysostosis, for pseudo-anodontia and hooked roots occur in this condition.
    c. Patients who have received therapeutic irradiation to the jaws and thus have a predisposition to osteoradionecrosis.
    d. Osteopetrosis, which causes extractions to be difficult and predisposes to chronic osteomyelitis.

REQUIREMENTS OF A PRE-EXTRACTION RADIOGRAPH

A pre-extraction radiograph must show the whole root structure and the alveolar bone investing the tooth. In most cases an intraoral periapical view will suffice, but sometimes an extraoral lateral oblique view of the mandible will be required to demonstrate the entire root, or the state, structure, and amount of supporting bone.

INTERPRETING A PREOPERATIVE RADIOGRAPH

A good radiograph is wasted unless it is carefully interpreted. The use of a hand lens and viewing box greatly aid interpretation and enable the following factors causing difficulty to be detected (Figs 5.1, 5.2).

1. Abnormal number of roots.
2. Abnormal shape of roots.
3. An unfavorable root pattern.
4. Caries extending into the root or root-mass.
5. Fracture or resorption of the root.
6. Hypercementosis of roots.

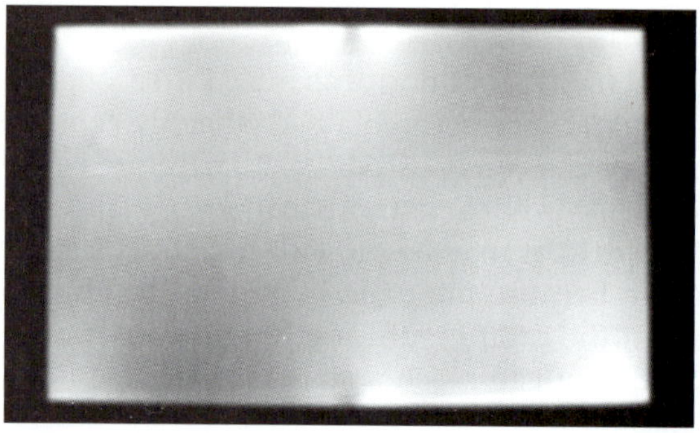

Fig. 5.1: The X-ray viewer.

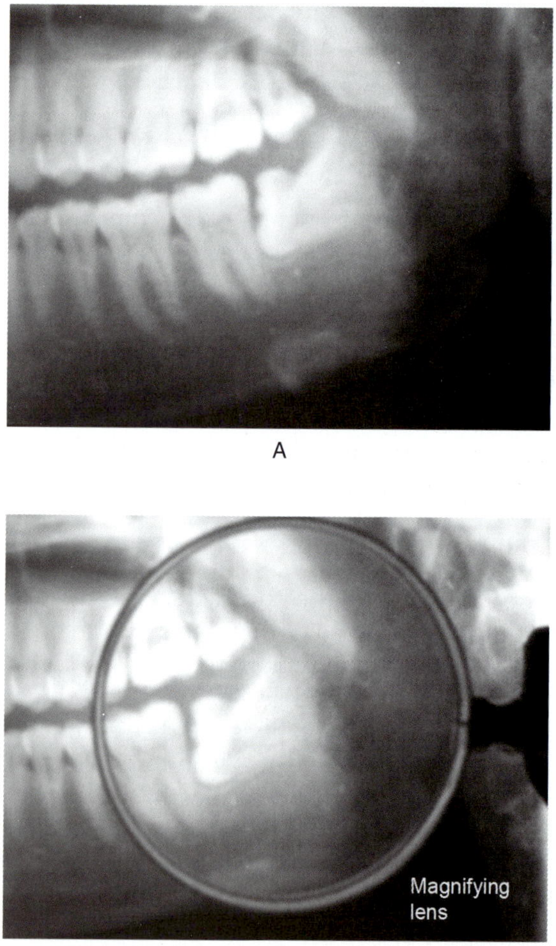

Fig. 5.2: Use of a magnifying lens can help in studying the proximity of the roots of the impacted mandibular third molar to the inferior alveolar canal.

7. Ankylosis.
8. Geminations.
9. Impacted teeth.
10. Bony sclerosis and pathological lesions.

Study the interpretations (as depicted in Fig. 5.3) on an orthopantomogram.

Careful interpretation of the radiograph may also reveal the possibility of the following complications:

a. Involvement of, and damage to, the inferior dental and mental nerves.
b. The creation of an oroantral or oronasal communication.
c. The retention of intrabony pathological lesions.
d. The displacement of a tooth or root into the maxillary antrum.
e. Fracture of the maxillary tuberosity.

THE RADIOLOGICAL PREDICTION OF INFERIOR ALVEOLAR NERVE INJURY DURING THIRD MOLAR SURGERY

The inferior alveolar nerve runs in a canal within the mandible usually near the apices of the third molar and, if the molar is impacted, a close relationship of the roots to the nerve is likely. Sometimes, during the surgical removal of a mandibular third molar, the inferior alveolar nerve is damaged leading to impairment of sensation in the lower lip; which is one of the most unpleasant postoperative complications. Pre-operative assessment must be carried out radiologically in an attempt to identify the proximity of the impacted tooth to the inferior alveolar canal (Fig. 5.3). This evaluation is the first stage in assessing the possible postoperative occurrence of labial sensory impairment and thus its prevention. A review of the literature revealed that seven radiological signs have been suggested as indicative of a close relationship between the mandibular third molar tooth and the inferior alveolar canal. Four of these signs are seen on the root of the tooth and the other three are changes in the appearance of the inferior alveolar canal.

Darkening of the Root

Usually the density of the root is the same throughout its length and this is not disturbed when the images of the tooth and inferior alveolar canal overlap. When there is impingement of the canal on the tooth root, there is

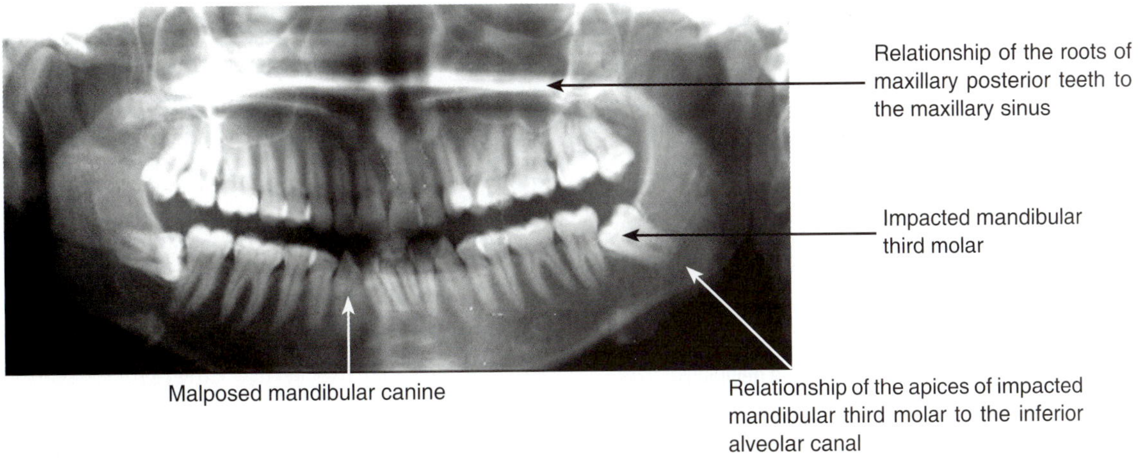

Fig. 5.3: Studying the interpretations carefully.

loss of density of the root; the root appears darker. Darkening of the root is attributed to the decreased amount of tooth substance or loss of the cortical lining of the canal between the source of X-rays and the film. Figure 5.4 gives a schematic representation of the relation between the apices of the impacted third molar and the inferior alveolar canal.

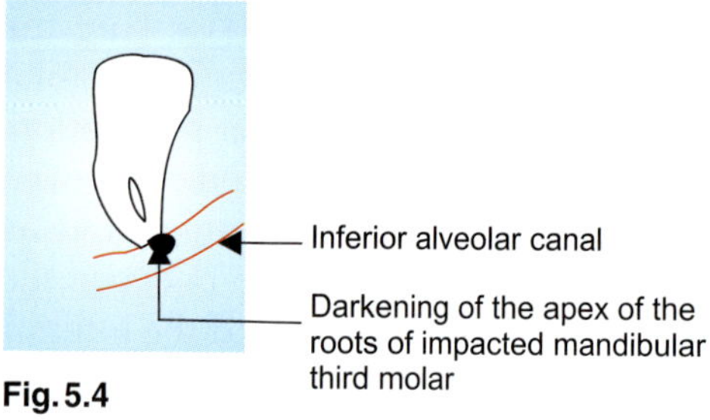

Fig. 5.4

Deflected Roots

Deflected roots or roots hooked around the canal are seen as an abrupt deviation of the root, when it reaches the inferior alveolar canal. The root may be deflected to the buccal or lingual side or to both sides so that it may completely surround the canal (Stockdale, 1959); or it may be deflected to the mesial or distal aspect (Waggener, 1959). The following is a schematic representation of the relation between the apices of the impacted third molar and the inferior alveolar canal.

Figure 5.5. is a schematic representation of the relation between the apices of the impacted third molar and the inferior alveolar canal.

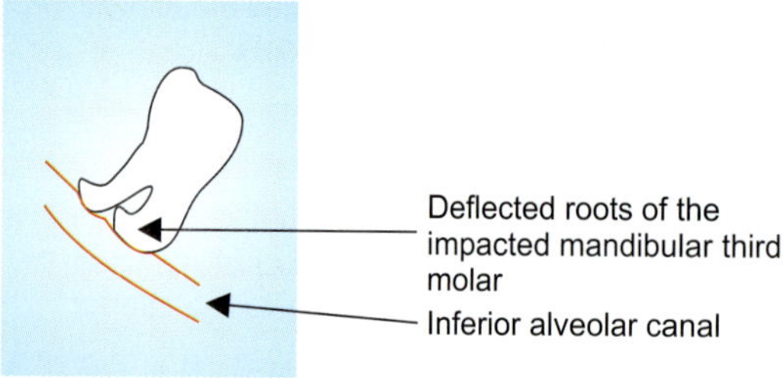

Fig. 5.5

Narrowing of the Root

Seward (1963) stated, If there is narrowing of the root where the canal crosses it, it implies that the greatest diameter of the root has been involved by the canal or that there is deep grooving or perforation of the root. Figure 5.6 is a schematic representation of the relation between the apices of the impacted third molar and the inferior alveolar canal.

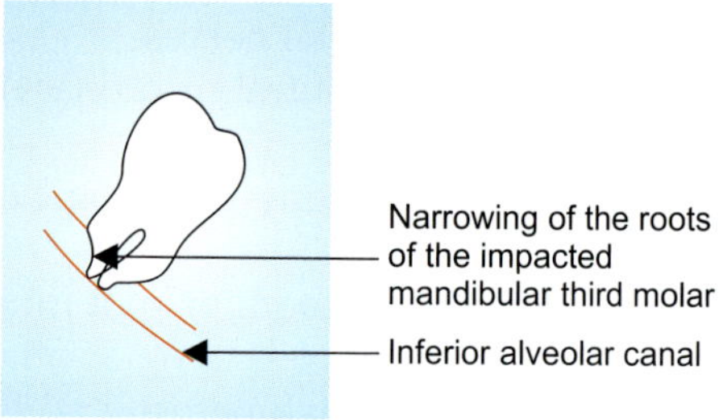

Fig. 5.6

Dark and Bifid Root

This sign (Fig. 5.7) appears when the inferior alveolar canal crosses the apex and is identified by the double periodontal membrane shadow of the bifid apex (Seward, 1963).

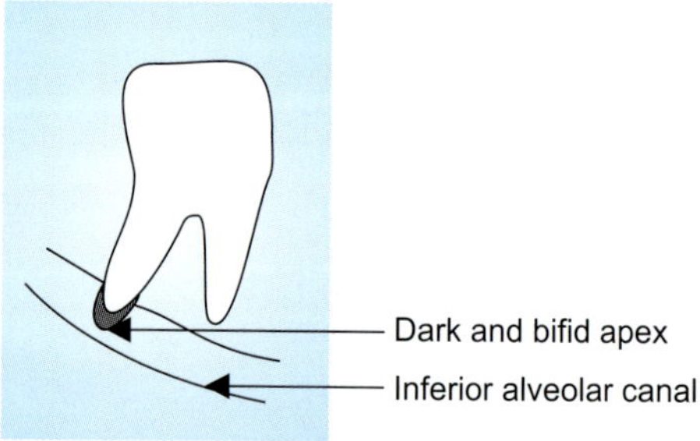

Fig. 5.7

Interruption of the White Line(s)

The white lines are the two radio-opaque lines that constitute the 'roof' and 'floor' of the inferior alveolar canal. These lines appear on a radiograph due to the rather dense structure of the canal walls (Durbeck, 1957). The white line is considered to be interrupted if it disappears immediately before it reaches the tooth structure; either one or both lines may be involved (Howe & Poyton, 1960; KiUey & Kay, 1975; MacGregor, 1976; Kipp et al, 1980; Rud, 1983b). The interruption of the white line(s) is considered to indicate deep grooving of the root if it appears alone or perforation of the root if it appears with the narrowing of the inferior alveolar canal (Seward, 1963; Howe, 1985). The interruption is considered by some to be a 'danger sign' of a true relationship between tooth root and canal (Summers, 1975) as shown in Figure 5.8.

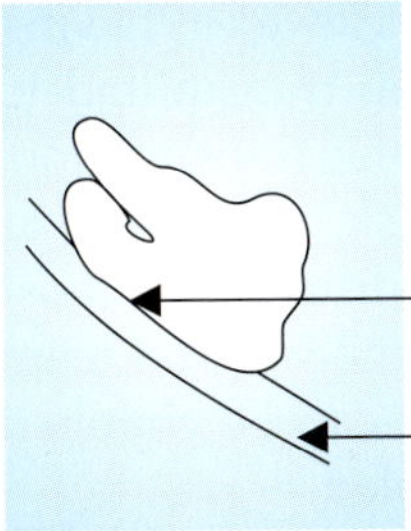

Fig. 5.8

Diversion of the Inferior Alveolar Canal

The canal is considered to be diverted if, when it crosses the mandibular third molar, it changes its direction, (Miles & West, 1954; MacGregor, 1976; KipI et al, 1980; Rud, 1983a). Seward (1963) attributed an upward displacement of the inferior alveolar canal to the contents of the canal passing through the root and hence, during eruption of the third molar, the contents are dragged upwards with it. Rud (1983a) reported a 1% incidence of an upward deflection of the canal where it overlapped the root and 4% when the root was grooved. Figure 5.9 is a schematic representation of the relation between the apices of the impacted third molar and the inferior alveolar canal.

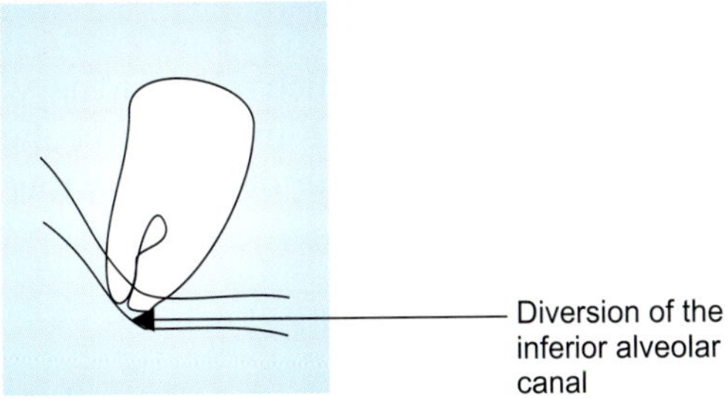

Fig. 5.9

Narrowing of the Inferior Alveolar Canal

The inferior alveolar canal is considered to be narrowed if, when it crosses the root of the mandibular third molar, there is a reduction of its diameter (Poyton, 1982). This narrowing (Fig. 5.10) could be due to the downward displacement of the upper border of the canal (Kipp et al 1980; Rud, 1983a) or the displacement of the upper and lower borders toward each other with the hourglass appearance (Cogswell, 1942; Rud, 1983a). The hourglass form indicates a partial encirclement of the canal (Seward, 1963; Mac Gregor, 1976) or a complete encirclement (Waggener, 1959; Killey & Kay, 1975; Summers, 1975; Howe, 1985); or it may mean either of these alternatives (Cogswell, 1942; Austin, 1947; Miles & West, 1954; Uotila & Kilpinen, 1968). Howe and Payton (1960) reported 33.7% of teeth in a true relationship with the canal to have this sign.

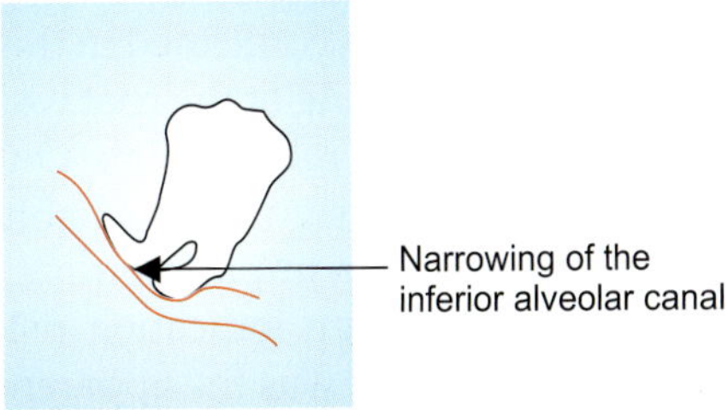

Fig. 5.10

Signs Related to Nerve injury

The most significant sign which related to nerve injury was diversion of the inferior alveolar canal followed by darkening of the root; then interruption of the white line.

Signs Unrelated to Nerve Injury

The signs found to be unrelated statistically to nerve injury were

i. narrowing of the root,
ii. dark and bifid root,
iii. narrowing of the inferior alveolar canal,
iv. deflected root.

Rud (1983a) found that there was a significant relation between the diversion of the canal and grooved roots. In this study a significant relation was found between the diversion of the canal and nerve injury (P < 0.001). One in three patients exhibiting this sign on preoperative X-rays will suffer impairment of labial sensation.

> ***"Diversion of the inferior alveolar canal was shown to be the most reliable sign indicating the impingement of the impacted third molar upon the canal".***
>
> Howe and Payton (1960) found that
>
> ***"Darkening of the root on X-rays was the most reliable indication of a true relationship between the third molar and the inferior alveolar canal."***

Kipp et al (1980) and Rud (1983a) found a significant relationship between root darkening and nerve injury and this was confirmed in this study (P < 0.001); and darkening of the root was found to be the second most reliable sign. Out of four patients having this sign, one is liable to experience labial sensation impairment.

The third most reliable sign indicating risk of postoperative nerve injury was the apparent interruption of white line on the radiograph were it crossed the impacted third molar. Howe and Payton (1960) considered it a reliable sign to indicate the true relationship of the tooth with the canal. Kipp et al (1980) and Rud (1983a) found this sign to be significantly related to nerve injury, and this was corroborated in the present study (P < 0.001). One in four patients exhibiting this sign on preoperative radiographs will experience impairment of labial sensation.

PREPARATION OF THE SURGEON AND THE PATIENT PRIOR TO THE EXTRACTION PROCEDURE

Surgeons must prevent inadvertent injury or transmission of infection to their patients or to themselves. The concept of universal precautions states that all patients must be viewed as having blood-borne diseases that can transmitted to the surgical team. To prevent this transmission, surgical gloves, surgical mask, and eyewear with shields are required. Additionally, most authorities recommend that the surgical team wear long-sleeved gowns at can be changed when they become visibly soiled.

If the surgeon has long hair, it is essential that the hair held in position with barrettes or other holding devices or be covered with a surgical cap. It is a major breach in aseptic technique to allow the surgeon's hair to hang over the patient's face and mouth. Before the patient undergoes the surgical procedure, a minimal amount of draping is necessary. A sterile drape should be put across the patient's chest to decrease the risk of contamination. Before the extraction, patients should vigorously rinse their mouths with an antiseptic mouth rinse, such as chlorhexidine. This reduces the gross bacterial contamination in the patient's mouth, which helps to reduce the incidence of postoperative infection.

To prevent teeth or fragments of teeth from falling to the mouth and potentially being swallowed or pirated into the lungs, many surgeons prefer to place 4 × 4 inch gauze loosely into the back of the mouth. This oral partition serves as a barrier so that, should a tooth slip from the forceps or shatter under the pressure of the forceps, it will be caught in the gauze rather than be swallowed or aspirated. The surgeon must take care that the gauze is not positioned so far posteriorly that it makes the patient gag. The surgeon should explain the purpose of the partition to gain the patient's acceptance and cooperation for allowing the gauze to be placed.

CHAIR POSITION FOR FORCEPS EXTRACTION

The positions of the patient, chair, and operator are important for successful completion of the extraction. The position is one that is comfortable for both the patient and surgeon and allows the surgeon to have maximum control of the force that is being delivered to the patient's tooth through the forceps. The correct position allows the surgeon to keep the arms close to the body and provides stability and support; it also allows the surgeon to keep the wrists straight enough to deliver the force with the arm and shoulder and not with the hand. The force delivered can thus be controlled in the face of sudden loss of resistance from a root or bone fracture.

For a maxillary extraction the chair should be tipped backward so that the maxillary occlusal plane is at an angle of about 60 degrees to the floor. The height of the chair should be such that the height of the patient's mouth is at or slightly below the operator's elbow level. ***When a maxillary tooth is being extracted, the chair should be adjusted so that the site of operation is about 8 cm (3 inches) below the shoulder level of the operator.*** For extraction of teeth in the maxillary anterior portion of the arch, the patient should be looking straight ahead. The position for the maxillary left portion of the arch is similar, except that the patient's head is turned slightly toward the operator.

For the extraction of mandibular teeth, the patient should be positioned in a more upright position so that when the mouth is opened widely, the occlusal plane is parallel to the floor. A bite block should be used to stabilize the mandible when the extraction forceps is used. Even though the surgeon will support the jaw, the additional support provided by the bite block will result in less stress being transmitted to the jaws. The chair should be lower than for extraction of maxillary teeth and the surgeon's arm is inclined downward to approximately 120 degree angle at the elbow. ***During the extraction of mandibular tooth the chair height should be adjusted so that the tooth to be extracted is about 16 cm. below the level of the operator's elbow.*** During removal of the right posterior teeth, the patient's head turned severely toward the surgeon to allow adequate access to the jaw and the surgeon should maintain the proper arm and hand position. When removing teeth in the anterior region of the mandible, the surgeon should rotate around to the side of the patient. When operating on the left posterior mandibular region, the surgeon should stand in front of the patient, but the patient's head should not turn quite so severely toward the surgeon.

MECHANICAL PRINCIPLES INVOLVED IN TOOTH EXTRACTION

The removal of teeth from the alveolar process employs the use of the following mechanical principles and simple machines: Lever, wedge, and wheel and axle.

Elevators are used primarily as levers. A lever is a mechanism for transmitting a modest force, with the mechanical advantages of a long lever arm and a short effector arm, into a small movement against great resistance. When an elevator is used for tooth extraction, a purchase point can be made and a crane pick can be used to elevate the tooth or a tooth root from the socket. The small, straight elevator is frequently used to help mobilize teeth in a similar fashion without the preparation of a purchase point.

The second machine that is useful is the wedge. It is useful in several different ways for the extraction of teeth. First the beaks of the extraction forceps are usually narrow at their tips; they broaden as they go superiorly. When the forceps is used, there should be a conscious effort made to force the tips of the forceps into the periodontal ligament space to expand the bone and force the tooth out of the socket. The wedge principle is also useful when a straight elevator is used to luxate a tooth from its socket. A small elevator is forced into the periodontal ligament space, which displaces the root toward the occlusion and therefore out of the socket.

The third machine used in tooth extraction is the wheel and axle, which is most closely identified with the triangular, or pennant-shaped, elevator. When one root of a multiple-rooted tooth is left in the alveolar process, the pennant-shaped elevator is positioned into the socket and turned. The handle then serves as the axle and the tip of the triangular elevator acts as a wheel and engages and elevates the tooth root from the socket.

PRINCIPLES OF FORCEPS USE

The primary instrument used for delivering a tooth from the alveolar process is the extraction forceps. The use of this instrument makes it possible to grasp the root portion of the tooth and dislocate the latter from its socket by exerting pressure on it. The forceps have blades and handles united by hinge joints. The larger the ratio between the length of the handles and the length of the blades, the greater the leverage which can be exerted upon the root. The length of the handles must be such that the forceps fit the operator's hand, for the greater the distance between the hinge joint and the operator's hand, the greater is the movement of the forceps within the hand.

Ideally the whole of the inner surface of the forceps blades should fit the root surface as shown in Figure 5.11 schematically.

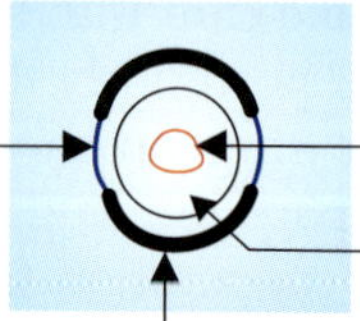

Fig. 5.11: Transverse section of the tooth at the root level showing the ideal fit of the beaks of the forceps on the tooth.

In practice, the size and shape of the roots vary so greatly that it is not possible to achieve this aim and the root is gripped by the edges of the blades— ***"two-point contact."*** See Figure 5.12 for schematic representation.

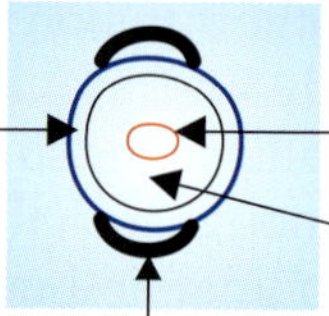

Fig. 5.12: Transverse section of the tooth at the root level showing the "two-point contact" of the beaks of the forceps on the tooth.

If there is only a single linear contact, "one-point contact" between root and forceps blade, the tooth will probably be crushed when it is gripped. See Figure 5.13 for schematic representation.

The Goal of Forceps use is Two-fold

1. Expansion of the bony socket by use of the wedge-shaped beaks of the forceps and the

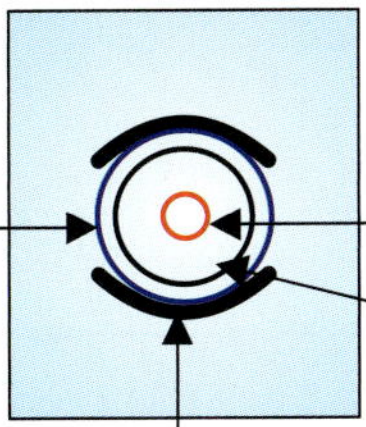

Fig. 5.13: Transverse section of the tooth at the root level showing the "one-point contact" of the beaks of the forceps on the tooth.

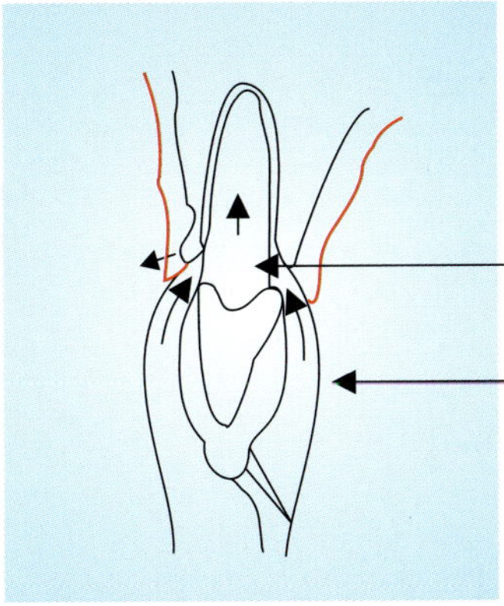

Fig. 5.14: Expansion of the bony socket following the application of the forceps.

movements of the tooth itself within the forceps.

2. Removal of the tooth from the socket.

The Forceps can Apply Five Major Motions to Luxate the Tooth and Expand the Bony Socket

1. *Apical pressure:* This accomplishes two goals.
   a. Bony expansion (Fig. 5.14).
   b. Centre of the tooth's motion is pushed apically. If the fulcrum is high, a larger amount of force is placed on the apical region of the tooth which increases the chance of fracturing of the root end. See Figure 5.15 for reference.

If the beaks of the forceps are forced into the periodontal ligament space, the centre of rotation is moved apically which results in greater movement of the expansion forces at the crest of the ridge and less forces moving the apex of the tooth lingually. This decreases the chance of apical root fracture (Fig. 5.16).

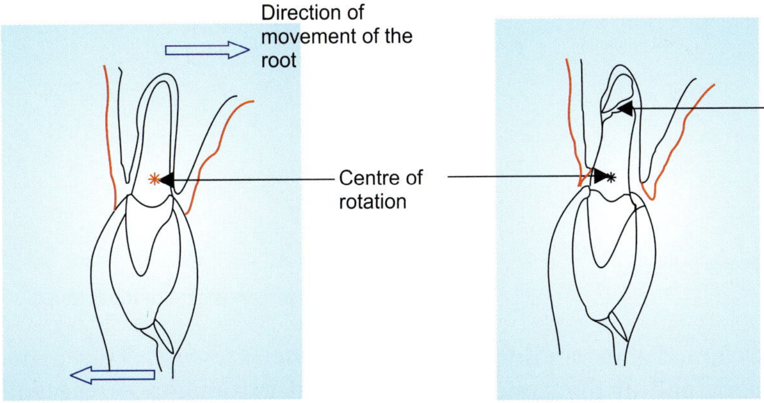

Fig. 5.15: Direction of movement of forceps.

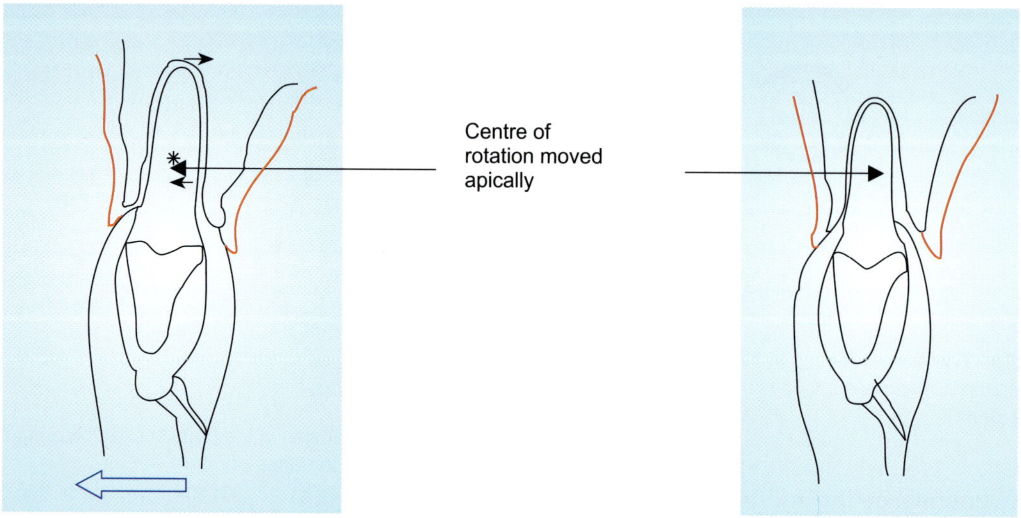

Fig. 5.16: Direction of movement of forceps.

2. *Buccal pressure:* The second major pressure or movement applied by the forceps is the buccal force. See Figure 5.17 for reference.

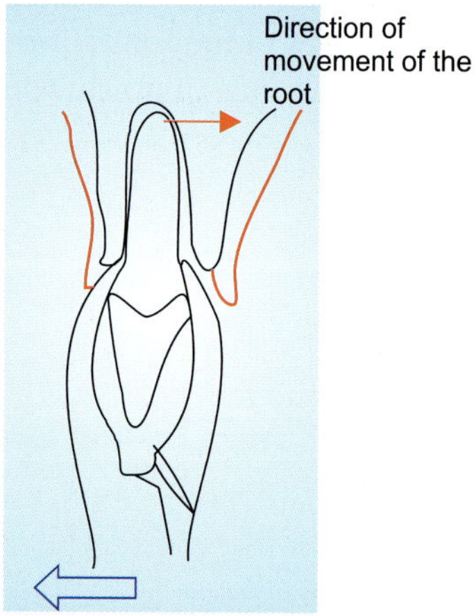

Fig. 5.17: Buccal movement of the forceps.

3. *Lingual pressure:* It is aimed at expanding the linguocrestal bone and at the same time avoiding the excessive pressures on the buccal apical bone. See Figure 5.18 for reference.

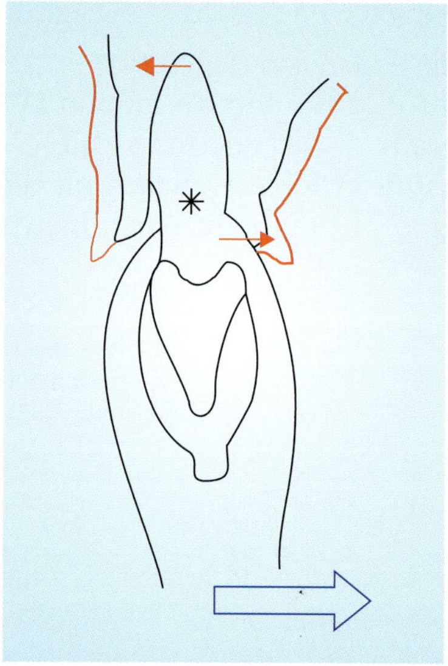

Fig. 5.18: Lingual movement of the forceps.

4. *Rotational pressure:* This causes some internal expansion of the socket. See Figure 5.19 for reference.

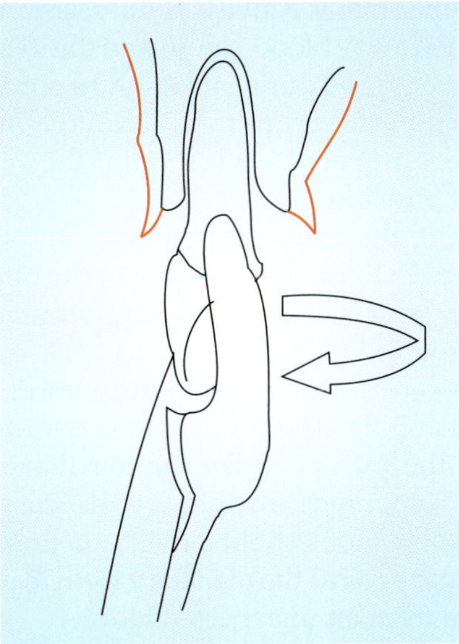

Fig. 5.19: Direction of rotation of the forceps.

5. *Traction forces:* They are useful for delivering the tooth from the socket once adequate expansion is achieved as shown in Figure 5.20.

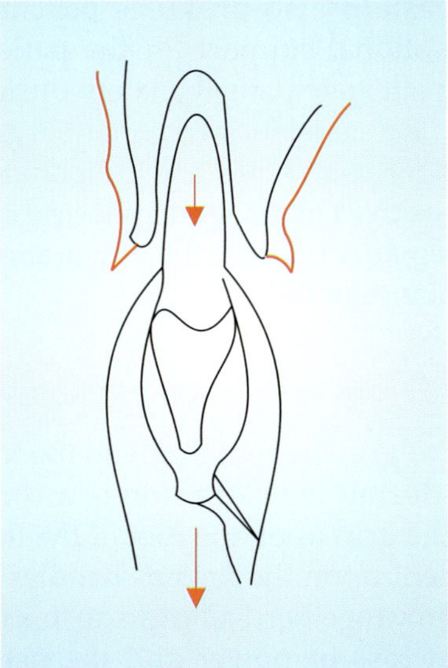

Fig. 5.20: Direction of tractional forceps.

PROCEDURE FOR CLOSED EXTRACTION

The correct technique for any situation should lead to an atraumatic extraction.

The three fundamental requirements for a good extraction are:

1. Adequate access and visualization of the field of surgery.
2. An unimpeded pathway for the removal of the tooth.
3. The use of controlled force to luxate and remove the tooth.

Steps for closed-extraction procedure

1. *Loosening of soft tissue attachment from the tooth.*

   Woodson periosteal elevator or the sharp end of the no. 9 periosteal elevator may be used for this purpose. The purpose of loosening the soft tissue from the tooth is two-fold:

   a. It allows the surgeon to ensure that profound anaesthesia has been achieved.
   b. To allow the tooth-extraction forceps to be positioned more apically without interference from or impingement on the soft tissue of the gingiva.
2. *Luxation of a tooth with a dental elevator.*
3. *Adaptation of the forceps to the tooth.*

   The forceps is seated onto the tooth so that the tips of the forceps beaks grasp the root underneath the loosened soft tissue. The lingual beak is usually seated first and then the buccal beak. Once the forceps has been positioned on the tooth, the surgeon grasps the handles of the forceps at the very ends to maximize mechanical advantage and control. The beaks of the forceps must be held parallel to the long axis of the tooth so that the forces generated by the application of pressure to the forceps handle can be delivered along the long axis of the tooth for maximal effectiveness in dilating and expanding the alveolar bone.

4. *Luxation of the tooth with the forceps.*

   The forceps must be apically seated as far as possible and reseated periodically during the extraction. The forces applied in the buccal and lingual direction should be slow, deliberate pressures and not jerky wiggles. The force should be held for several seconds to allow the bone time to expand.

5. *Removal of the tooth from the socket.*

Role of the Opposite Hand During Extraction Procedure

1. Reflecting the soft tissues of the cheeks, lips and tongue to provide adequate visualization of the area of surgery.
2. To protect other teeth from the forceps should it release suddenly from the tooth socket.
3. To stabilize the patient's head during the extraction process.
4. To support and stabilize the lower jaw when mandibular teeth are being extracted.
5. To support the alveolar process and provide tactile information to the operator concerning the expansion of the alveolar process during the luxation period.

Role of the Assistant During Extraction Procedure

1. The assistant helps the surgeon visualize and gain access to the operative area by reflecting the soft tissue of the cheeks and tongue so that the surgeon can have an unobstructed view of the surgical field. Even during a closed extraction, the assistant can reflect the soft tissue so that the surgeon can apply the instruments to loosen the soft tissue attachment and adapt the forceps to the tooth and tooth root in the most effective manner.
2. Another major activity of the assistant is to suction away blood, saliva, and the irrigating solutions used during the surgical procedure. This prevents fluids from accumulating and makes proper visualization of the surgical field possible.
3. During the extraction the assistant should also help to protect the teeth of the opposite arch, which is especially important when removing lower posterior teeth. If traction forces are necessary to remove a lower tooth, occasionally the tooth releases suddenly and the forceps strike the maxillary teeth and sometimes fracture a tooth cusp. The assistant should hold either a suction tip or a finger against the maxillary teeth to protect them from an unexpected blow.
4. During the extraction of mandibular teeth, the assistant may play an important role by supporting the mandible during the application of the extraction forces. A surgeon who uses the hand to reflect the soft tissue may not be able to support the mandible. If this is the case, the assistant plays an important role in stabilizing the mandible to prevent TMJ discomfort.
5. The assistant also provides psychologic and emotional support for the patient by helping alleviate patient anxiety during the surgery. The assistant is important in gaining the patient confidence and cooperation by using positive language and physical contact with the patient during the preparation and performance of the surgery.

Common Errors in Forceps Extraction

1. Failure to grip the root firmly in the forceps blades during the extraction is a common error. The grip upon the root of the tooth is dependent upon the forceps handles being held firmly together. Failure to do this results in great loss of power and the needless fracture of many teeth.

2. When there has been no movement in response to the application of moderate force, further attempts to move the root within its socket may result in its fracture and damage to the investing structures, which will delay healing and cause after-pain. The forceps should be put down and the patient allowed to rest while the operator decides whether the 'transalveolar' method of extraction should be employed.
3. Another common mistake is to grip the crown in the forceps blades instead of the root or root-mass. This often causes the crown to fracture, especially if it is either carious or heavily restored.
4. Incorrect alignment of the forceps blades to the long axis of the root is another frequent cause of failure, but perhaps the most common cause is hurry. Forceps extraction is a skilled and delicate procedure, and the good extractor works with an economy of movement and does not yield to the temptation to hurry if he is either uncertain of his anaesthesia or very busy.

If the forceps move upon the root, or if the operator tires, or is in a bad position, it always pays to stop and review the situation. After correcting the underlying error in technique, or having a short rest, the same forceps or a more suitable pair are reapplied to the tooth and the extraction completed.

POSTEXTRACTION CARE OF THE TOOTH SOCKET

Once the tooth has been removed from the socket, it is necessary to provide proper care. The socket should be debrided only if necessary. If a periapical lesion is visible on the preoperative radiograph and there was no granuloma attached to the tooth when it was removed, the periapical region should be carefully curetted to remove the granuloma or cyst. If any debris is obvious, such as calculus, amalgam, or tooth fragment remaining in the socket, it should be gently removed with a curette or suction tip. However, ***if neither periapical lesion nor debris is present, the socket should not be curetted.*** The remnants of the periodontal ligament and the bleeding bony walls are in the best condition to provide for rapid healing. Vigorous curettage of the socket wall merely produces additional injury and may delay healing.

The expanded buccolingual plates should be compressed back to their original configuration. Finger pressure should be applied to the buccolingual cortical plate to gently but firmly compress the plates to their origin a position or approximate them even more closely, if possible. This helps prevent bony undercuts that may have been caused by excessive expansion of the buccocortical plate.

If the teeth were removed because of periodontal disease, there may be an accumulation of excess granulation tissue around the gingival cuff. If this is the case, special attention should be given to removing this granulation tissue with a curette or hemostat. The arterioles of granulation tissue have little or no capacity to retract and constrict, which leads to bothersome bleeding if excessive granulation tissue is left.

Finally, the bone should be palpated through the overlying mucosa to check for any sharp, bony projections. If any exist, the mucosa should be reflected and the sharp edges smoothed judiciously with a bone file.

To gain initial control of hemorrhage, a moistened 2 × 2 inch gauze is placed over the extraction socket. The gauze should be positioned so that when the patient closes the teeth together, it fits into the space previously occupied by the crown of the tooth.

COMPLICATED EXODONTIA

The removal of most erupted teeth can be achieved by closed or forceps, delivery, but occasionally this technique does not suffice. The surgical, or open, extraction technique is the method used for recovering roots that were fractured during routine extraction or teeth that cannot be extracted by the routine closed methods for a variety of reasons.

INDICATIONS FOR HOSPITALISATION

1. Patients who are not cooperative.
2. Medically compromised patients such as patients with bleeding disorders, cardiac anomalies, diabetes, renal diseases.
3. Patients who have to undergo multiple extractions.
4. Patients with history of previous allergic reaction to anaesthetic agents.
5. Cases which are anticipated to be difficult extractions.

PRE-SURGICAL PREPARATION

Following hospitalization the complete work-up of the patient should be carried out and fitness obtained prior to surgical intervention.

PRINCIPLES OF FLAP DESIGN, DEVELOPMENT AND MANAGEMENT

The term flap indicates a section of soft tissue that:

- Is outlined by a surgical incision.
- Carries its own blood supply.
- Allows surgical access to underlying tissues.
- Can be replaced in the original position.
- Can be maintained with sutures and expected to heal.

Design Parameters for Soft Tissue Flaps

- When the flap is outlined,the base of the flap must be broader than the free margin to preserve an adequate blood supply.
- The flap must be of adequate size to provide adequate access, and facilitate instrumentation without undue stretching of the flap.
- The flap must be a full thickness mucoperi-osteal flap.
- The incision that outlines the flap must be made on intact bone that will be present after the surgical procedure is complete.
- The flap should be designed to avoid injury to the local vital structures in the area of surgery.
- Releasing incisions should be used only when necessary and not routinely. A vertical release incision should be made so that it does not cross bony prominences, such as the canine eminence.
- Vertical releasing incisions should cross the free gingival margin at the line angle of the tooth, not directly on the facial aspect of the tooth and not directly in the papilla.

PRINCIPLES AND TECHNIQUE OF SURGICAL EXTRACTION

As a general guideline, surgeons should consider performing an elective surgical extraction anytime they perceive a possible need for excessive force to extract a tooth. When surgically removing a tooth, the philosophy of "divide and conquer" results in the most efficient extraction.

Open Window Technique

A modification of the open technique can be performed to deliver the root fragment without removal of the entire buccal plate overlying the tooth. This technique is known as the "open-window" technique. A soft tissue flap is reflected in the usual fashion and the apex area of the tooth fragment is located. A dental bur is used to remove the bone overlying the apex of the tooth, exposing the root fragment. An instrument is then inserted into the window, and the tooth is displaced out of the socket. The preferred flap technique is the three-cornered flap, since there is a need for more extensive exposure of the apical areas. This approach is especially indicated when the buccal crestal bone must be left intact. An important and common example is the removal of maxillary premolars for orthodontic purposes, especially in adults (Figs 5.21 to 5.23).

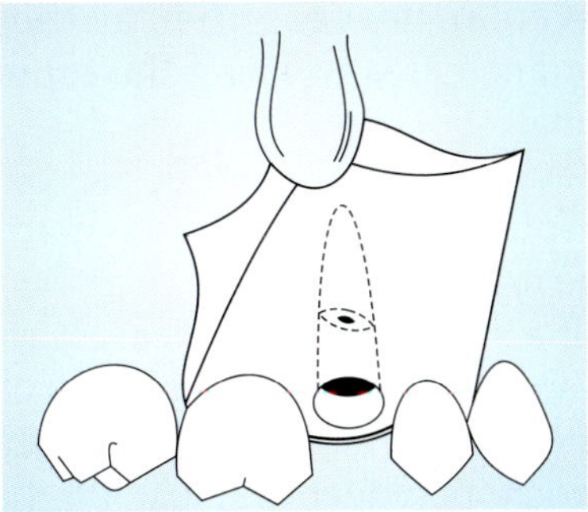

Fig. 5.21: Open window approach for retrieving the root is indicated when buccal crestal bone must be maintained.

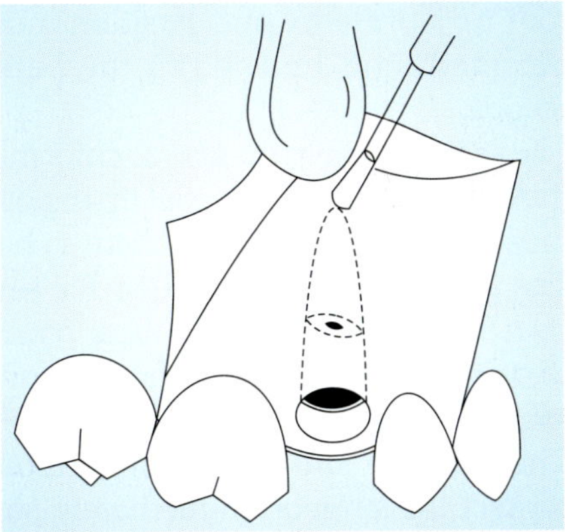

Fig. 5.22: Bur is used to uncover apex of root and allow sufficient access for insertion of straight elevator.

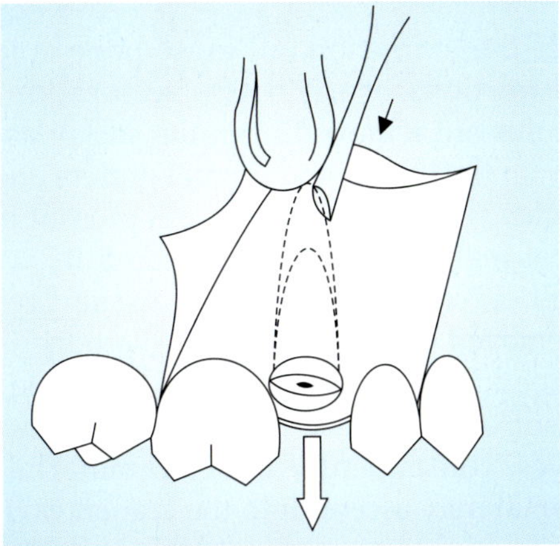

Fig. 5.23: Small straight elevator is used to displace tooth of Bur is used to uncover apex of root and allow sufficient access.

POLICY FOR LEAVING ROOT FRAGMENTS

When a root tip has fractured, and closed approaches of removal have been unsuccessful and the open approach may be excessively traumatic, the surgeon may consider leaving the root in place. As with any surgical approach, the surgeon must balance the benefits of surgery against the risks of surgery.

Three conditions must exist for a tooth root to be left in the alveolar process.

- The root fragment must be small, usually no more than 4 to 5 mm in length.
- The root must be deeply embedded in bone and not superficial.
- The tooth involved must not be infected, and there must be no radiolucency around the root apex.

The risk of surgery is considered greater if any of the three conditions exist.

- If removal of the root will cause excessive destruction of surrounding tissue, that is, excessive amounts of bony tissue will need to be removed to retrieve the root.
- If removal of the root endangers vital structures, most commonly the inferior

alveolar nerve, either at the mental foramen area or along the course of the canal.

- If attempts at recovering the root tip can displace the root into tissue spaces or into the maxillary sinus.

If a surgeon elects to leave a root tip in place, a strict protocol must be observed.

- The patient must be informed that in the surgeon's judgement, leaving the root in its position will do less harm than the surgery.
- Radiographic documentation of the root tip's presence and position must be obtained and retained in the patient's record.
- The fact that the patient was informed of the decision to leave the root tip in position must be recorded in the patient's chart.
- The patient must be recalled for several routine periodic follow-ups over the ensuing years to track the fate of this root.
- The patient should be instructed to contact the surgeon immediately should any problems develop in the area of the retained root.

POSTEXTRACTION PROCEDURE

After the extraction, all loose bone spicules and portions of the tooth, restoration and calculus are removed from the socket as well as from the buccal and lingual gutters and the tongue. If pathological tissue is present in the apical region, it is removed carefully with a small curet. The granulation tissue "velvet" is removed or broken up but the bone is not scraped. This is not done in the maxillary incisor area because the veins here have no valves; consequently infected material and thrombi may ascend into the cranial cavity to form a cavernous sinus thrombosis. If a recent radiograph does not show apical radiolucency, it is wise not to put a curet into any socket since this will only inoculate the socket with organisms and debris from the free gingival margin if the original curet is used.

The socket must be compressed by the fingers to reestablish the normal width present before the plate was surgically expanded. In the case of multiple extractions the sockets can be overcompressed by one-third which will eliminate the need for alveoloplasty in many borderline cases.

The wound is closed with interrupted sutures.

The socket is covered with a 7.6 × 7.6 cm gauze sponge that has been folded into quarters and moistened slightly at its centre with cold water. This is done to prevent the haemorrhage from the socket from penetrating the gauze at that point, which would be torn away from the remainder of the clot when the gauze is removed, resulting in new bleeding. The side of the gauze placed over the wound is not touched by the operator for aseptic reasons. When the covering sponge is in place, the sponge originally placed over the tongue is removed. Saliva and debris are kept out of the socket by this method. The patient is asked to bite on the sponge for 5 minutes. After that time has elapsed, a postoperative radiograph is made if there is any question about the extraction, and another moistened gauze is placed, to be retained until the patient arrives home. A printed instruction sheet is given to the patient, together with a prescription if pain is anticipated. Analgesic drugs should be started as soon as the patient returns home, well before the local anaesthetic effect wears away. An appointment for postoperative examination is given.

IMPACTED TEETH

Removal of impacted teeth is one of the most common surgical procedures performed by oral and maxillofacial surgeons, and most surgeons cite third molar removal as the operation most likely to humble them. Extensive training, skill, and experience are necessary to perform this procedure with minimal trauma. In many situations this decision is made based on clinical experience and professional judgment; in others the decision is clear cut based on available and dental practices demand evidence based decision-making, and the surgeon is called on more and more frequently to justify surgical procedures, including the removal of third molars.

INDICATIONS FOR REMOVAL OF AN IMPACTED TOOTH

An impacted tooth can cause the patient mild to serious problems if it remains in the unerupted state. Not every impacted tooth causes a problem of clinical significance, but each does have that potential. The indications for removal of impacted teeth are as follows.

1. For prevention or treatment of pericoronitis.
2. Prevention of dental disease like dental caries or periodontal problems.
3. Orthodontic considerations.
   a. If the orthodontist is attempting to move the buccal segments posteriorly, removal of the impacted third molar may facilitate treatment and allow predictable outcomes.
   b. When maxillary or mandibular osteotomies are planned, presurgical removal or the third molars may facilitate the planned surgery.
4. Prevention of odontogenic cysts and tumours.
5. Prevention of root resorption of adjacent teeth.
6. Prior to fabrication of a prosthesis.
7. Prevention of jaw fracture.
8. Management of unexplained pain.

When a patient presents with this type of complaint, the surgeon must make sure that all other sources of pain are ruled out before suggesting surgical removal of the third molar. In addition, the patient must be informed that removal of the third molar may not relieve the pain completely.

CONTRAINDICATIONS FOR REMOVAL OF IMPACTED TEETH

The decision to remove a given impacted tooth must be based on a careful evaluation of the potential benefits versus risks. The general contraindications for removal of impacted teeth can be grouped into three primary areas: Advanced patient age, poor health, and surgical damage to adjacent structures.

1. *Advanced patient age:* As a patient becomes older, there is decreased healing response which may result in a greater bony defect postoperatively than was present because of the impacted tooth. Additionally, the surgical procedure grows more and more difficult as the patient ages owing to more densely calcified bone, which is less flexible and more likely to fracture. As patient ages, the response to surgical insult is tolerated less easily and the recuperation period grows longer.

2. *Compromised medical status:* As age increases, so does the incidence of moderate to severe cardiovascular disease, pulmonary disease and other health problems.

THE CLINICAL EXAMINATION

1. A conscious assessment of the general size and build of the patient should be made.
2. The patient's attitude and emeanour is important and may give valuable clues as to the way he or she ill respond to the stress of surgery and therefore the type of anaesthesia and/or sedation which will be required.
3. The presence of facial swelling and enlarged, tender, lymph nodes of course indicates the presence of active infection and used to preclude an operation until it had been treated. However, with antibiotic cover, postoperative morbidity in such cases is not increased.
4. The size of the oral cavity, the size of the tongue, the degree to which the patient can open his or her mouth, the size of the rima oris and the extensibility of the lips and checks all contribute to surgical access.
5. A general inspection of the mouth reveals much about the patient's oral hygiene habits, the general state of the dentition, and the degree to which it has required previous dental care.
6. The health of the 1st and 2nd molars may affect the decision to remove the wisdom teeth. Large crowns, inlays or amalgams in 2nd molars can be dislodged during elevation of the wisdom tooth even when care is being exercised. Teeth which are loose due to advanced periodontal disease and crowns on anterior teeth should be mentioned to the anaesthetist if a general anaesthetic is required.
7. Attention is then focused on each 3rd molar in turn, observing how much of the crown is visible, or palpable if it is unerupted. Partially erupted teeth should be explored with a probe to determine which is the occlusal surface (which feels rough) and which a mesial or distal surface (which will feel smooth) for at times it is not easy to differentiate horizontal,vertical and disto-angular impactions by inspection alone.
8. If no part of the 3rd molar crown is visible, the gingival crevice distal to the 2nd molar should be explored with a periodontal probe to see if there is a pocket leading down to the crown of the 3rd molar.
9. The depth of any visible crown below the occlusal plane and its general relation to the level of the alveolar crest is noted, as is the distance between the distal surface of the 2nd molar and the anterior border of the ascending ramus.
10. The external and internal oblique ridges of the mandible are palpated. If the external oblique ridge is low, relatively vertical and relatively posterior to the tooth, there will be thin alveolar bone buccal to the 3rd molar. If the external oblique-ridge lies high and well forward relative to the tooth the thick cortex of the ridge will form the bone buccal to the 3rd molar.
11. The condition of the soft tissues over the wisdom itself is noted. Are they scarred and indented by the upper 3rd molar? Is there active pericoronitis present or pus beneath the gum flap? Both conditions require treatment and there may be a delay before operation. A non-tender flap from beneath which a whitish, creamy material resulting from desquamated follicular epithelium can be milked is not a contraindication to surgery provided the flap is cleaned preoperatively with a sucker and povidone iodine or other suitable antiseptic introduced under it. Of importance to the future health of the gingivae around the lower 2nd molar is the relationship of the masticatory mucoperiosteum to that tooth. If there is a broad zone of gingival mucoperiosteum buccal to the 2nd molar which extends distally, there are good prospects that there

will be a normal gingival margin around the distal aspect after the 3rd molar wound has healed

12. The position and condition of the upper 3rd molar is checked and its occlusal relationships to the lower 3rd and 2nd molars noted. If the tooth is in a position which makes it difficult to keep clean, if it is already carious, if it does not, and will not, occlude with a tooth which is to be retained, and particularly if it is over-erupted, it should be extracted. Indeed if it bites on the gum flap of the lower 3rd molar its extraction may cut short an attack of pericoronitis permitting more latitude in the timing of lower 3rd molar surgery. Lastly, consideration should be given to its possible future use as a denture or bridge abutment.
13. If the lower 3rd molar on one side is considered for extraction the other side also should be examined, particularly if it is likely that the operation will be carried out under a general anaesthetic. Finally, the related lymph nodes should be palpated to determine the extent of any infection.

Similar protocol is followed for other impacted teeth.

RADIOGRAPHIC EXAMINATION

1. Periapical radiographs are taken whenever possible because the detail which they reveal is better than with any other technique .
2. An occlusal film should be taken for all difficult teeth and particularly where the tooth is completely unerupted so as to complete the two views at right angles necessary for an understanding of the problem in three dimensions.
3. Orthopantomograms have largely displaced oblique lateral jaw views but they lack the valuable details seen on a periapical radiograph.
4. When the proximity of the third molar to the inferior alveolar canal is anticipated a CT scan may prove valuable in studying the case.

RADIOLOGICAL ASSESSMENT

Assessment in relation to the surgical removal of lower third molars means estimating how much work will need to be done at the operation and what technical difficulties will need to be overcome.

1. **The orientation of the tooth:** Lower third molars may be mesioangularly, vertically, distoangularly inclined, horizontal or ectopic in position (Fig. 5.24).

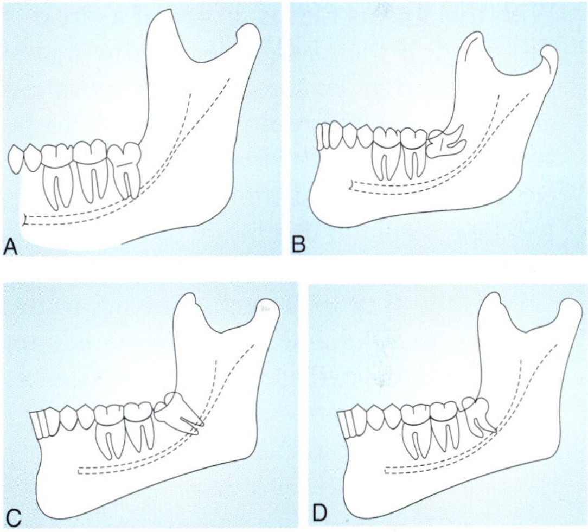

Fig. 5.24: (A) Vertical impaction **(B)** Horizontal impaction **(C)** Mesioangular impaction **(D)** Distoangular impaction.

2. **The depth of the tooth***:* An assessment of the depth of the tooth indicates the amount of bone which must be removed to uncover the tooth. Depth is measured first from the alveolar crest to the level of the greatest diameter of the crown and secondly from the neck of the tooth to the greatest diameter of the root if the latter is bulbous.

3. **The degree of impaction of the tooth:** This together with root shape indicates whether tooth division is optional as a means of facilitating the extraction of the tooth and so reducing bone removal, or whether it is obligatory. Mesioangular and mesially facing horizontal teeth are impacted against the 2nd molar. In general such teeth must be tilted upwards, rotating them about a point close to the apex of a single-rooted tooth or the distal apex of a two-rooted tooth until the mesial surface of the third molar will clear the crown of the second molaras it is ejected from the socket. To test whether this can be permitted by bone removal alone a line is drawn from the apex of the distal root of the third molar to the tip of its mesial cusp. With this line as radius an arc of a circle is described. If this passes clear of the image of the crown of the second molar, elevation after simple bone removal is likely to be successful. If the arc cuts the image of the crown of the second molar, tooth division will be essential if this mode of elevation is used (Figs 5.25 and 5.26).

With the split bone technique a varying amount of distal and lingual bone is split away. Elevation of the tooth is by application of the force to the cervical enamel just under the crown of the tooth and from the buccal side.

The tooth rotates about the apices and is displaced lingually and upwards. If a good occlusal radiograph can be obtained the likely success of this manoeuvre can be tested because this time the radius of the arc of the movement joins the lingual edge of the distal root apex to the tip of the mesiobuccal cusp.

If the mesiobuccal cusp will clear the tooth in front as the tooth rotates lingually, simple elevation will be successful; if not tooth division will be required (Fig. 5.27).

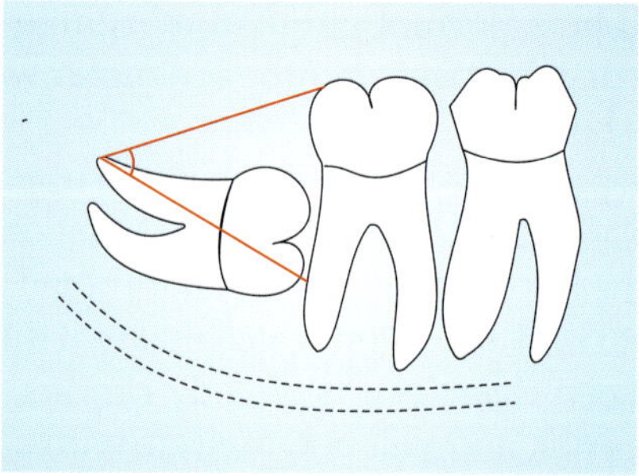

Fig. 5.26: The arc drawn passes through the crown of the second molar and so the sectioning of the third molar is obligatory in this case.

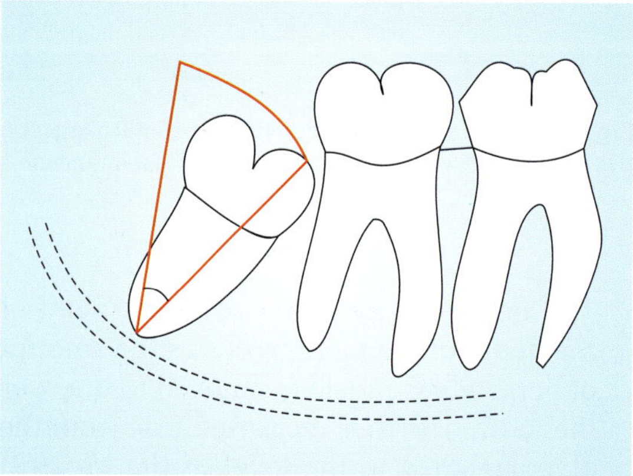

Fig. 5.25: The arc drawn is well away from the crown of the second molar and so the sectioning of the tooth may be optional.

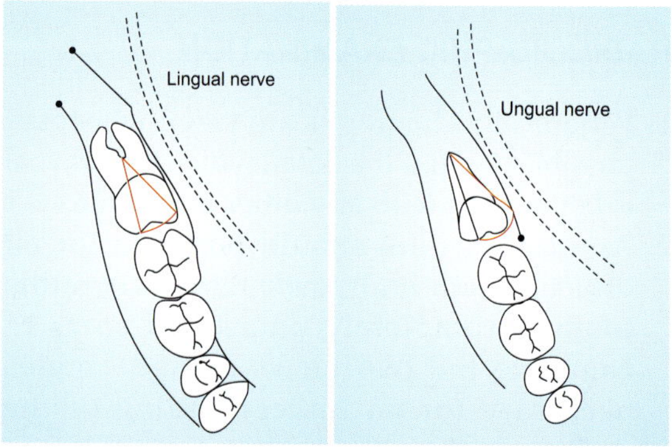

Fig. 5.27: **(A)** the arc drawn intersects the distal aspect of the 2nd molar. **(B)** the arc does not intersect the distal aspect of the second molar.

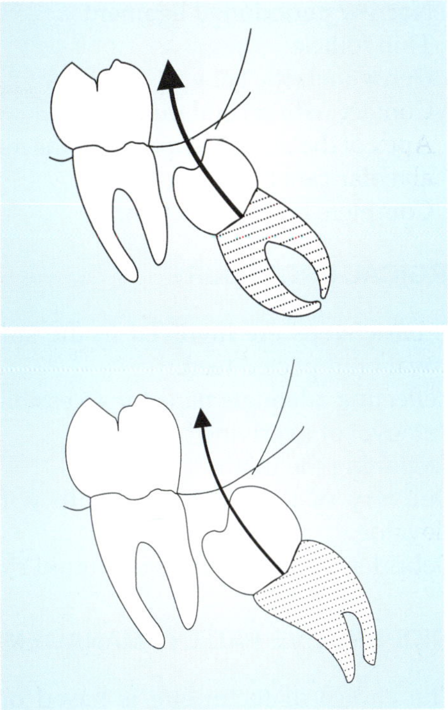

Fig. 5.28: Unfavourable root curvatures.

4. **Root shape:** This may be either favourable or unfavourable. Roots may be unfavourable in that their curvature opposes the initial distal tilting movement which most impacted teeth require. When there are two or more roots they may either converge or diverge, locking the tooth in bone and this again is unfavourable and often demands tooth division (Fig. 5.28).
5. **Bone removal to form a path of elevation:** Bone has to be removed to provide space into which the tooth can be tilted in preparation for the application of a force dislocating it from the socket. The relationship of the mandibular canal as it curves downwards through the bone to the site of distal bone removal should be noted to avoid damage to the nerve if a substantial amount of distal bone is to be removed.
6. **Bone removal to permit application of elevators:** Usually a channel must be created down to the follicular space beneath the mesial surface of the crown at the amelo-cemental junction. If the follicular space is narrow it must be widened to accommodate the elevator blade. Another common point of application of the elevator is buccally at the bifurcation of a two-rooted tooth or under the buccal bulbosity of the crown of a single-rooted one.
7. **Bone density:** This affects the ease with which bone may be removed. It may be assessed by noticing the thickness and the number of medullary trabeculae. The thickness of the medullary cortex at the lower border will also give some indication of the density to be expected in the external oblique ridge, as will the relative radiopacity of the latter in a periapical film, given a standard exposure.
8. **The relationship to the inferior alveolar canal.**

WINTER'S LINES

In this method, three imaginary lines (traditionally described by number or colour) are drawn on a geometrically accurate periapical radiogaph, as follows (Fig. 2.29).

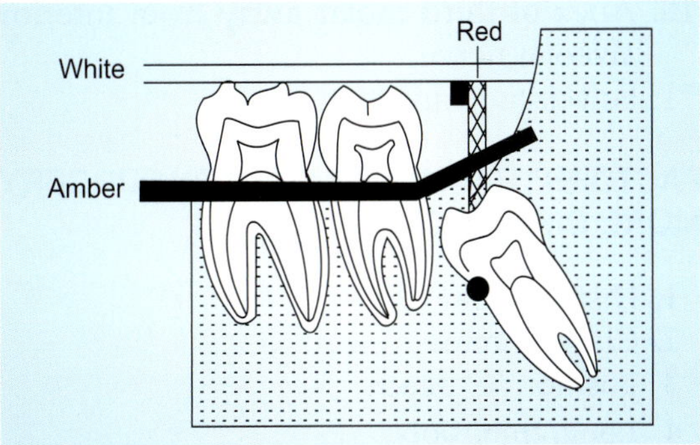

Fig. 5.29: Illustrating Winter's lines.

1. The first or white line is drawn along the occlusal surfaces of the erupted first and second molars.
2. The second or amber line is drawn along the crest of the interdental bone between the first and second molars, extending distally along the internal oblique ridge, not the external oblique ridge. This line indicates the margin of the alveolar bone surrounding the tooth.
3. The third line or the red line is a perpendicular dropped from the white line to the point of application for an elevator, but is measured from the amber line to this point. This line measures the depth of the third molar within the mandible. As a general rule if the red line is 5 mm or more in length the extraction is considered sufficiently difficult for the tooth to be removed under general anaesthesia or using local anaesthetic and sedation.

FACTORS THAT MAKE IMPACTION SURGERY LESS DIFFICULT

1. Mesioangular position
2. Class 1 ramus.
3. Position 'A' depth
4. Roots 1/3 to 2/3 formed
5. Fused conical roots
6. Wide periodontal ligament
7. Large follicle
8. Elastic bone
9. Separated from second molar
10. Apex of third molar away from inferior alveolar nerve
11. Soft tissue impaction.

FACTORS THAT MAKE IMPACTON SURGERY MORE DIFFICULT

1. Distoangular
2. Class 3 ramus
3. Position 'C' depth
4. Long, thin roots
5. Divergent curved roots
6. Narrow periodontal ligament
7. Thin follicle
8. Dense inelastic bone
9. Contact with second molar
10. Apex of the third molar close to the inferior alveolar canal
11. Complete bony impaction.

SURGICAL PROCEDURE

Five basic steps are involved in the surgical removal of impacted teeth:

1. Reflecting adequate flaps for accessibility.
2. Removal of overlying bone
3. Sectioning the tooth
4. Delivery of the sectioned tooth with an elevator
5. Debridement of wound and wound closure

PERIOPERATIVE PATIENT MANAGEMENT

a. The choice of technique is based on the surgeon's preference. The goals are to achieve a level of patient comfort that allows the surgeon to work rapidly and efficiently and that limits the patient experience to the minimal number of unpleasant effects.
b. Prescription consisting of potent analgesics and antibiotics for 3–4 days.
c. Administration of steroids either preoperatively or postoperatively to combat the swelling associated with the third molar surgery.

Patients can expect a modest amount of swelling in the area of surgery for 3 or 4 days with the swelling completely dissipating by about 10 days. A modest amount of discomfort usually follows the procedure. Patients usually require analgesics for 2 or 3 days on a routine basis and intermittently for several more days.

Patients who have had third molars surgically removed frequently have mild to moderate trismus. This inability to open the mouth interferes with the patient's normal oral hygiene and eating habits. Patient's should be warned that they will be unable to open their mouths normally following surgery. The trismus gradually resolves and the ability to open the mouth should return to normal by 10–14 days after surgery.

ADVANTAGES OF BUR TECHNIQUE

1. The placement of the handpiece in the patients mouth is a familiar experience, common to everyone who has occupied the dental chair, as contrasted to the use of the chisel and mallet.
2. The physical blows and pressures associated with the chisel and mallet technique are eliminated.
3. Since the surgical handpiece technique eliminates the need for an assistant to do the malleting, fewer personnel are required in the operatory.
4. The surgical field is irrigated to reduce the heat caused by the bur. This creates a continuously washed field in which to work.
5. The operator has the ability to trench around the impaction in a delicate and controlled fashion in order to remove osseous tissue so that an instrument purchase can be obtained. This feature of the bur technique is particularly useful for the recovery of mandibular molar root tips lying close to the mandibular canal and maxillary root tips lying close to the maxillary sinus. This eliminates apically directed forces such as occur in the case of an elevator purchase under or next to an impacted fragment. The instrument purchase can be enhanced when a notch is made with a bur on the remaining portion of the tooth.

RADIOLOGICAL PREDICTION OF INFERIOR ALVEOLAR NERVE INJURY DURING THIRD MOLAR SURGERY

The inferior alveolar nerve runs in a canal within the mandible usually near the apices of the third molar, and if the third molar is impacted, a close relationship of the roots to the nerve is likely. Seven radiological signs have been mentioned predictive of inferior alveolar nerve injury following third molar surgery.

1. Darkening of the root.
2. Deflected roots.
3. Narrowing of the roots.
4. Dark and bifid root.
5. Interruption of the white line(s).
6. Diversion of the inferior alveolar canal.
7. Narrowing of the inferior alveolar canal.

Of these seven signs, the most significant signs related to nerve injury were:

- Diversion of the inferior alveolar canal.
- Darkening of the root.
- Interruption of the white line.

REFERENCES AND BIBLIOGRAPHY

1. *The Extraction of Teeth*, 2nd edn; Geoffrey L. Howe.
2. *Contemporary Oral and Maxillofacial Surgery*, 4th edn; Larry J. Peterson, Edward Ellis, James R. Hupp, Myron R. Tucker.
3. The Radiological Prediction of Inferior Alveolar Nerve Injury during Third Molar Surgery; *British Journal of Oral and Maxillofacial Surgery*; 1990; 28; 20-25.

Chapter 6

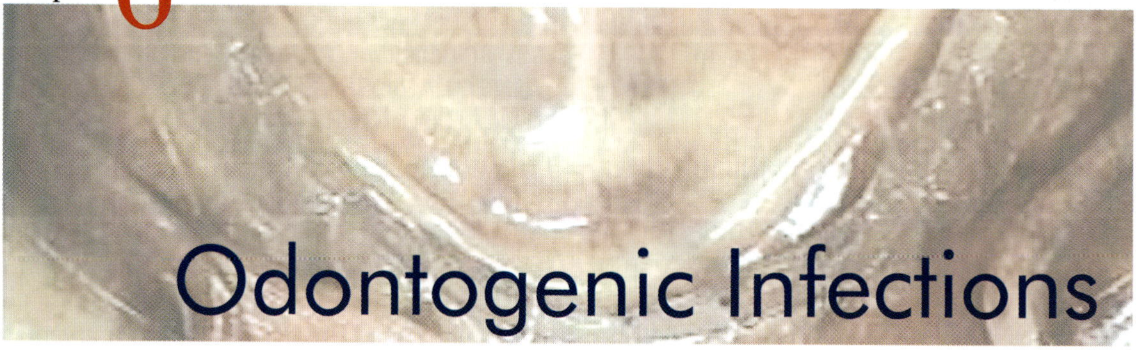

Odontogenic Infections

Odontogenic infections are usually mild and are easily treated. These infections may require only the administration of an antibiotic, may be more complex, requiring incision and drainage, or may be very complicated requiring that the patient be admitted to the hospital. Some infections that occur in the oral cavity are preventable if the surgeon uses appropriate antibiotic prophylaxis.

MICROBIOLOGY OF ODONTOGENIC INFECTIONS

The bacteria that cause infection are most commonly part of the indigenous flora. Odontogenic infections are caused by bacteria that comprise the plaque, that are found on the mucosal surfaces and those found in the gingival sulcus. They are primarily aerobic gram-positive cocci and anaerobic gram-positive cocci and anaerobic gram-negative rods. These bacteria cause a variety of common diseases such as dental caries, gingivitis and periodontitis. When these bacteria gain access to the deeper underlying tissues, as through a necrotic dental pulp or through a deep periodontal pocket, they cause odontogenic infections.

Microorganisms Causing Odontogenic Infections

Aerobic

Gram-positive cocci.
- *Streptococci*
- *Staphylococci*
- *Eikenella*

Gram-negative cocci
- *Neisseria*

Gram-positive rods
- *Corynebacterium*

Gram-negative rods
- *Haemophilus*

Miscellaneous and undifferentiated.

Anaerobic

Gram-positive cocci
- *Streptococci*
- *Peptococci*
- *Peptostreptococci*

Gram-negative cocci
- *Veilonella*

Gram-positive rods
- *Eubacterium*
- *Lactobacillus*
- *Actinomyces*
- *Clostridia*

Gram-negative rods

Bacteroides

Fusobacterium.

PRINCIPLES OF THERAPY OF ODONTOGENIC INFECTIONS

Principle 1

Determine the Severity of Infection

The history of the patient's infection follows the same guidelines as any history. The onset, duration and progress of the patient's symptoms should be noted. The patient's symptoms should be elicited. These signs and symptoms include rubor, calor, dolor, tumor, and functiolaesa.

Physical Examination

The first step in the physical examination is to collect the patients vital signs: temperature, pulse rate, respiration rate and blood pressure. Patients with systemic involvement of infection will have elevated temperatures. The pulse rate will increase as the temperature increases. The vital sign that varies the least with infection is the blood pressure.

Only if there is significant pain will there be mild elevation in systolic blood pressure. The patient's respiratory rate should be closely monitored. The major consideration in most odontogenic infections is the potential for upper airway obstruction as extension of the infection into fascial spaces in the pharynx.

The patient should be examined for any swelling and erythema.

Character of the Swelling

It varies from very soft and almost normal (doughy feeling) to a firm or hard swelling (indurated swelling).

Swelling Texture

Fluctuance is the feeling of a fluid filled swelling and it mostly means that there is collection of pus in the underlying tissues.

	Cellulitis		*Abscess*
1.	Acute, severe and generalized	1.	Chronic, localized
2.	Large	2.	Small
3.	Diffuse borders	3.	Well circumscribed
4.	Doughy to indurated	4.	Fluctuant
5.	No collection of pus	5.	Collection of pus
6.	More serious condition due to spreading nature	6.	Less severe due to its localized nature

RADIOGRAPHIC EXAMINATION

Intraoral periapical radiographs may be adequate in less severe cases but in more severe cases, which are showing signs of trismus, extraoral radiographs may be advised such as the lateral oblique, orthopantomograms etc (Fig. 6.1). In very extensive cases ultrasonography or CT scan may be advised.

Laboratory Investigations

For less severe cases, examination of the complete blood count, bleeding and clotting time may be sufficient but in cases which are medically compromised evaluation of the necessary tests is mandatory prior to the aggressive therapy.

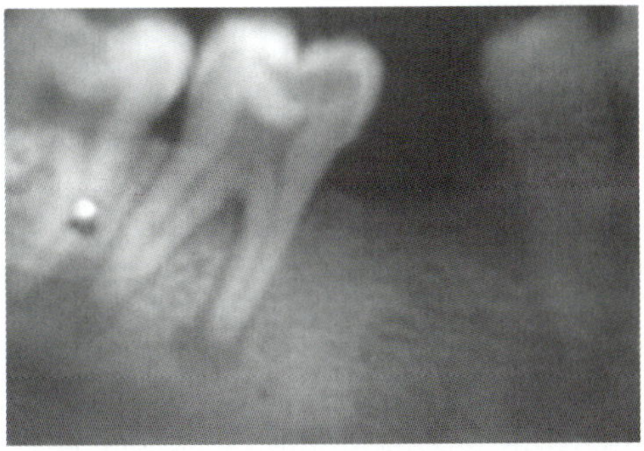

Fig. 6.1: Intraoral radiograph showing periapical abscess in relation to mandibular second molar.

Principle 2

Evaluate the State of Patient's Host Defence Mechanisms

The different host defence mechanisms are:
1. Local defences
   a. Intact anatomic barrier
   b. Indigenous bacteria
2. Humoral defences
   a. Immunoglobulins
   b. Complement
3. Cellular defences
   a. Phagocytes
      Granulocytes
      Monocytes
   b. Lymphocytes

There are a certain conditions which compromise the host defences. These are as follows:
1. Uncontrolled metabolic diseases
   a. Uremia
   b. Alcoholism
   c. Malnutrition
   d. Severe diabetes
2. Suppressing diseases
   a. Leukemia
   b. Lymphoma
   c. Malignant tumours
3. Suppressing drugs
   a. Cancer chemotherapeutic agents
   b. Immunosuppressives

Principle 3

Treat the infection Surgically

The primary goal in surgical management of infection is to provide drainage of accumulated pus and necrotic debris. A secondary goal is to remove the cause of infection, which is most commonly a necrotic pulp or deep periodontal pocket (Fig. 6.2).

The abscess is drained via an incision. Once the incision is completed, a closed curved haemostat is inserted through the incision into the abscess cavity and opened in several directions to break up any small loculation or cavities of pus. Next a small rubber drain is inserted to maintain the opening. The drain should remain in place until all the drainage from the abscess cavity has stopped, usually 2 to 5 days.

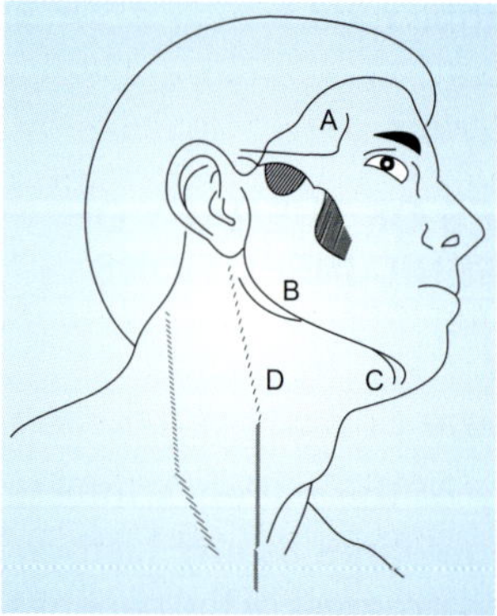

Fig. 6.2: Typical incision and drainage sites for various fascial space infections. (A) Superficial and deep temporal space. (B) Submandibular masseteric and pterygomandibular spaces. (C) Submental space. (D) Lateral pharyngeal and retropharyngeal spaces.

Principle 4

Support the Patient Medically

Patients with odontogenic infections may have depressed host defence mechanisms as the result of the pain and swelling associated with the infection. Because of the pain from the infection the patients frequently have not taken adequate fluid intake, nutritional intake or rest. During the immediate postincision and drainage period, patients should be encouraged to drink a lot of water or juice and take high calorie nutritional supplements. They should also be prescribed adequate analgesics for relief of pain so that they can rest.

Principle 5

Choose and Prescribe the Appropriate Antibiotic

Choosing the appropriate antibiotic for treating odontogenic infection must be done carefully.

While appropriate use may result in dramatic resolution and cure of patients with infection, misuse of antibiotics provides little benefit to offset the associated risks and expense of antibiotic administration.

Indications for the use of antibiotics:
1. Acute onset of infection
2. Diffuse swelling
3. Compromised host defences
4. Involvement of fascial spaces
5. Severe pericoronitis
6. Osteomyelitis.

To begin with the management of patients with infections, empirical antibiotics are prescribed and the pus sample collected during incision and drainage is sent for culture and antibiotic sensitivity.

Indications for culture and antibiotic sensitivity testing:
1. Rapidly spreading infection
2. Post-operative infection
3. Non-responsive infection
4. Recurrent infection
5. Compromised host defences
6. Osteomyelitis
7. Suspected actinomycosis

Principle 6

Administer the Antibiotic Properly

Once the decision is made to prescribe an antibiotic to the patient, the drug should be administered in the proper dosage and at the proper dosage interval.

Principle 7

Evaluate the Patient Frequently

Once the patient has been treated by surgery and antibiotic therapy has been prescribed, the patient should be followed up carefully to monitor response to treatment and complications. In most situations the patient should be asked to return for follow up 2 days after the initial therapy.

If therapy is successful there is a dramatic decrease in swelling and pain. Check the incision and drainage site to determine if the drain can be removed at this time. Other parameters such as temperature, trismus, swelling, and patient's subjective feeling of improvement should be investigated.

However, sometimes the treatment that has been rendered does not relieve the patient of his/her symptoms and several causes have been sited for treatment failure. A few of them are as follows:
1. Inadequate surgery
2. Depressed host defences
3. Foreign body
4. Antibiotic problems
   a. Patient non-compliance
   b. Drug not reaching the site
   c. Drug dosage too low
   d. Wrong bacterial diagnosis
   e. Wrong antibiotic

	Penicillin V	Erythromycin	Clindamycin	Cephalexin
Bactericidal or bacteriostatic	Bactericidal	Bacteriostatic	Both	Bactericidal
Spectrum	Streptococci, oral anaerobes	Gram-positive cocci, oral anaerobes	Gram-positive cocci, anaerobes	Gram-positive cocci, some gram-negative rods, oral anaerobes.
Dose-interval	250–500mg qid	250–500mg qid	150–300mg qid	500mg qid
Metabolized	Kidney	Liver	Liver	Kidney

PRINCIPLES OF PREVENTION OF METASTATIC INFECTION

Metastatic infection is defined as infection that occurs at a location physically separate from the portal of entry of the bacteria. The classic and most widely accepted example of this phenomenon is bacterial endocarditis which arises from bacteria that are introduced into the blood stream as a result of any procedures associated with bleeding.

Factors Necessary for Metastatic Infection

1. Distant susceptible site
2. Haematogenous bacterial seeding
3. Impaired local defences

Prophylaxis of Infective Endocarditis

Infective endocarditis may be caused by bacteria introduced into the circulation as a result of oral surgery attaching to a sterile vegetation that exists on an abnormal heart valve. The valvular lesions that may predispose toward endocarditis are:

1. Prosthetic heart valve
2. Congenital heart malformations
3. Rheumatic valve disease
4. Mitral valve prolapse with insufficiency
5. Previous episode of bacterial endocarditis

However, not all the dental procedures require antibiotic prophylaxis. A few of the examples of operative procedures which do not require antibiotic prophylaxis are:

1. Supragingival prophylaxis
2. Restorative tooth preparation
3. Placement of orthodontic appliances
4. Conservative endodontic therapy

Patients at risk for bacterial endocarditis should have a comprehensive prophylaxis programme. This includes excellent oral hygiene with excellent periodic professional care.

ANTIBIOTIC REGIMEN FOR PROPHYLAXIS OF BACTERIAL ENDOCARDITIS

1. *Standard regimen*
   A. Oral penicillin V
      Preoperatively 2 gm orally 1 hour before surgery.
      Postoperatively 1 gm orally 6 hours after first dose
   B. Parenteral: Penicillin G
      Preoperatively 2 million units aqueous penicillin G i.v or i.m 30 to 60 min before surgery
      Postoperatively 1 million units 6 hours after first dose
2. *Penicillin allergic patient*
   A. Oral: Erythromycin
      Preoperatively 1 gm 1 hour before surgery
      Postoperatively 500mg 6 hours after initial dose
3. *Paediatric dose (children less than 60 pounds)*
   A. Oral: Penicillin V
      Preoperatively 1 gm orally 1 hour before surgery
      Postoperatively 500 mg orally 6 hours after first dose
   B. Oral: Erythromycin
      Preoperatively 20 mg/kg 1 hour before surgery
      Postoperatively 10 mg/kg 6 hours after first dose
   C. Parenteral: Penicillin G
      Preoperatively 50,000μ/kg i.m or i.v 30 to 60 min before surgery.
      Postoperatively 25,000μ/kg 6 hours after initial dose.

REFERENCE AND BIBLIOGRAPHY

1. Contemporary Oral and Maxillofacial Surgery, 4th edn; Larry J. Peterson, Edward Ellis, James R. Hupp, Myron R. Tucker.

Chapter 7

Oral and Maxillofacial Trauma

One of the most rewarding and demanding aspects of surgical practice is the management of a patient who has suffered facial trauma. The abruptness of the injury can cause intense emotional distress even when only minor injuries are present. The perception of the injury by the patient or family and their reaction to trauma may seem out of proportion to the degree of injury. The patient and the family may be highly anxious and fearful and they depend heavily on the clinician to make an accurate diagnosis, communicate that diagnosis to them, offer hope for a successful outcome, and perform the treatment necessary to repair the injury. Therefore the patient must deal effectively with both the patient's physical injuries and the patient's emotional state. Whenever a maxillofacial injury is sustained, the patient goes abruptly from a normal state to a state of tissue disruption.

ETIOLOGY OF FACIAL FRACTURES

The major causes of facial fractures include motor vehicle accidents and altercations. Other causes of injuries include falls, sports related incidents, and work related accidents (Fig. 7.1).

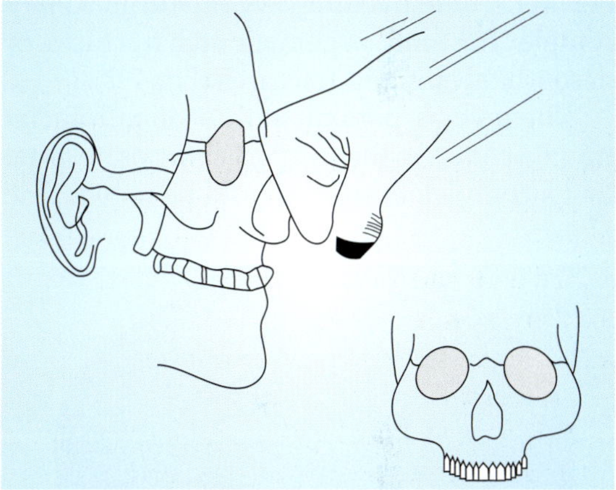

Fig. 7.1: Schematic representation of how the direction of force can influence the nature of injury.

Mandibular Fractures

Depending on the type of injury and the direction and force of the trauma, fractures of the mandible commonly occur in several different locations. Fractures are designated as occurring in the condylar, angle, body, symphyseal, alveolar, ramus, and coronoid process areas. Another system of classification of mandibular fractures categorizes the type of fracture as greenstick, simple, comminuted, and compound fractures. These categories describe the condition of the bone fragments at the fracture site and possible communication with the external environment. Fractures of the mandible are referred to as favourable or unfavourable, depending on the angulation of the fracture and force of the muscle pull proximal and distal to the fracture. In a favourable fracture, the fracture line and the muscle pull resist displacement of the fracture. In an unfavorable fracture, the muscle pull results in the displacement of the fracture.

Midface Fractures

Midfacial fractures include fractures affecting the maxilla, the zygoma, and the nasoorbital ethmoid complex. fractures can be classified as LeFort I, II or III fractures, zygomaticomaxillary complex fractures, zygomatic arch fractures, or nasoorbital ethmoid fractures (Fig. 7.2).

Whenever a patient with a maxillofacial trauma comes to the surgical clinic or hospital first a complete history should be noted. One must ask the following questions to the patient, parent or any reliable respondent.

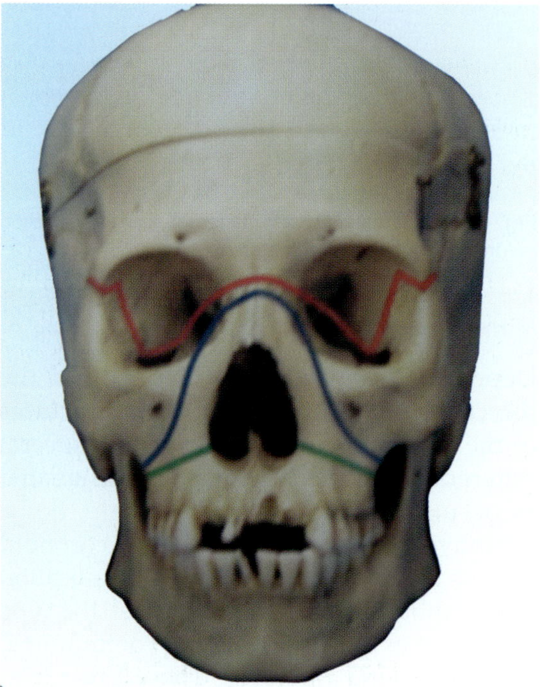

Fig. 7.2: Le Fort lines of fracture marked on the skull.

Who is the Patient?

Included here is the patient's name, age, address, phone and other pertinent demographic data.

When did the Injury Occur?

The time of the injury should be noted. This may be important from the medicolegal point of view.

Where did the Injury Occur?

This is important to ascertain the bacterial and chemical contamination.

How did the injury Occur?

The nature of the trauma provides valuable insight into what the resultant tissue injury is likely to be. The circumstances of the injury is valuable information and should make the clinician investigate the possibility of further injuries. If the patient cannot remember what happened, a pre-existing medical condition such as a seizure disorder may have caused the accident producing the injury.

What Treatment has been Provided Since the Injury?

It provides important information regarding the original condition of the injured area.

Did Anyone Note Tooth or Pieces of Teeth at the Site of the Accident?

Before an accurate diagnosis and treatment plan are made, it is imperative that each tooth the patient had before the accident be accounted for. If during the clinical examination, a tooth or crown is found missing and no history suggests that it was lost at the scene, a radiographic examination of the perioral soft tissues and the chest and abdomen regions is necessary to rule out the missing piece's presence within the tissues or other body cavities.

What is the General Health of the Patient?

A history that touches on drug allergy, heart murmur, bleeding disorder, other systemic disease and current medication should be taken before treatment.

Did the Patient have Nausea, Vomiting, Unconsciousness, Amnesia, Headache, Visual Disturbances or Confusion After the Accident?

An affirmative answer to any of these may indicate intracranial injury and direct the surgeon to obtain medical consultation immediately after completing treatment.

Is there a Disturbance in the Bite?

An affirmative answer to this question may indicate tooth displacement, or dentoalveolar or jaw fracture.

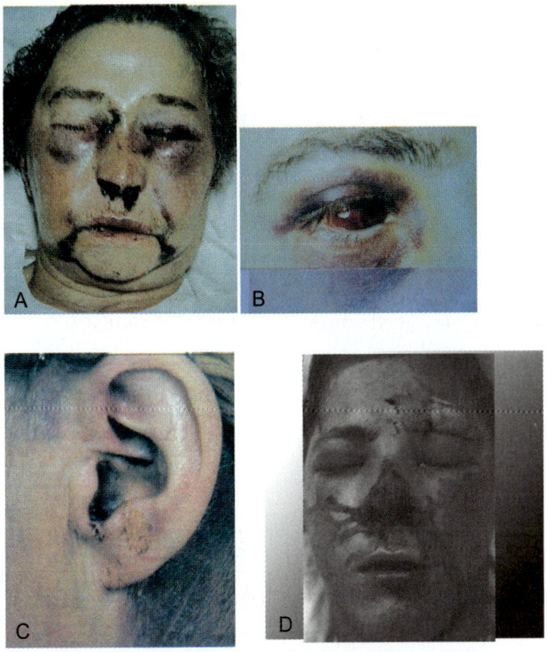

Fig. 7.3: A bilateal circumorbital ecchymosis: (A) Panda facies; Raccoon eyes, (B) Subconjunctival haemorrhage, (C) Battle's sign, (D) The tram line effect.

CLINICAL EXAMINATION

Examination should not be restricted only to the site of the maxillofacial injury but other systems of the body should also be assessed to rule out abdominal injury, chest trauma or concomitant cervical injury.

Vital signs such as pulse rate, blood pressure, and respiration should be measured.

The mental state of the patient is also assessed throughout the taking of the history and while performing the clinical examination by observation of the manner in which the patient reacts to the examination and responds to the questioning. During the clinical examination the following areas should routinely be examined.

1. Extraoral Soft Tissue Wounds

Lacerations, abrasions and contusions of the skin are all common with dentoalveolar injuries. If a laceration is present, its depth should also be noted. Are there any vital structures crossing the line of the laceration such as the parotid duct or the facial nerve?

2. Intraoral Soft Tissue Wounds

Before a thorough examination, it may be necessary to remove blood clots, irrigate with sterile saline and cleanse the oral cavity. Soft tissue injuries should be noted and an examination should ascertain whether there are any foreign bodies, such as tooth crowns or teeth, within the substance of the lips, floor of the mouth, cheeks or other areas.

3. Fractures of the Jaws or the Alveolar Process

Fractures of the jaws are most readily found on palpation.

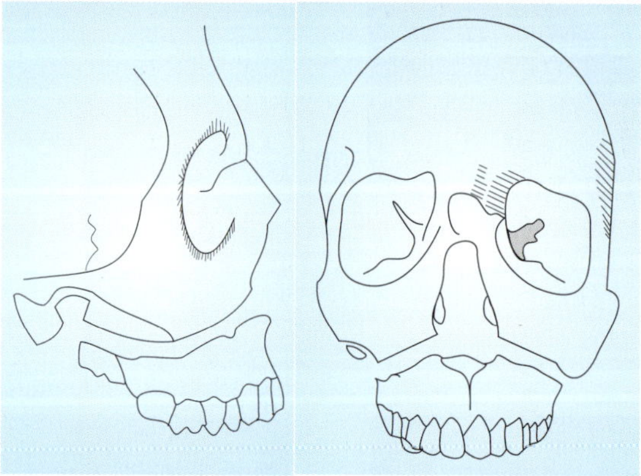

Fig. 7.4: Schematic representation of the Le Fort I fracture line.

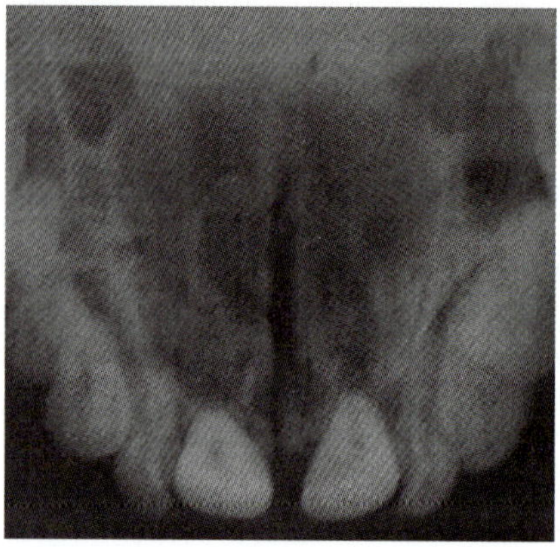

Fig. 7.6: The maxillary occlusal view showing midpalatal split.

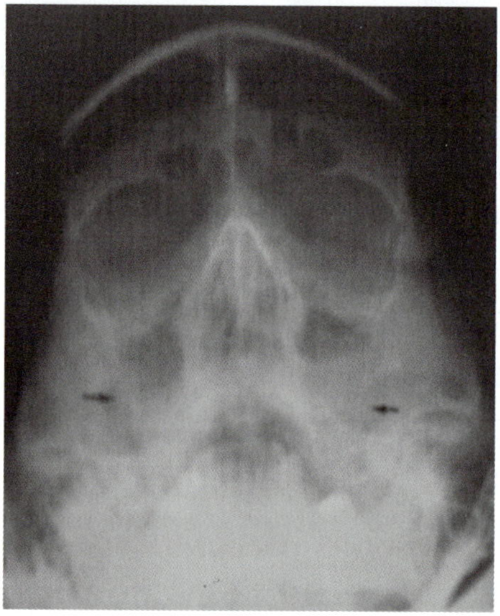

Fig. 7.5: PA Water's view showing Le Fort I fracture of the face.

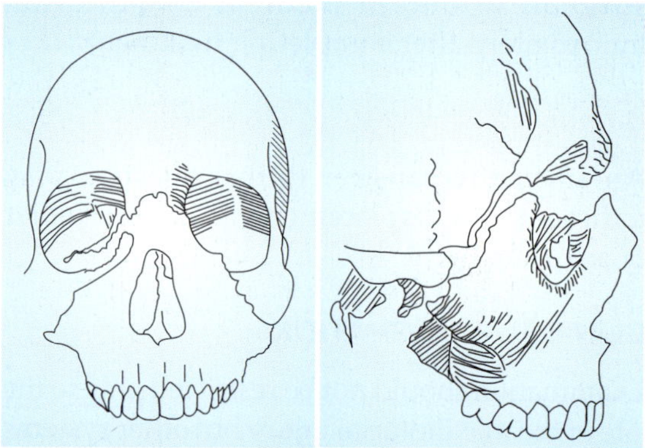

Fig. 7.7: Schematic representation of LeFort II fracture of the middle third of face.

Le Fort I Fracture

Introduction

- Low level #
- Extension: Lateral border of the pyriform aperture—above the alveolus—below zygomatic buttress—maxillary tuberosity—pterygoid plates
- Occ: Nasal septum, midpalatal split (Fig. 7.4).

Clinical Features

- Swelling of the mid face
- Displacement of the maxilla
- Anterior open bite due to posterior gagging
- Buccal sulcus ecchymosis
- Guerin's sign
- Parasthesia
- Mid palatal split.

Radiographic Features

- Clouding of the maxillary sinus—Water's view (Fig. 7.5).

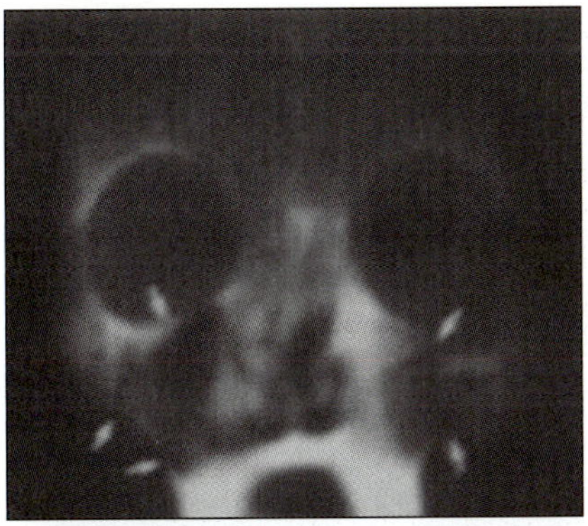

Fig. 7.8: Radiographic view showing Le Fort II fracture of the middle third of face.

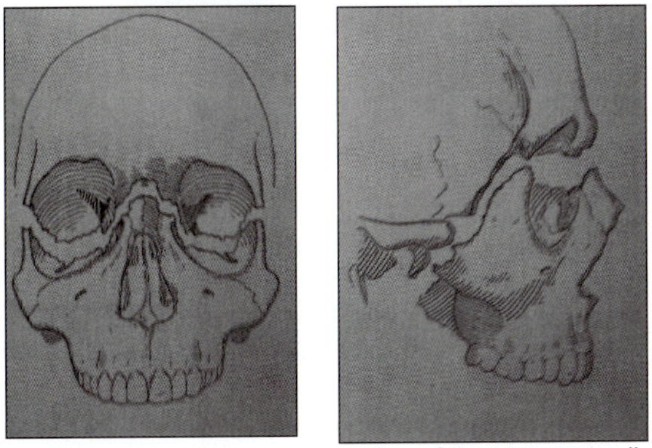

Fig. 7.9: Schematic representation of the pterygomaxillary dysjunction.

- Sharp line of cleavage through the sinus and pterygoid plates—lateral view
- Canted maxilla, anterior open bite
- Discontinuity in the lateral wall of maxillary sinus (Fig. 7.6).

Le Fort II Fracture

Clinical Features (Fig. 7.7)

- Gross oedema of the face
- Bilateral peri orbital oedema—raccoon sign
- Elongation of the face
- Epistaxis
- Circumorbital ecchymosis/panda facies
- Occlusal derangement
- CSF rhonorrhoea.

Radiographic Signs (Fig. 7.8)

- Increased width of frontonasal suture.
- Step defect along the infraorbital margin.
- Separation of the zygomaticomaxillary suture
- Haziness of sinus due to haemorrhage
- Disruption of pterygoid plates–lateral view.

Le Fort III Fracture

Extension of the Fracture Line

- Frontonasal suture—depth of ethmoid—cribriform plate of ethmoid—optic foramen.
- Backwards across the ptergomaxillary fissure—pterygoid plates (Fig. 7.9).
- Laterally—lateral wall of orbit—separating the zygomatic bone at the frontozygomatic suture.

Clinical Features

- Massive facial oedema
- Subconjunctival haemorrhage
- CSF rhinorrhoea, Otorrhoea
- Altered consciousness
- Increased facial height
- Occlusal derangement.

Radiographic Features (Figs 7.10, 7.11)

- Widening of frontonasal suture
- Widening of frontomaxillary suture
- Enlargement of zygomaticotemporal suture
- Cleavage line in the frontal process of maxilla
- Cleavage through the pterygoid plates
- Haziness of the sinus
- CT scan is mandatory.

Zygomatic Complex Fracture

Clinical Features

- *Flattening of cheek*
- *Tenderness/step deformity*

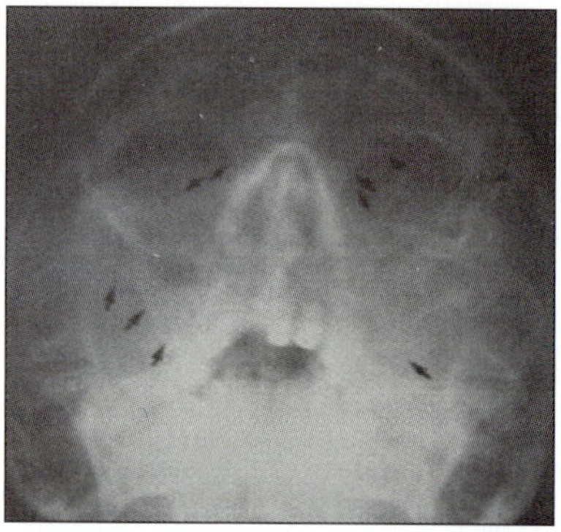

Fig. 7.10: PA Water's view showing the pterygomaxillary dysjunction.

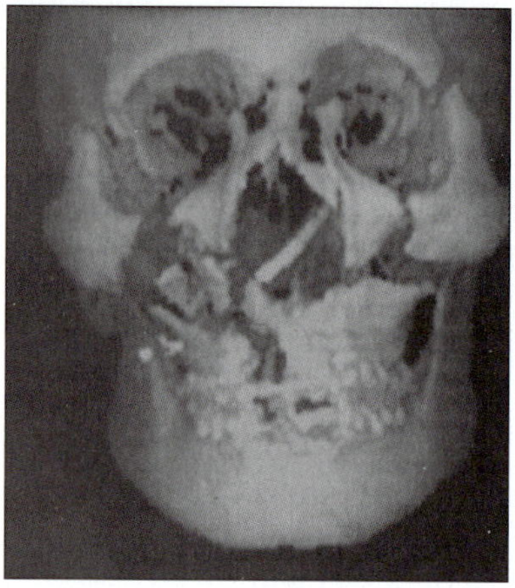

Fig. 7.11: CT Scan with 3-D facial reconstruction is more useful for studying panfacial trauma.

- *Circum orbital ecchymosis*
- *Diplopia*
- *Enopthalmosis*
- *Posterior Gagging of occlusion*
- *Trismus*
- In the case of fractured zygoma the **PA Water's** will show the following (Fig. 7.12):
  - Opacification of sinus
  - Diastasis of frontozygomatic and zygomaticotemporal sutures
  - Discontinuity in the maxillary line
  - Rotation of the displaced zygoma—***rail road track sign***
  - Fracture of infra orbital rim.

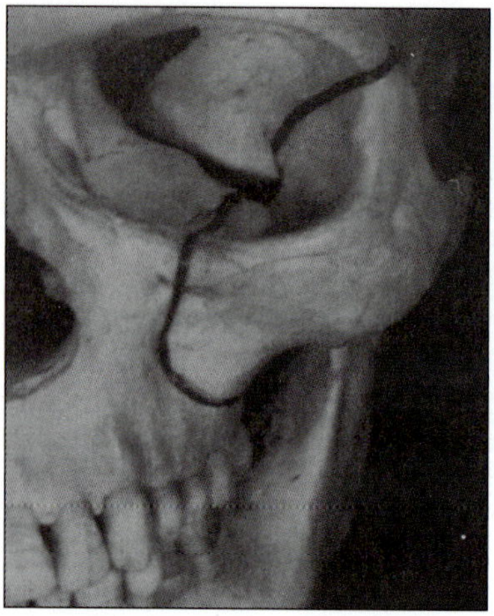

Fig. 7.12

Other views which can be taken in the case of fracture zygoma are:

1. PA Caldwell.
2. Submentovertex or the jug handle view.

THE 4 'S'—A USEFUL APPROACH TO EVALUATE FACIAL FRACTURES

- Symmetry
- Sharpness
- Sinus
- Soft tissues—swelling, foreign bodies, emphysema.

RADIOGRAPHIC EXAMINATION

Once the history has been noted and a thorough clinical examination has been carried out radiographic examination may be carried out to confirm the diagnosis anticipated by the history and the examination.

A host of radiographic techniques are available to evaluate dentoalveolar trauma. Most commonly a combination of occlusal and periapical radiographs are used. The radiographic examination should provide the following information:

1. Presence of root fracture.
2. Degree of extrusion or intrusion.

3. Presence of pre-existing periapical disease
4. Extent of root development
5. Size of the pulp chamber and root canal
6. Presence of jaw fractures
7. Tooth fragments and foreign bodies lodged in soft tissues

INDICATIONS OF RADIOGRAPHIC VIEWS

The ***lateral skull view*** can be indicated for the following:

- Fractures of cranial vault
- Middle third fractures.
- Fractures of nasal bones
- Pterygoid plates
- Ant open bite due to post gagging
- CSF leaks — to demonstrate fluid levels in the sphenoid, maxillary sinuses

The ***PA Water's view*** can be indicated for the following:

- Orbital fracture
- Zygomatic arch fracture
- Nasal bone fracture
- Le Fort fracture

The ***Lateral cervical view*** is indicated for the following:

- Cervical spine injury (C_7–T_1)
- Swimmer's view—for patient's with short neck
- Retropharyngeal/subcutaneous air

The ***PA Caldwell view*** is indicated for the following:

- Orbits
- Blow out fracture
- Pyriform aperture
- Lamina papyracea
- Frontal sinuses.

Radiographic Signs

The following radiographic signs may be suggestive of a fracture in the craniomaxillofacial region:

- XL line with sharply defined margins
- Change in the normal outline, asymmetry
- Step deformity in the smooth outline
- Occlusal step
- Increased density of the bone
- Trap door sign—blow out fracture of orbit
- Bright light sign — free bony fragment in the sinus
- Rail road track sign — PA Water's, Caldwell view.

Signs of Sinus Involvement

- Generalised haziness due to mucosal oedema
- Well defined mass due to sub mucosal/intra mucosal haematoma
- Opacification due to mucosal tear
- Discontinuity in the walls
- Trap door sign
- Bright light sign

Radiographic evaluation for foreign bodies within the soft tissues of the lips or cheeks are taken with the radiographic film placed inside the soft tissues to be examined, labial to the alveolus. A reduced radiographic exposure time is used (approximately one-third normal). Foreign bodies in the floor of the mouth are viewed with cross-sectional occlusal radiographs also with reduced radiographic exposure time.

MANAGEMENT OF DENTOALVEOLAR INJURIES

The goal in the treatment of dentoalveolar injuries is re-establishing normal form and function of the masticatory apparatus.

Crown Fracture

The treatment of crown fracture is determined by the depth of tissue involvement. For fractures that are only through the enamel or those with minimal amounts of dentin involvement, no treatment other than smoothing of the sharp edges is warranted.

If a considerable amount of dentin is exposed, measures to promote secondary dentin deposition by the pulp are undertaken. Restorative procedures are adopted and the tooth is managed conservatively. If the pulp is exposed, the aim of the treatment is to preserve the pulp in a vital healthy state. Periodic follow-up examinations are mandatory after any pulpal procedure. The final restorative decision will be based on the pulpal health of the tooth. Since the prognosis is guarded, endodontic treatment may be necessary if the pulp degenerates.

Crown-Root Fracture

The treatment of crown—root fractures depends on the location of the fracture and local anatomic variance. Depending on the apical extent of the fracture, it may be necessary to perform periodontal procedures to make the apical margin of the fracture accessible for restorative procedures. If the pulp is involved and the tooth is restorable, endodontic treatment is implemented. If on the other hand the tooth is not restorable, removal is indicated.

Horizontal Root Fractures

When a horizontal or oblique fracture of the root occurs, the main factor in determining the prognosis and therefore directing treatment is the position of the fracture in relation to the gingival crevice. If the fracture is above or close to the gingival crevice, the tooth should either be removed or the coronal fragment should be removed and endodontic treatment be performed on the root. The root can then be restored with a post and core restoration. Fractures in the middle and apical third of the root have a good prognosis for survival of the pulp and healing of the root fragments to one another. Immobilisation period of 2–3 months is needed for bridging of the fracture.

Sensitivity (Concussion)

No acute treatment is recommended other than symptomatic relief such as relieving the tooth from occlusal contact.

Mobility

If only mildly mobile, relieving the occlusal contact is effective treatment. Most mobile teeth stabilize with time. If the tooth is extremely mobile, splinting it to adjacent teeth is recommended.

Intrusion

Some clinicians favour surgically repositioning and splinting the intruded teeth, others feel that the intruded teeth should be left alone and allowed to re-erupt. Some use orthodontic forces to assist re-eruption of intruded teeth. Whether to perform endodontic treatment is based on the follow-up findings. However, if intrusion has occurred in a apically mature tooth, pulpal degeneration is likely and endodontic treatment should be performed.

If a deciduous tooth has been intruded to the point of it touching the follicle of the succedaneous tooth, a period of observation should be followed, since re-eruption is common.

Extrusion

Extruded teeth can usually be manually seated back into their socket if the injury was very recent. After replacement of the tooth within the socket splinting for several weeks is essential.

Lateral Displacement

Manual repositioning followed by splinting for several weeks is indicated. Soft tissue lacerations are sutured.

Avulsion

The factors most important for determining how successful treatment measures will be are:

a. Time the tooth has been out of the socket
b. State of the tooth and periodontal tissues
c. Manner in which the tooth was preserved before replantation

The various transport medium to hold the tooth during the extra-alveolar period are:

a. Patient's saliva
b. Saline
c. HBSS
d. Milk

The avulsed tooth is gently cleansed of debris and the socket is gently irrigated for removal of bulk of the clot. Stabilisation of an avulsed tooth can be achieved by a number of materials:

a. Wires
b. Arch bars
c. Splints

The period of stabilization should be as short as possible for the tooth to become re-attached, usually 7–10 days.

Alveolar Fractures

The treatment of this type of injury is to place the segment in into its proper position and then to stabilize it until osseous healing occurs.

The flap used for access should not jeopardize the blood supply to the dentoosseous segment. The soft tissues must be left attached to the lingual portion of the alveolar process, with exposure on the facial aspect. The teeth in the dentoalveolar fragment should be examined. Endodontic treatment in 1–2 weeks to help prevent inflammatory root resorption and infection should be performed if the apical blood supply to the teeth has obviously been interrupted. The segment should then be manipulated with digital pressure to determine where areas of resistance exist. If an irregular area of bone is sprung and inhibits repositioning, it may be removed with rongeurs or bur. Slight misalignment along the base of the alveolar segment is acceptable as long as the occlusal relationship is accurate. The dento-osseous segment should be stabilized for a period of 4 weeks to allow osseous healing. The dentoalveolar segment can be stabilized with any of the following methods: arch bar, acid-etched arch wire, cold-cured acrylic splint.

SOFT TISSUE INJURIES

Soft tissue injuries frequently accompany dento-alveolar injuries and maxillofacial trauma. Their management is outlined as follows.

Abrasion

An abrasion is a wound caused by friction between an object and the surface of the soft tissue.

If the abrasion is not particularly deep, re-epithelisation occurs without scarring. If the abrasions are deep enough, they should be thoroughly cleansed to remove foreign material. Once the wound is free of debris, topical application of an antibiotic ointment is adequate treatment. Systemic antibiotics are usually not indicated.

Contusion

A contusion is more commonly called a bruise. It indicates that some amount of tissue disruption has occurred within the tissues, resulting in subcutaneous or submucosal haemorrhage without a break in the soft tissue surface. The importance of contusions from a diagnostic point of view is that when they are seen, a search for osseous fractures should be made.

A contusion usually requires no surgical treatment. If a contusion is seen early, the application of ice or pressure dressing may help constrict the blood vessels and therefore decrease the amount of haematoma that forms. When there has been no break in the surface of the soft tissue, infection is unlikely and systemic antibiotics are not indicated. If, however, the contusion is secondary to dentoalveolar trauma, there is a good chance of communication existing between the oral cavity and the submucosal haematoma. In this case systemic antibiotics are warranted since coagulated blood represents an ideal culture medium.

Laceration

A laceration is a tear in the epithelial and subepithelial tissues. Some involve the external surface only, but others extend deeply into the tissue, disrupting the nerves, blood vessels, muscle and other anatomic cavities and structures. There are four major steps in the surgical management of lacerations, cleansing, debridement, haemostasis and closure.

FACIAL FRACTURES

Whenever facial structures are injured, the goals of treatment should be maximal rehabilitation of the patient. For facial fractures, goals of treatment include the following.

a. Rapid bone healing.
b. A return of normal ocular, masticatory and nasal function.
c. Restoration of speech.
d. An acceptable facial and dental esthetic result.
e. Minimise the adverse effect on the patient's nutritional status and achieve treatment goals with the least amount of discomfort and inconvenience possible.

In order to achieve these goals the following basic principles should serve as a guide for treatment.

a. Reduction of the fracture.
b. Fixation and stabilization of the bony segments.
c. Immobilisation of the segments at the fracture site.
d. The preoperative occlusion must be restored and infection in the area of the fracture must be eradicated or prevented.

Presurgical Evaluation

The timing of facial fractures depends on many factors.

In many cases patients have other injuries that demand more immediate treatment. An injury such as severe neurologic trauma that precludes presurgical stabilization of the patient and increases anaesthetic and surgical risks should be managed before facial fractures. In some cases a delay of one or two days results in the presence of tissue oedema, making a further wait of 3–4 days necessary for elimination of the oedema and easier fracture treatment.

Treatment of facial fractures should begin from "bottom-up" and "inside-out".

Mandibular Fractures

The first and most important thing in the treatment of mandibular fracture is to reduce the fracture properly or place the individual segments into the proper relationship to each other along with establishing a proper occlusal relationship.

Establishing a proper occlusal relationship by wiring the teeth together is termed intermaxillary fixation or maxillomandibular fixation. Maxillomandibular fixation can be done with the help of arch bar or ivy loops or continuous loop wiring.

In the case of fracture of an edentulous patient, the mandibular dentures can be wired to the mandible with circummandibular wiring, and the maxillary denture can be secured to the maxilla using either wiring techniques or bone screws to hold the denture in place. A splinting technique that can be used for dentulous patients involves the use of a lingual or occlusal splint. This is particularly useful in treatment of mandibular fractures in children in whom placement of arch bars is difficult because of the configuration of the deciduous teeth and because patient understanding and cooperation is difficult to obtain.

Postoperative care to be taken following closed reduction

a. Check for the occlusion.
b. Check if any of the wires is impinging on the mucosa.
c. Advise proper oral hygiene techniques. Use a toothbrush and tooth paste to clean teeth. Avoid cleaning teeth with finger as the wires may cause trauma.
d. Regular follow-up of the patient is important to check if any wires have become loose.
e. Antibiotics and analgesics should be prescribed to prevent infection. Mouthwashes should also be prescribed.
f. Patient's diet will be affected because of the maxillomandibular fixation. Hence he should be prescribed protein supplements and should be encouraged to take plenty of juices and other liquids to maintain the diet.
g. Maxillomandibular fixation is maintained for 4–6 weeks and in the case of subcondylar fractures for 3 weeks followed by elastics for two weeks.
h. Arch bars are removed after 4–6 weeks of immobilization.

Postoperative care to be taken following open reduction

a. Check for the occlusion.
b. Check if any of the wires is impinging on the mucosa.
c. Advise proper oral hygiene techniques. Use a toothbrush and tooth paste to clean teeth. Avoid cleaning teeth with finger as the wires may cause trauma.
d. Regular follow-up of the patient is important to check if any wires have become loose.
e. Antibiotics and analgesics should be prescribed to prevent infection. Mouthwashes should also be prescribed.
f. Patient is advised to have soft diet for a period of 4–6 weeks.
g. Arch bars are removed after a period of 4–6 weeks of immobilization.

REFERENCES AND BIBLIOGRAPHY

1. *Contemporary Oral and Maxillofacial Surgery*, 4th edn; Larry J. Peterson, Edward Ellis, James R.Hupp, Myron R. Tucker.
2. *Diagnostic radiology*; White and Pharaoh.

Chapter 8

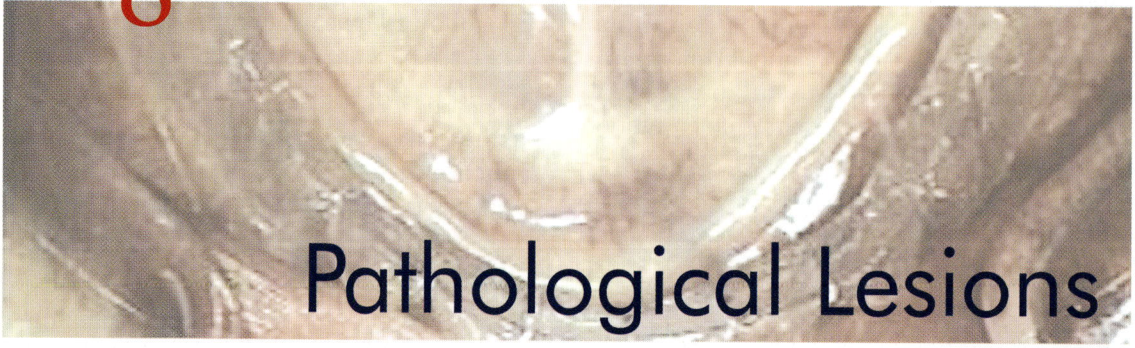

Pathological Lesions

CYSTS

A cyst is defined generally as an epithelium-lined sac filled with fluid or soft material. The prevalence of cysts in the jaws can be related to the abundant epithelium that proliferates in bone during the process of tooth formation, and along the lines where the surfaces of embryologic jaw processes fuse. Cysts of the jaws may be divided into two types—those arising from odontogenic epithelium and those arising from oral epithelium that is trapped between the fusing processes during embryogenesis.

Residual fragments of cyst membrane tend to produce recurrent cysts. This necessitates complete excision of the epithelial lining of the cyst at the time of the operation. Some cysts such as the keratocysts behave more aggressively in both destructive characteristics and recurrence rates. Cysts have been known to destroy large portions of the jaws and to push teeth into remote areas of the jaws. Enlargement of the cysts is caused by a gradual expansion and most are discovered on routine dental radiographs.

Choice of Anaesthesia

The cysts can be treated under local anaesthesia. At times, sedation may be chosen and if the cyst is large and in close proximity of vital structures then patient may be operated under general anaesthesia. Also the general and medical condition of the patient are to be considered when choosing the type of anaesthesia.

Investigations

After the complete case history has been noted and the examination of the patient carried out investigations in support of the diagnosis may be ordered.

Blood Investigations

Complete blood count.

Bleeding time and coagulation time.

However, if the patient is to be operated under sedation or under general anaesthesia or if the medical condition of the patient warrants, then the following investigations may also be ordered.

Complete coagulation profile.
Liver function test.
Renal function test.
HBsAg and VDRL and HIV

Radiographic Examination

If incidentally a cyst is located on an intraoral radiograph, an extraoral view such as a PA Water's or a lateral oblique view or an orthopantomogram should be ordered to compare similar areas on the other side and to exactly delineate the extent of the lesion. At times the cortical plates may be perforated and then a CT scan or a MRI may be a useful aid to study the soft tissue involvement.

Aspiration Biopsy

The contents of the swelling should be aspirated to rule out a haemorrrhagic lesion.

Incisional Biopsy

Once a haemorrhagic lesion has been ruled out an incisional biopsy may be done to confirm the diagnosis and to rule out any ameloblastomatous changes or carcinogenic changes taking in the cyst lining.

MODALITIES OF TREATMENT

Cysts of the jaws are treated in one of the four basic methods:

1. Enucleation
2. Marsupialisation
3. A staged combination of the two procedures.
4. Enucleation with curettage.

Enucleation (Figs 8.1 and 8.2)

It is the process by which the total removal of the cystic lining is achieved.

Enucleation of cysts should be carried out with care in an attempt to remove the cyst in one piece without fragmentation. This reduces the chances of recurrence by increasing the likelihood of total removal.

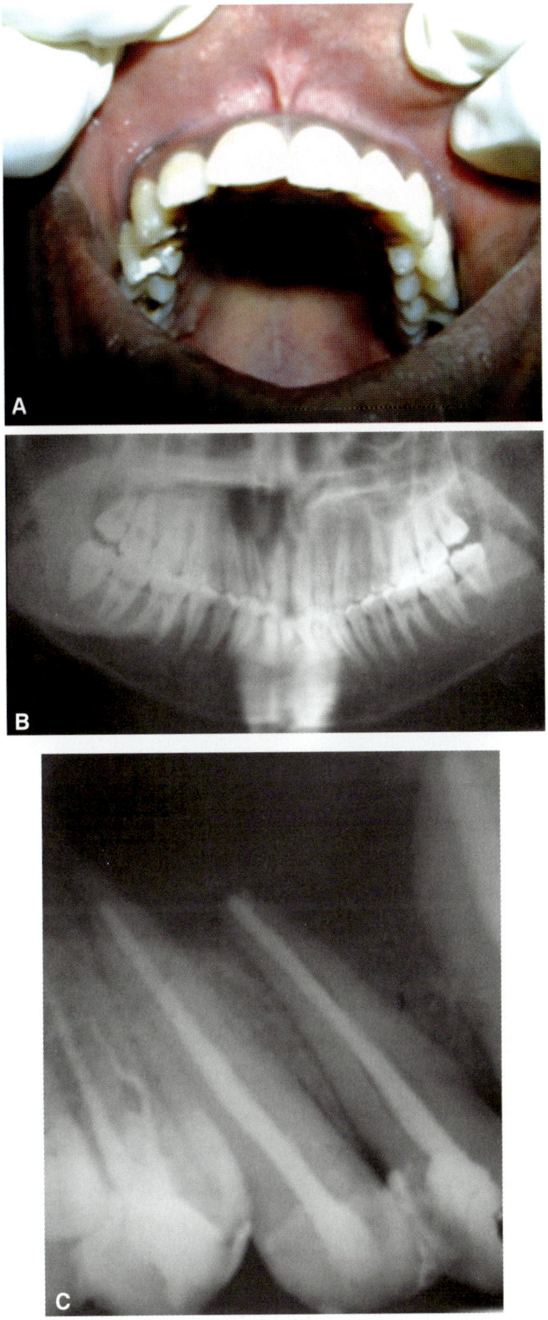

Fig. 8.1: Surgical steps in the management of a radicular cyst. (A) Intraoral view of the affected teeth, (B) Orthopantomogram of the patient outlining the extent of the lesion, (C) Endodontic treatment of the affected teeth is carried out.

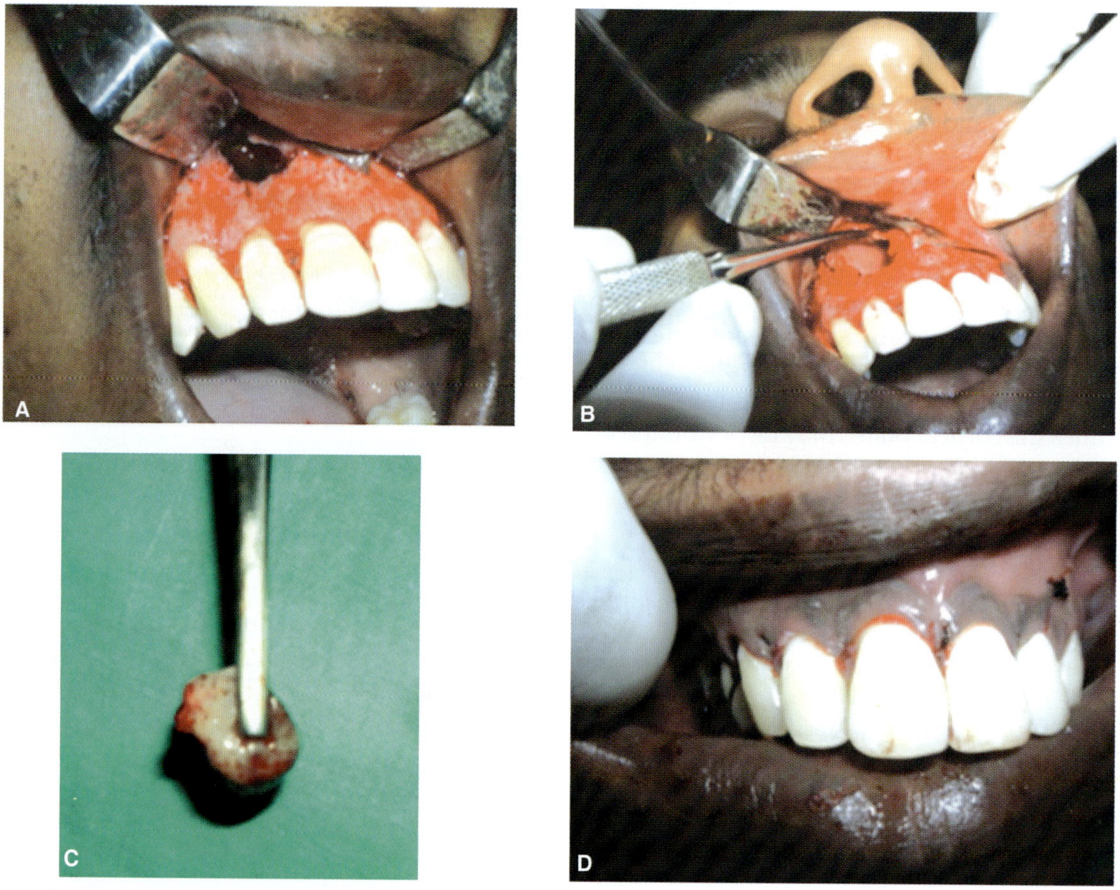

Fig. 8.2: Surgical steps in the management of a radicular cyst, (A) Mucoperiosteal flap is reflected to expose the perforation in the labial cortical plate, (B) Cystic lining is enucleated, (C) Cyst enucleated in one piece, (D) Wound sutured with 3-0 black silk interrupted sutures.

Indications

Should be employed for any cyst of the jaw which can be safely removed without unduly sacrificing the adjacent structures.

Advantages

Pathologic examination of the entire cyst can be undertaken.

Chances of recurrence are minimized.

Disadvantages

Normal tissue may be jeopardized.

Fracture of the jaw could occur.

Devitalisation of teeth could result.

The impacted tooth has to be removed.

Marsupialisation

Marsupialisation, decompression and Partsch operation all refer to creating a surgical window in the wall of the cyst; evacuating the contents of the cyst and maintaining continuity between the cyst and the oral cavity; maxillary sinus or nasal cavity (Fig. 8.3).

Indications

The following factors should be considered

before deciding whether a cyst should be removed by marsupialisation.

1. Amount of tissue injury.
2. Surgical access.
3. Assisstance of eruption of teeth.
4. Extent of surgery.
5. Size of the cyst.

Advantages

1. Simple procedure.
2. It may spare vital structures from damage should immediate enucleation be attempted.

Disadvantages

1. Pathologic tissue is left in situ without thorough histologic examination.
2. Patient is inconvenienced in several respects.

Marsupialisation followed by Enucleation

Marsupialisation is frequently followed by enucleation at a later date. Initial healing is rapid after marsupialisation, but the size of the cavity may not decrease appreciably past a certain point. Now the enucleation may be undertaken without injury to adjacent structures.

Indications

Anticipation of the amount of tissue injury enucleation would cause the degree of access one might have for enucleation, whether or not impacted teeth associated with the cyst would benefit from eruption guidance with marsupialisation, the medical condition of the patient and the size of the lesion.

Advantages

1. Protection of the adjacent vital structures.
2. The development of a thickened cystic lining which makes the secondary enucleation an easier procedure.

Disadvantages

The complete pathologic tissue is not removed in the first step.

Enucleation with Curettage

Enucleation with curettage means that after enucleation a curette or bur is used to remove 1–2 mm of bone around the entire periphery of the cystic cavity. Its purpose is to remove any remaining epithelial cells that may be present in the periphery of the cyst wall or bony cavity. These cells could proliferate into a recurrence of the cyst.

Indications

There are two instances in which the clinician should perform curettage with enucleation.

a. Removal of an odontogenic keratocyst.
b. Any cyst that recurs after what was deemed a thorough removal.

Advantages

If enucleation leaves epithelial remnants, curettage may remove them, thereby decreasing the likelihood of recurrence.

Disadvantages

Curettage is more destructive of adjacent bone and other tissues. The dental pulps may be stripped of their neurovascular supply when curettage is performed close to the root tips.

POSTOPERATIVE CARE

When a patient has been treated for marsupialisation of a cyst, the following care should be taken.

a. The diet of the patient should be high in protein content.
b. Patient should be advised to maintain good oral hygiene. Mouthwashes should be prescribed.

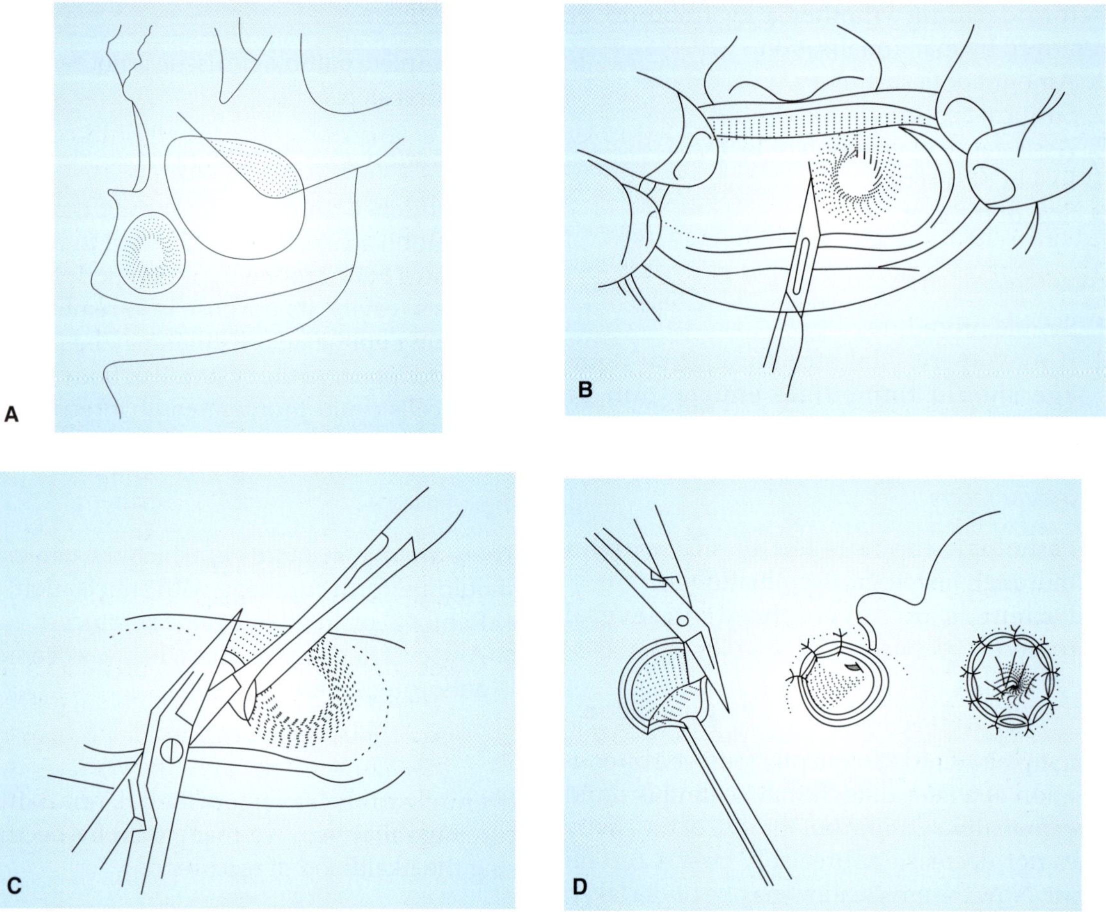

Fig. 8.3: Illustration of the marsupialisation technique. (A) Cyst within maxilla, (B) Incision through oral mucosa and cyst wall into center of the cyst, (C) Scissors used to complete excision of window of mucosa and cyst wall, (D) Oral mucosa and mucosa of cyst wall sutured together around the periphery of opening.

c. Antibiotics should be prescribed to prevent infection. Analgesics should also be prescribed in the initial phase.
d. If possible a surgical stent should be constructed to cover the defect.
e. Periodic follow up of the patient is essential along with serial radiographs to study the healing of the wound.

When a patient has undergone enucleation of a cyst, the following perioperative care is essential.

a. The diet of the patient should be high in protein content.
b. Patient should be advised to maintain good oral hygiene. Mouthwashes should be prescribed.
c. Antibiotics should be prescribed to prevent infection. Analgesics should also be prescribed in the initial phase.
d. Periodic follow up of the patient is essential along with serial radiographs to study the healing of the wound.

TUMOURS

Lesions of the oral cavity and perioral areas must be identified and characterized so that specific therapy can lead to elimination of the lesion. When a lesion is discovered, several important, orderly steps should be undertaken to identify and characterize it. These steps include the health history, history of the specific lesion, clinical examination, radiographic examination, laboratory investigation, and, if indicated, surgical procedures to obtain a specimen for pathologic examination.

HISTORY OF THE LESION

When a patient presents to the surgeon with a lesion in the maxillofacial region, he should be thoroughly questioned for the following.

1. *How long has the lesion been present?*
   The duration of the lesion may provide valuable clues to the nature of the lesion. A lesion that has been present for several years may be congenital.
2. *Has the lesion changed in size? If so, at what rate and to what magnitude?*
   A rapidly growing lesion has more chances of being aggressive, whereas a slow growing lesion may indicate a more benign process.
3. *Has the lesion changed in character, i.e. did a lump become an ulcer; did an ulcer begin as a vesicle?*
4. *What symptoms are associated with the lesion, i.e. pain, abnormal sensations, anaesthesia, a feeling of swelling, bad taste or smell, dysphagia, swelling or tenderness of adjacent lymph nodes? If painful, what is the character of the pain? What exacerbates and what relieves the pain?*
   Pain is most often associated with lesions that contain an inflammatory component. Numbness in the distribution of one of the sensory nerves usually indicates an inflammatory or malignant process, unless other physical causes can be ascertained. Swelling may be one of the more common symptoms associated with the oral lesions. In general tender lymph nodes indicate an inflammatory or infectious cause of the lesion.
5. *Are there any associated constitutional symptoms, i.e. fever, nausea and anorexia?*
   This questions provides an insight into the systemic condition of the patient.
6. *Is there any historical reason for the lesion, i.e. trauma to the area, a recent toothache?*
   Frequently lesions in and around the oral cavity are caused by habits, hard or hot foods, application of medicines not intended for topical use and recent trauma. Additionally, the dentition should always be examined very carefully when a lesion is found in the general area, since a large percentage of such lesions have some relationship to the teeth.

CLINICAL EXAMINATION

When a lesion is discovered, it must be carefully examined for clues to its nature. Furthermore, a thorough examination of the areas around the lesion, including the regional lymph nodes, is mandatory. An examination classically includes inspection, palpation, percussion and auscultation. The following are some of the more important points to be evaluated.

1. *The anatomic location of the mass.* Lesions may arise from any tissue within the oral cavity, including epithelium, subcutaneous and submucosal connective tissue, muscle, tendon, nerve, bone, blood vessels and salivary glands (Fig. 8.4).
2. *The overall physical character of the lesion.* The lesion should be described in proper

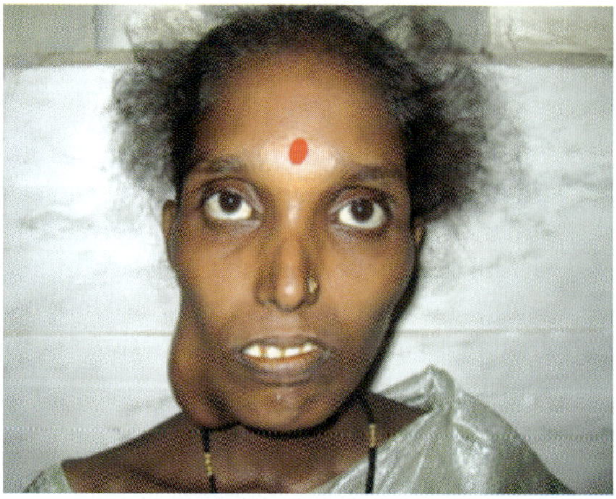

Fig. 8.4: Patient with a swelling in the region of the angle of the mandible.

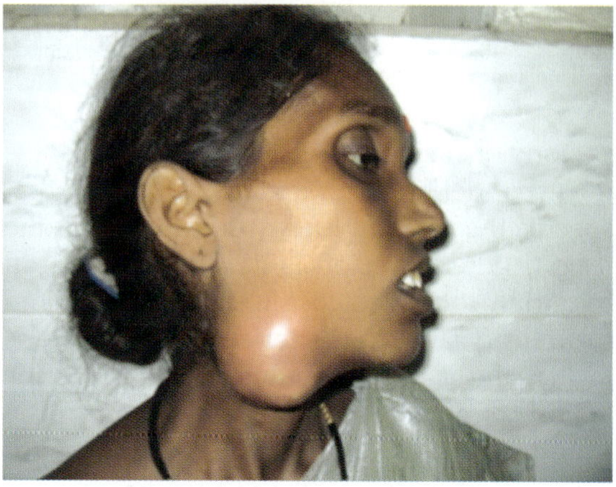

Fig. 8.5: Patient with a secondarily infected tumour in the region of the angle of the mandible. Note the shiny skin over the swelling

medical terminology such as either a macule, nodule, papule, plaque, pustule, scale, ulcer, vesicle.

3. *The size and shape of the lesion.* Accurate recordings of these two basic physical characteristics should be made for further reference.
4. *Single versus multiple lesions.*
5. *Surface of the lesion.* The surface may be smooth, lobulated, or irregular. If ulceration is present, the characteristics of the ulcer base should be recorded. Ulcer beds can be smooth, full of granulation tissue, covered with a slough, membrane or scab, or fungating, such as is seen in some malignancies (Fig. 8.5).
6. *The colour of the lesion.* A bluish swelling that blanches on pressure indicates a vascular lesion whereas a bluish lesion that does not blanch on pressure may indicate a mucous containing lesion. A pigmented lesion of the oral mucosa may carry more importance than a lesion of normal colour. Some lesions may have more than one colour and this should be noted in detail.
7. *The sharpness of the boundaries of the lesion.* If a mass is present, is it fixed to surrounding deeper tissues or is it freely movable? The margin of an ulcer may be flat, raised or rolled.
8. *The consistency of the lesion to palpation.* The consistency of the lesions is described as soft, as in the case of a lipoma; firm which is the consistency of a fibroma; or hard as in the case of an osteoma or tori. Indurated simply means firm or hard.
9. *Presence of fluctuation.* Fluctuation is the term given to a wave-like motion felt on palpating a mass or cavity with non-rigid walls containing fluid. It usually indicates fluid within the mass.
10. *Presence of pulsation.* Palpation of a mass may reveal a pulsatile quality, which indicates a large vascular component.
11. *Lymph node examination.* No evaluation of an oral lesion is complete without a thorough regional lymph node examination. In recording findings, five characteristics should normally include: *location size, tenderness, degree of fixation, texture.*

The standard examination of the lymph nodes requires only simple inspection and palpation. It is always useful to compare sides, using the middle three fingers for palpation. This examination is methodical and proceeds downward as follows (Fig. 8.6):

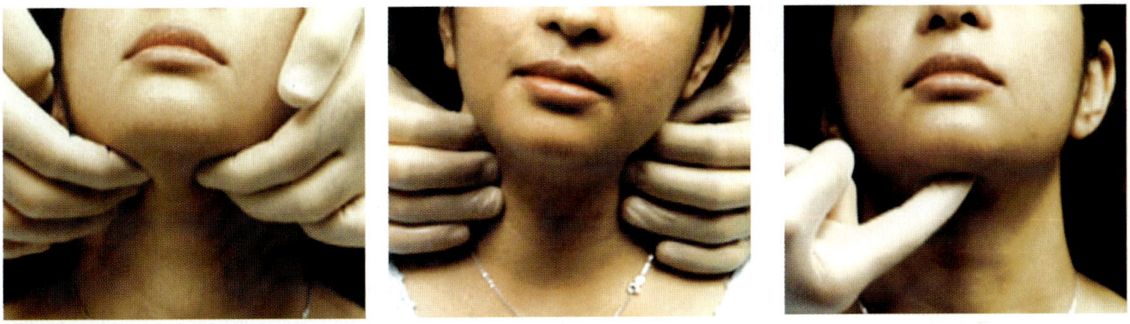

Fig. 8.6: Examination of the lymph nodes: Submandibular, cervical and submental nodes.

1. Occipital and post-auricular.
2. Submandibular and submental.
3. Anterior cervical triangle.
4. Downward along sternocleidomastoid muscle.
5. Posterior triangle.
6. Supraclavicular.

RADIOGRAPHIC EXAMINATION

Radiographs are useful as diagnostic adjuncts to the clinical examination and history of lesions within or adjacent to bone. A variety of radiographic projections may be used, depending on the anatomic location of the lesion. Most pathologic conditions of the mandible and the maxilla can be satisfactorily demonstrated by routine radiography, but occasionally special imaging techniques are required to elucidate some particular facet of the case under investigation (Figs 8.7, 8.8). In special instances radiopaque dyes or instruments can be useful in conjunction with routine or special radiographs.

LABORATORY INVESTIGATION

Several oral lesions may be manifestations of systemic diseases. For instance, multiple lytic lesions and loss of lamina dura suggest the possibility of hyperparathyroidism. Serum levels of calcium, phosphorus and alkaline phosphatase should identify this metabolic abnormality. A patient with multiple radiolucencies of the jaws or other bones may also have multiple myeloma.

SURGICAL SPECIMEN FOR PATHOLOGICAL EXAMINATION

In most instances the data obtained from the history and the clinical and radiographic examination provide enough information for a tentative diagnosis. Lesions that appear traumatic in origin may be initially treated non-surgically by elimination of any continued source of irritation. Observation for 10–14 days will verify the presumptive diagnosis in these cases, that is the lesion should heal if trauma is the cause.

Indications for a Biopsy

a. Any lesion that persists for more than 2 weeks with no apparent aetiologic basis.
b. Any inflammatory lesion that does not respond to local treatment after 10–14 days (that is after removing local irritant).
c. Persistent hyperkeratotic changes in the surface tissues.
d. Any persistent tumescence, either visible or palpable beneath relatively normal tissue.
e. Inflammatory changes of unknown cause that persist for long periods.
f. Lesions that interfere with local function.
g. Bone lesions not specifically identified by clinical and radiographic findings.

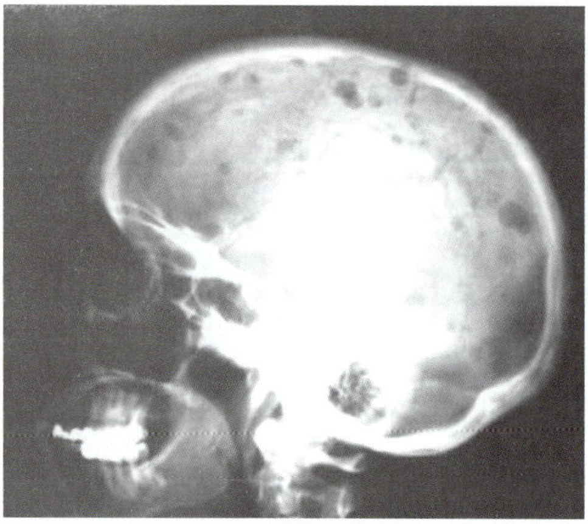

Fig. 8.7: The true lateral view showing multiple radiolucent lesions in the skull.

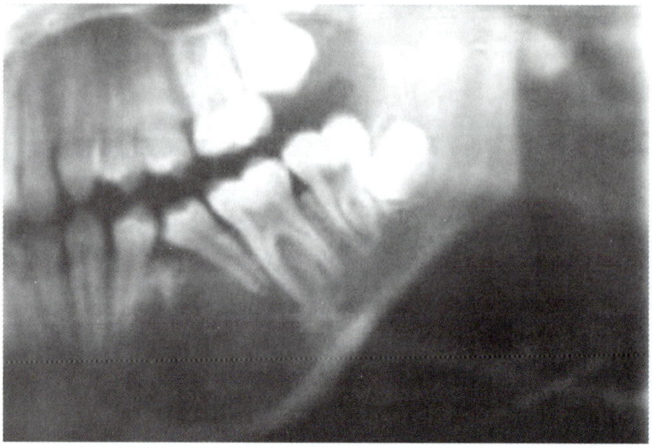

Fig. 8.8: The lateral oblique view showing a lesion causing displacement of the roots of the premolars.

h. Any lesion that has the characteristics of malignancy.

The specific surgical techniques for the management of oral pathologic conditions can be as varied as those for surgical management of any other entity.

The basic surgical goals are the following.

Eradication of the Pathologic Condition

The therapeutic goal of any extirpative surgical procedure is to remove the entire lesion, leaving no cells that could proliferate and cause a recurrence of the lesion. The methods used to achieve this goal vary tremendously and depend on the nature of the pathologic condition with which one is dealing.

Functional Rehabilitation of the Patient

Although eradication of disease may be the most important goal of treatment, by itself it is frequently inadequate in the comprehensive treatment of patients. The second goal of any treatment used for eradication of disease is an allowance for the functional rehabilitation of the patient. After the primary objective of eradicating a lesion has been achieved, the most important consideration is dealing with the residual defects resulting from the extirpative surgery.

SURGICAL OPERATIONS USED FOR THE REMOVAL OF JAW TUMOURS

Enucleation and/or Curettage

Local removal of a tumour by instrumentation in direct contact with the lesion. Used for very benign type of the lesions (Fig. 8.9).

Resection

Removal of a tumour by incising through uninvolved tissues around the tumour, thus delivering the tumour without direct contact during instrumentation.

Marginal (segmental) Resection

Resection of a tumour without disruption of the continuity of the bone.

Partial Resection

Removal of a tumour by removing a full-thickness portion of the jaw.

Total Resection

Removal of a tumour by removal of the involved bone, e.g. maxillectomy and mandibulectomy.

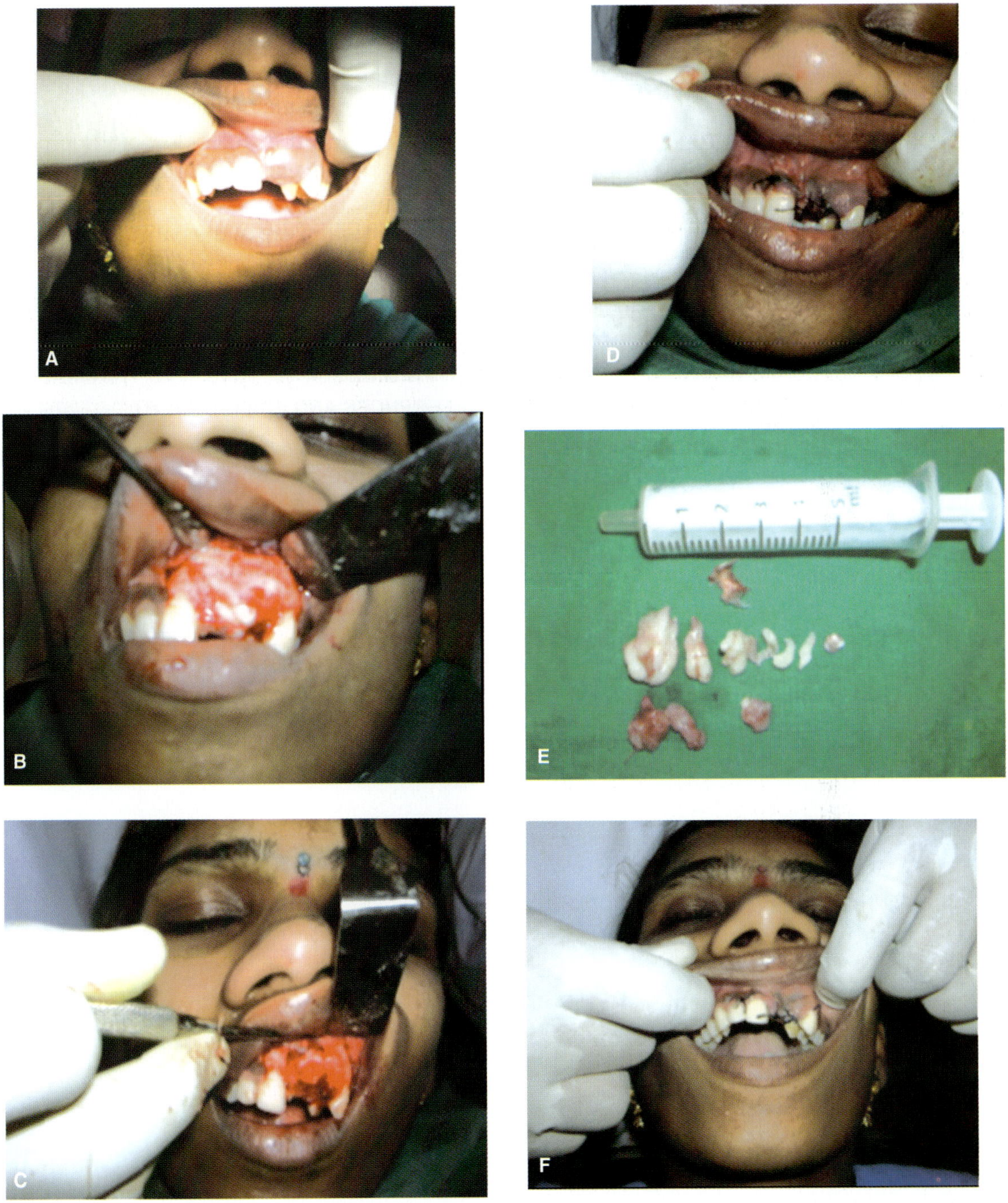

Fig. 8.9: Surgical removal of compound composite odontome. (A) Preoperative view, (B) Mucoperiosteal flap has been reflected thereby exposing a part of the compound composite odontome, (C) The compound composite odontome is removed, (D) Wound sutured with 3-0 black silk interrupted sutures, (E) The calcified masses with tooth-like appearance, (F) Postoperative view after 7 days.

Composite Resection

Resection of a tumour with bone, adjacent soft tissues and contiguous lymph node channels.

FACTORS THAT MUST BE EVALUATED BEFORE SURGERY

1. Aggressiveness of the lesion.
2. Anatomic location of the lesion.
3. The confinement of the lesion to bone.
4. The duration of the lesion.
5. Possible methods for reconstruction following surgery.

POSTOPERATIVE CARE OF THE PATIENTS OPERATED FOR TUMOURS OF THE ORAL CAVITY

1. The patient should be encouraged to maintain oral hygiene.
2. The diet of the patient should be such that it should not cause disturbance to the wound but at the same time the health of the patient should also be maintained.
3. Antibiotics and analgesics should be prescribed to prevent the wound from getting infected.
4. Periodic follow-up of the patient along with serial radiographs is essential to study the healing of the wound.

   Patient with a swelling in the region of the angle of the mandible.

REFERENCES AND BIBLIOGRAPHY

1. *Contemporary Oral and Maxillofacial Surgery,* 4th edn; Larry J. Peterson, Edward Ellis, James R. Hupp, Myron R. Tucker.
2. Killey and Kay's *Outline of Oral Surgery;* 2nd edn; Gordon R. Seward, Malcolm Harris, David A. McGowan.

Chapter 9

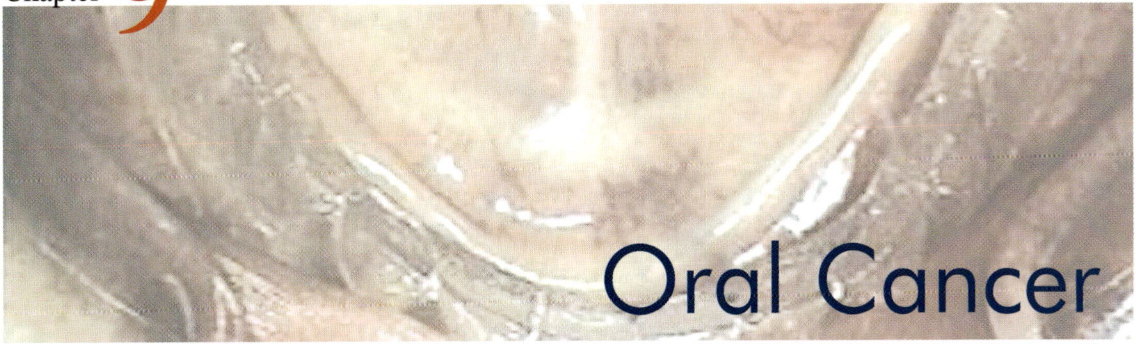

Oral Cancer

Malignancies of the oral cavity may arise from a variety of different tissues such as salivary gland, muscle, and blood vessels, or may even present as metastases from distant sites. Most common, however, are epidermoid carcinoma of the oral cavity. Oral cancer is a serious problem in many countries. Not only does it account for significant mortality, but it is also responsible for extensive disfigurement, loss of function, behavioural changes, and financial and sociologic hardships.

REASONS FOR DELAYED DETECTION AND TREATMENT

1. The public is generally unaware of oral cancer and its risk factors.
2. Approximately 50% of the public does not have routine dental or oral examinations and care.
3. Most early oral cancers are symptomless.
4. In the cancers that do produce symptoms, the symptoms are common to those produced by common dental diseases.
5. A significant number of clinicians may not perform a thorough systematic oral, face and neck examination.
6. A significant number of clinicians are not able to recognize pre-malignant lesions or early oral cancer.
7. Unnecessary delays occur among lesion detection, diagnosis and treatment.
8. Some practitioners treat oral cancer only occasionally. This means that the treatment received by the patient is inferior to that rendered by a practitioner who treats oral cancer on a regular basis.

PREMALIGNANT LESIONS AND PREDISPOSING CONDITIONS

Some oral lesions show a propensity to become cancerous as time progresses. Some predisposing systemic conditions increase the risk of oral cancer (Fig. 9.1).

Premalignant Lesions

a. Erythroplakia
b. Speckled leukoplakia and erythroleukoplakia
c. Leukoplakia (homogenous type) (Fig. 9.2)
d. Lichenoid dysplasia
e. Proliferative verrucous leukoplakia
f. Candidal infection

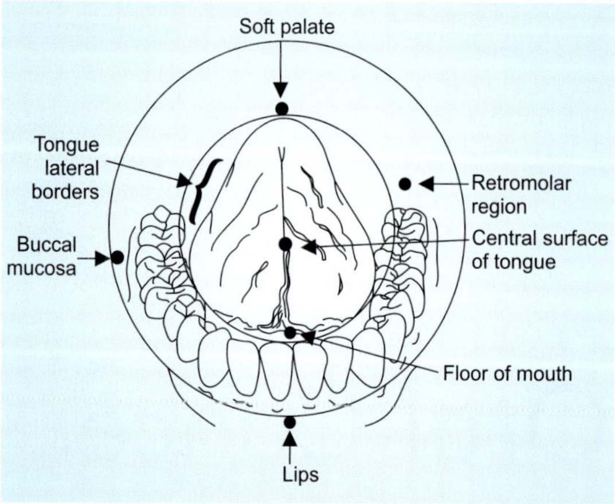

Fig. 9.1: High risk oval identifies the most frequent sites of oral squamous cell carcinoma.

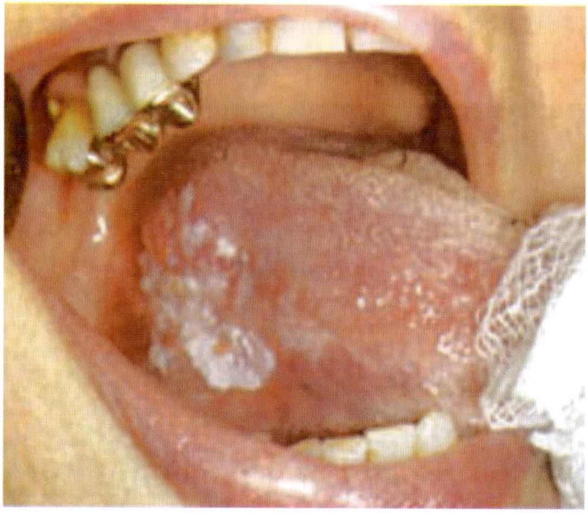

Fig. 9.2: Leukoplakic patch of the right lateral border of the tongue caused due to chronic irritation from the sharp posterior teeth.

Predisposing Conditions

a. Submucous fibrosis
b. Immune deficiency states
c. Dyskeratosis congenita
d. Syphilitic glossitis
e. Ethnic and family history of oral cancer
f. Atrophic, erosive or bullous lichen planus
g. Diets low in fresh vegetables, fruits or grains

SYMPTOMS AND SIGNS OF ORAL CANCER

1. Lump or swelling
2. Rough spot
3. Crust
4. Pain or tenderness
5. Bleeding
6. Change in bite
7. Loose tooth or teeth
8. Malfitting denture
9. Neck lump or swelling
10. Restriction of the tongue
11. Change in jaw movement
12. Dysgeusia (change in taste)
13. Change in sensation. (hyperaesthesia, parasthesia or anaesthesia)
14. Paresis or paralysis
15. Diplopia
16. Chronic cough
17. Speech change
18. Voice change
19. Dysphagia
20. Symptoms of distant primary tumour.

CLINICAL APPEARANCES OF ORAL CANCER (Figs 9.3, 9.4)

1. Patch or plaque.
   i. Red
   ii. Red and white
   iii. White
2. Exophytic (rough) surface.
   i. Red
   ii. White
   iii. Pink
   iv. Multicoloured
   v. Ulcerated
   vi. Non-ulcerated.
3. Ulcer
4. Crust
5. Bluish, brownish or black lesion
6. Bleb.

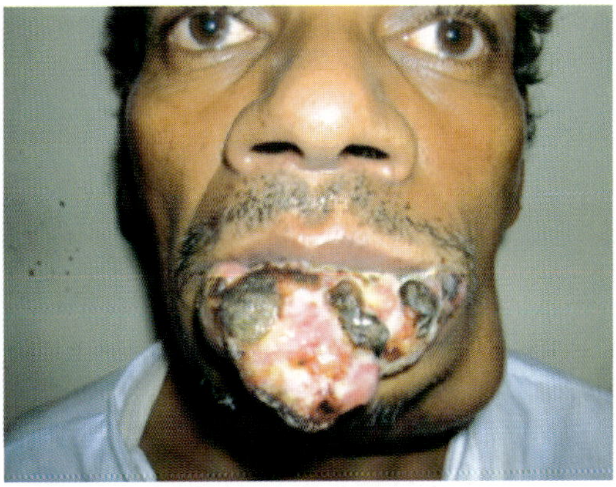

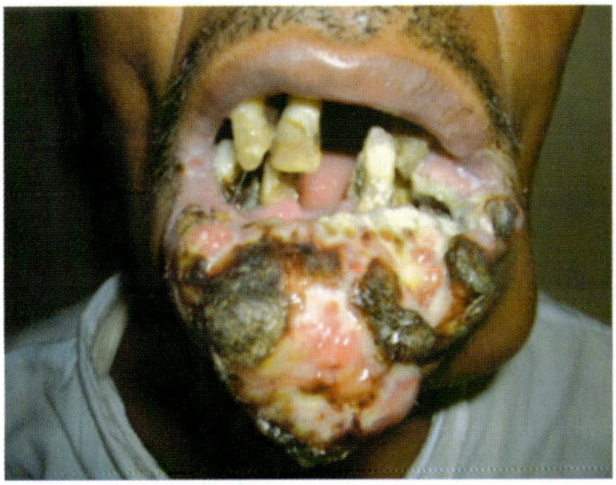

Fig. 9.3: Exophytic carcinoma of lip.

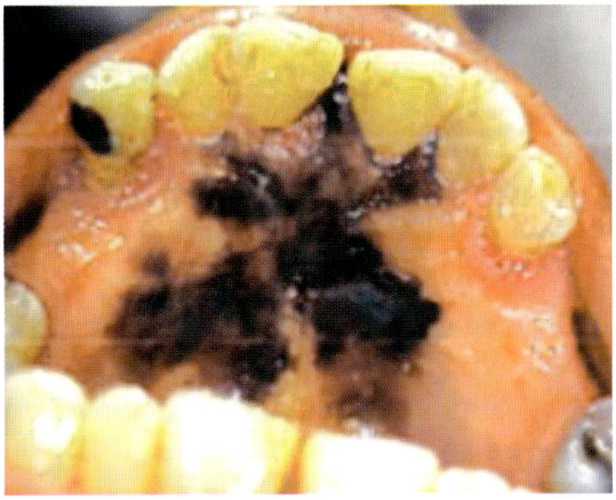

Fig. 9.4: Melanoma of the palate.

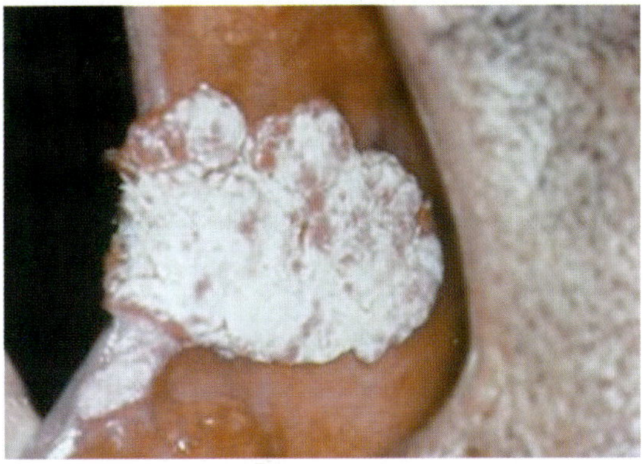

Fig. 9.5: Verrucous carcinoma of the commissure.

RADIOGRAPHIC APPEARANCE OF ORAL CANCER

1. Radiolucency with ragged and vague borders.
2. Bandlike widening of the periodontal ligament.
3. Combined radiolucent—radiopaque lesion with a vague pattern.
4. Radiopacity with vague borders.
5. Sunburst appearance from the border of the bone, possibly combined with changes in the first three appearances.
6. Onionskin appearance from the border of the bone, possibly combined with changes in the first three appearances.

TYPES OF INTRAORAL MALIGNANCIES

1. Primary
   a. Squamous cell carcinoma (90% to 95%)
   b. Malignant salivary gland tumour
   c. Mesenchymal, osteogenic sarcoma, chondrosarcoma and others.
   d. Melanoma
   e. Verrucous carcinoma (Fig. 9.5).
2. Systemic
   a. Metastatic carcinoma
   b. Multiple myeloma.
3. Lymphoma and leukemia
4. Kaposi's sarcoma.

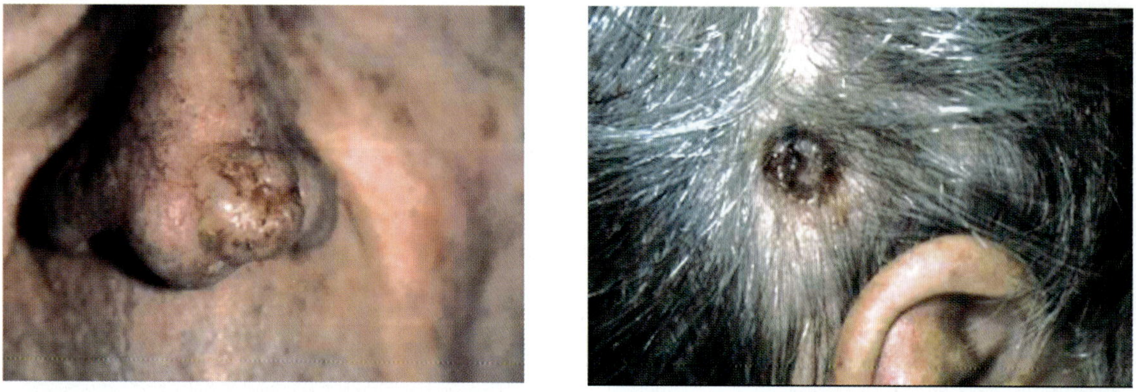

Fig. 9.6: Basal cell carcinoma. (A) Nodular type. (B) Pigmented type.

PERIORAL MALIGNANCIES

1. Cervical lymph node metastasis.
2. Salivary cancers of the parotid and submandibular glands.
3. Basal cell carcinoma of the face (Fig. 9.6).
4. Malignancy of the maxillary sinus.

TRIAGE OF LESIONS

1. Low suspicion index: Treat and follow to observe disappearance within 2 weeks; upgrade if appropriate.
2. Moderate suspicion index: Refer immediately.
3. High suspicion index: Refer immediately.

TUMOUR CLASSIFICATION

First the lesion is staged using the TNM system. The TNM classification has been used for many years. Microscopic evaluation of the degree of anaplasia at the deep invading borders is used to supplement this system.

The location or site of the lesions is factored in to render a composite formula of ***STNMP***, in which **S** means "site" and **P** means "histodifferentiation".

TNM Classification

*The **T** (primary tumour) categories:*

- $\mathbf{T_1}$—Greatest diameter of the primary tumour is 2 cm or less.
- $\mathbf{T_2}$—Greatest diameter of the primary tumour is more than 2 cm but no more than 4 cm.
- $\mathbf{T_3}$—Greatest diameter of the primary tumour is more than 4 cm.
- $\mathbf{T_4}$—Massive tumour of more than 4 cm involves adjacent structures.

*The **N** (cervical lymph node) categories:*

- $\mathbf{N_0}$—No clinically positive nodes.
- $\mathbf{N_1}$—Single clinically positive homolateral node 3 cm or less in diameter.
- $\mathbf{N_2}$—Single clinically positive homolateral node more than 3 cm but no more than 6 cm in diameter or multiple clinically positive homolateral nodes, none more than 6 cm in diameter.
- $\mathbf{N_3}$—Massive homolateral node(s), bilateral nodes, or contralateral node(s).

*The **M** (distant metastasis) categories:*

- $\mathbf{M_0}$—No (known) distant metastasis.
- $\mathbf{M_1}$—Distant metastasis present.

TREATMENT MODALITIES FOR MALIGNANCIES

Malignancies of the oral cavity are treated with surgery, radiation, chemotherapy or a combination of these modalities. The treatment for any given case depends on several factors, including, the histopathologic diagnosis, the location of the tumour, the presence and degree of metastasis, the radiosensitivity and chemosensitivity of the tumour, the age and the general physical condition of the patient, the experience of the treating clinicians and the wishes of the individual. In general, if a lesion can be completely excised without mutilating the patient, this is the preferred modality. If spread to regional lymph nodes is suspected, radiation may be employed before or after surgery to help eliminate small foci of malignant cells in the adjacent areas. If widespread systemic metastasis is detected, or if a tumour, such as lymphoma, is especially chemosensitive, chemotherapy is used with or without surgery and radiation.

Modes of Cancer Treatment

1. Surgery
2. Irradiation (external or interstitial)
3. Chemotherapy (seldom used alone)
4. Immunotherapy
5. Combinations of all of these

Most head and neck tumour boards also include a general dentist, a maxillofacial prosthodontist, a nutritionist, a speech pathologist, and because of the potential mutilative nature of surgery, a sociologist/psychiatrist.

RADIOTHERAPY

Radiotherapy (Fig. 9.7) for treatment of malignant neoplasms is based on the fact that tumour cells in stages of active growth are more susceptible to ionizing radiation than adult tissue. The faster the cells are multiplying, or the more undifferentiated the tumour cells, the more likely that radiation is to be effective. Radiation prevents the cells from multiplying by interfering with their nuclear material.

Radiation can be delivered to the patient in several different forms, including implantation of radioactive material into the tumour. The patient's host tissues in the immediate area of the tumour are spared of the total effect of the radiation by two mechanisms of delivery: fractionation and multiple ports.

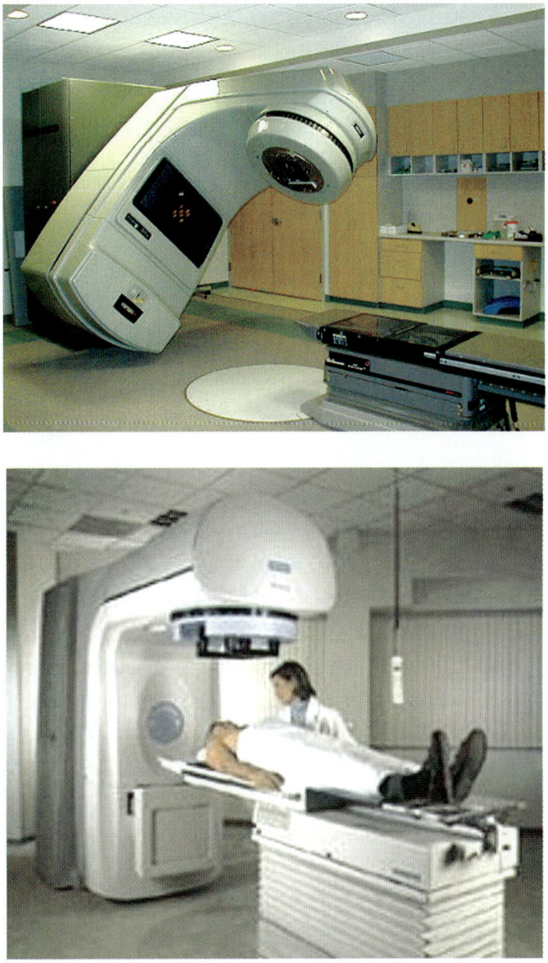

Fig. 9.7: Chemotherapy equipment.

CHEMOTHERAPY

Chemicals that act by interferring with rapidly growing tumour cells are used for treating many types of malignancies. These chemicals affect the normal cells to some extent. Most of these agents are given intravenously, but recently injections into the arteries feeding the tumour have been used. Because the agents are delivered systemically, they adversely affect many different body systems. Most affected is the haematopoietic system because of its rapid rate of cell turnover.

To reduce the toxicity of a single agent given in large quantities, multiple-agent therapy is frequently administered.

Chemotherapeutic Agents

- 5-fluorourasil
- Cisplatin
- Methotrexate
- Cyclophosphamide
- Vinblastine
- Doxorubicin (Adriamycin)
- Bleomycin

SURGERY

The surgical procedures for excision of oral malignancies varies with the type and extent of lesion. Small epidermoid carcinomas that are in accessible areas (for instance the lower lip) and are not associated with palpable lymph nodes can be excised. A larger lesion associated with palpable lymph nodes or a similar lesion in the area of the tonsillar pillar may need extensive surgery for adequate removal of it and it's local metastases. Malignancies of the oral cavity that have either suspected or proven lymph node involvement are candidates for composite resection, in which the lesion, surrounding tissues and lymph nodes of the neck are removed in toto. This procedure may produce extensive loss of soft tissues, making functional and aesthetic rehabilitation a long, involved process.

Surgical Modalities for Oral Cancer

1. Blade
2. Laser
3. Electrosurgery
4. Cryosurgery

MAJOR COMPLICATIONS OF ORAL CANCER TREATMENT

- Surgical defects with loss of aesthetics and function.
- Xerostomia and mucositis.
- Radiation caries and dental infection.
- Soft tissue infections.
- Osteoradionecrosis.

REFERENCE AND BIBLIOGRAPHY

1. *Differential Diagnosis of Oral and Maxillofacial Lesions*, 5th edn; Norman K.Wood, Paul W. Goaz.

Chapter 10

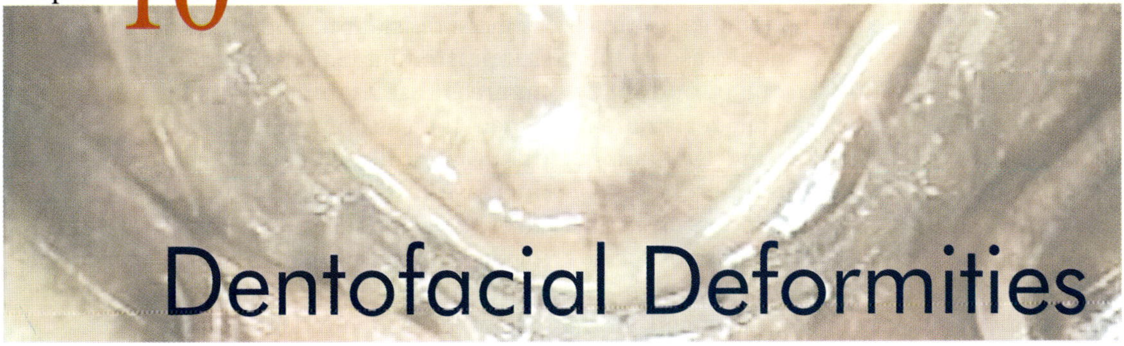

Dentofacial Deformities

Patients with congenital or acquired abnormalities of facial bones and soft tissue generally require the assistance of many medical and dental specialists to achieve maximal rehabilitation. Patients with malocclusions and facial abnormalities resulting from an abnormal growth of facial bones usually require the services of general dentists, prosthodontists, periodontists, orthodontists and oral and maxillofacial surgeons.

EVALUATION OF DENTOFACIAL DEFORMITY PATIENTS

Many areas of dental practice, in addition to orthodontics and surgery, must be integrated to address the complex problems of patients with dental deformities. This integrated approach, used throughout the evaluation and presurgical and postsurgical phases of patient care, provides the best possible results for these patients.

The most important phase in patient care centers on evaluation of the existing problems and definition of treatment goals. At the initial appointment a thorough interview should be conducted with the patient to discuss his or her perception of the problems as well as the goals of any possible treatment that may be accomplished. The patient's current health status and any medical and psychologic problems that may affect treatment are also discussed.

The involved orthodontist and oral and maxillofacial surgeon should conduct a thorough examination of facial structure with consideration of full-face as well as profile aesthetics. Evaluation of facial aesthetics in the full-face view should assess the presence of asymmetries and evaluate overall facial balance. The evaluation should include assessment of the position of the forehead, eyes, infraorbital rims, paranasal areas, malar eminences, configuration and width of the alar base, lip morphology, relationship of the lips to the incisors and overall proportional relationships of the face in the vertical and transverse dimension. The profile evaluation allows an assessment of the anteoposterior and vertical relationships of the components of the face. The nasolabial angle and the soft tissue configuration of the throat should also be evaluated. Photographic documentation of the pre-treatment condition of the patient should be a standard part of the evaluation.

A complete dental examination should include assessment of the dental arch form, symmetry, tooth alignment and occlusal abnormalities in the transverse, anteroposterior, and vertical dimensions. The muscles of mastication and TMJ function should also be evaluated. A screening periodontal examination, including probing, should assess the patient's hygiene and current periodontal health status. Impressions and bite registration for dental cast construction and evaluation should also be obtained at this time.

Lateral cephalometric and panoramic radiographs as well as posteroanterior facial films and TMJ films, when indicated, are an important part of the initial assessment. It is important to note, however, that cephalometric radiographs are only a part of the evaluation process. Cephalometric evaluation should be combined with clinical assessment of the patient's facial structure and occlusion when the nature of the deformity is determined and possible treatment is planned. After careful clinical assessment and evaluation of the diagnostic records, a problem list and treatment plan should be developed.

PRESURGICAL TREATMENT PHASE

Periodontal Considerations

As the first step in treatment, gingival inflammation must be controlled and the patient's cooperation ensured. In patients who are unwilling or unable to clean their teeth properly before the placement of orthodontic appliances, oral hygiene procedures will be even less effective when complicated by orthodontic band placement. Periodontal therapy including oral hygiene instructions, scaling and root planing; in certain instances, flap surgery to gain access for root planning may be needed to provide proper tissue health. Whenever possible, it is desirable to delay comprehensive treatment until adequate patient compliance and control of inflammation are achieved.

As a result of the periodontal examination findings and proposed orthodontic—surgical plan, mucogingival surgery is often accomplished during this initial phase of therapy to provide a zone of attached keratinized tissue, which is more resistant to potential orthodontic and surgical trauma. Soft tissue grafting is indicated in areas that have no keratinized gingiva or where there is only a thin band of keratinized tissue with little or no attachment when an increase in the amount of tissue trauma is likely. Such trauma to these areas includes labial orthodontic movement of teeth or a surgical procedure such as a genioplasty or segmental osteotomies in interdental areas.

Restorative Considerations

During the pre-surgical restorative phase, the patient is evaluated for carious lesions and faulty restorations. Teeth should be evaluated endodontically and periodontally for restorability, and any non-restorable teeth should be extracted before surgical intervention. All carious lesions should be restored early in the presurgical treatment phase. Existing restorations must function for 18—24 months during the orthodontic and surgical treatment phases, requiring that more durable restorative materials are employed, even though they may be replaced during the definitive post-surgical treatment phase. It is wise to delay final restorative treatment until the proper skeletal relationships are achieved and the finishing orthodontics completed.

In the edentulous or partially edentulous patient, particular attention is paid to residual ridge shape and contour in denture-bearing areas. The distance between the maxillary tuberosity, posterior mandible and ramus areas must be evaluated to ensure that adequate space is present for partial or complete dentures. Teeth that serve as removable partial denture abutments should be evaluated for potential retentive undercuts. If undercuts can be enhanced by minor orthodontic movement, this information is conveyed to the orthodontist.

Presurgical Orthodontic Considerations

It is obvious that not all malocclusions need to be corrected with surgery. When the skeletal discrepancy is minimal and orthodontic compensation does not adversely affect dental or facial aesthetics or post-treatment stability, orthodontic treatment alone is the treatment of choice. However, when orthodontic compensation for a skeletal abnormality results in an adequate occlusion but poor facial or dental aesthetics or a poor long term prognosis for post-treatment retention, surgery should be combined with orthodontic treatment (Fig. 10.1).

Treatment Timing

Treatment of the stable adult deformity can be started without delay, but questions often arise about how to best manage the growing child who is identified as having a developing dentofacial deformity. If the facial pattern is favourable and adequate growth potential remains, growth modification with functional appliances may be the preferred approach to dentofacial problems. Surgery usually is reserved for patients who do not respond to growth modification. As a general guideline, orthognathic surgery should be delayed until growth is complete in patients who have problems of excess growth, although surgery can be considered earlier for patients with growth deficiencies.

Orthodontic Treatment Objectives

Dental compensations for the skeletal deformity are corrected before surgery by orthodontically repositioning teeth properly over the underlying skeletal component without considerations for the bite relationship to the opposing arch. The essential steps in orthodontic preparation are to align the arches individually, achieve compatibility of the arches or arch segments, and establish the proper anteroposterior and vertical position of the incisors. The amount of

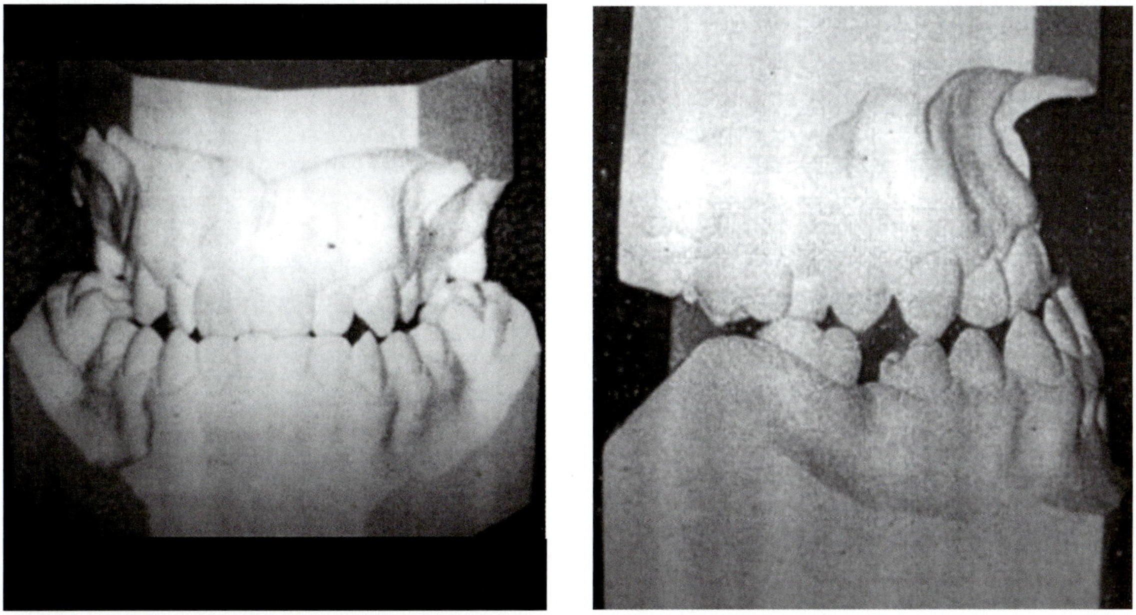

Fig. 10.1: Pretreatment models are made to study the dental as well as skeletal relationships.

presurgical orthodontics can vary, ranging from only appliance placement in a few patients to approximately 12 months of appliance therapy in those with severe crowding and incisor malposition. As the patient is approaching the end of orthodontic preparation for surgery, It is helpful to take impressions and examine the hand-articulated models for occlusal compatibility. Minor interferences that exist can be corrected easily with arch wire adjustment, significantly enhancing the post-surgical occlusal result. After any final orthodontic adjustments have been made, large stabilizing arch wires are inserted into the brackets. These provide the strength needed to withstand the forces resulting from intermaxillary fixation.

SURGICAL TREATMENT PHASE

After the completion of the presurgical periodontics, restorative dentistry and orthodontics, the patient returns to the oral and maxillofacial surgeon for final presurgical planning. At this appointment the evaluation completed at the initial patient examination is repeated. The patient's facial structure and the malocclusion are re-examined. Presurgical photographs, radiographs and presurgical models are taken, and a centric relation bite registration and face bow recording for model mounting are completed.

Mock surgery on a duplicated set of presurgical dental casts determines the exact surgical movements necessary to accomplish the desired postoperative occlusion. Prediction tracings coordinated with dental casts determine the desired postoperative facial aesthetic result. After completion of the model surgery and prediction tracings, the orthodontist and the general dentist are consulted to ensure that the predicted occlusal result is acceptable to all practitioners involved in the patient's treatment. Any orthodontic or restorative changes necessary to improve postsurgical position should be planned at this time.

PERIOPERATIVE CARE OF THE ORTHOGNATHIC SURGICAL PATIENT

Patients undergoing orthognathic surgery are admitted to the hospital the day before or the day of surgery. Before surgery a complete physical examination, preoperative laboratory tests and radiographic examinations and consultations with the anaesthesiologist are completed. Orthognathic surgery is accomplished in the operating room with the patient under general anaesthesia. After surgery the patients are taken to the recovery room for an appropriate period of time and returned to their hospital rooms later. Postoperative progress is continually monitored by a nursing staff trained and experienced in the postoperative care of the surgery patient. As soon as is feasible, postoperative radiographs are obtained to ensure that the predicted bony changes have taken place. The patient is discharged when feeling comfortable, taking food and fluid orally without difficulty and ambulating well. The postsurgical hospital stay generally ranges from 2 to 4 days. The importance of postoperative nutrition should be discussed with patients and their families before the hospital admission for surgery. Immediately after the intermaxillary fixation is released, the interocclusal splint used at the time of surgery can be wired to either the upper or lower jaw. Light elastics are then placed on the surgical wires and the combination of the splint and elastics serve to guide the jaw into the new postsurgical occlusion. After an adequate accommodation period the occlusal splint is removed and the patient returned to the orthodontist's care.

POSTSURGICAL TREATMENT PHASE

Completion of Orthodontics

When satisfactory range of jaw motion and stability of the osteotomy sites are achieved, the orthodontic treatment can be finished.

The heavy surgical arch wires are removed and replaced with light orthodontic wire. Final alignment and positioning of teeth is accomplished, as is closure any residual extraction space. The light vertical elastics are left in place at this time to override proprioceptive impulses from the teeth, which otherwise would cause the patient to seek a new position of maximum intercuspation. The settling process proceeds rapidly, rarely taking longer than 6 months. Retention after surgical orthodontics is no different than for other adult patients, and definitive periodontal and prosthetic treatment can be initiated immediately after the final occlusal relationships have been established.

The treatment of patients with dentofacial deformity involves the evaluation and treatment of many types of dental and skeletal problems. These problems require that all practitioners involved in patient care interact in a multidisciplinary team approach to treatment. This sequential team approach yields the most satisfying results.

REFERENCE AND BIBLIOGRAPHY

1. *Contemporary Oral and Maxillofacial Surgery* 4th edn; Larry J. Peterson, Edward Ellis, James R. Hupp, Myron R. Tucker.

Chapter 11

Preprosthetic Surgeries

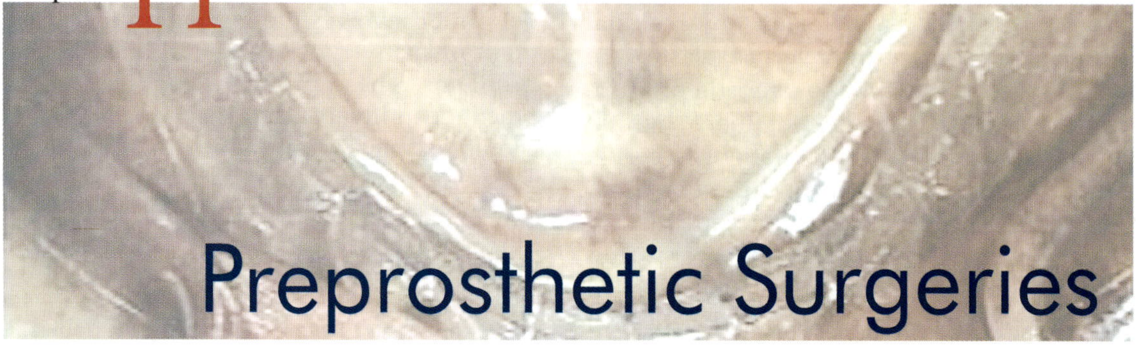

In spite of dentistry's improved ability to maintain dentition, there continues to be a large portion of the population that requires replacement of some or all of their teeth. Surgical improvement of the denture bearing area and surrounding tissues offers an exciting and demanding challenge in the area of surgical practice. Many minor modifications of the alveolar ridge and vestibular areas can greatly improve denture stability and retention.

The prosthetic replacement of lost or congenitally absent teeth frequently involves surgical preparation of the remaining oral tissues to support the best possible prosthetic replacement. Often oral structures, such as frenal attachments and exostosis, have no significance when teeth are present but become obstacles to proper prosthetic appliance construction after tooth loss. The challenge of prosthetic rehabilitation of the patient includes restoration of the best masticatory function possible, combined with restoration or improvement of dental and facial aesthetics.

OBJECTIVES OF PREPROSTHETIC SURGERY

The objective of preprosthetic surgery is to create proper supporting structures for subsequent placement of prosthetic appliances. The best denture support has the following characteristics.

1. No evidence of intraoral or extraoral pathologic conditions.
2. Proper jaw relationship in the antero-posterior, transverse and vertical dimensions.
3. Alveolar processes that are as large as possible and of the proper configuration. (The ideal shape of the alveolar process is a broad U-shaped ridge with the vertical component as parallel as possible.)
4. No bony or soft tissue protuberances or undercuts.
5. Adequate attached keratinized mucosa in the primary denture bearing area.
6. Adequate vestibular depth.

PRINCIPLES OF PATIENT EVALUATION AND TREATMENT PLANNING

Before any surgical or prosthetic treatment, a thorough evaluation outlining problems to be solved and a detailed treatment plan should be developed for each patient. It is imperative that no preparatory surgical procedure be undertaken without a clear understanding of the desired design of the final prosthesis.

Preprosthetic surgical treatment must begin with a thorough history and physical examination of the patient. An extremely important aspect of the history is to obtain a clear idea of the patient's chief complaint and expectations of surgical and prosthetic treatment. Aesthetic and functional goals of the patient must be assessed carefully and a determination made as to whether these expectations can be met. Psychologic factors and the adaptability of patient's are important determinants of their ability to function equately with full or partial dentures. Information on success or failure with previous prosthetic appliances may be helpful in determining the patient's attitude towards adaptability to prosthetic treatment. The history should include important information such as the patient's risk factors for surgery, with a particular emphasis on systemic diseases that may affect bone or soft tissue healing.

An intraoral and extraoral examination should include an assessment of the following:

a. The existing tooth relationships, if any remain.
b. Amount and contour of remaining bone.
c. Quality of soft tissue overlying the primary denture bearing area.
d. Vestibular depth.
e. Location of muscle attachments.
f. Jaw relationships.
g. Presence of soft tissue or bony pathologic conditions.

EVALUATION OF SUPPORTING BONY TISSUES

Evaluation of the supporting bone should include visual inspection, palpation, radiographic examination, in some cases evaluation of models. Abnormalities of the remaining bone can often be assessed during the visual inspection; however, because of bony resorption and location of muscle or soft tissue attachments, many abnormalities may be obscured. Palpation of all areas of the maxilla and mandible, including the primary denture bearing area and the vestibular area, is necessary.

Evaluation of the denture-bearing area of the maxilla includes an overall evaluation of the bony ridge form. No bony undercuts or gross bony protuberances that block the path of denture insertion should be allowed to remain in the area of the alveolar ridge, buccal vestibule or palatal vault. Adequate post-tuberosity notching must exist for posterior denture stability and peripheral seal.

The remaining mandibular ridge should be evaluated for overall ridge form and contour, gross ridge irregularities, tori, and buccal exostosis. The location of the mental foramen and mental neurovascular bundle can be palpated in relation to the superior aspect of the mandible and neurosensory disturbances noted.

Evaluation of the interarch relationship of the maxilla and the mandible is extremely important and includes an examination of the anteroposterior and vertical relationships as well as any possible skeletal asymmetries that may exist between the maxilla and the mandible. Careful attention must be paid in the interarch distance, particularly in the posterior areas. Any vertical excess of tuberosity, either bony or soft tissue, may impinge on space necessary for placement of a prosthesis that is properly constructed.

Proper radiographs are an important part of the initial diagnosis and treatment planning. Panoramic radiographs provide the most information on the assessment of the underlying bony structure and pathologic conditions. Radiographs should disclose bony pathologic lesions, impacted teeth, portions of remaining roots, bony pattern of the alveolar ridge, and the size and pneumatization of the maxillary sinus.

EVALUATION OF SUPPORTING SOFT TISSUE

Assessment of the quality of tissue of the primary denture bearing area overlying the alveolar ridge is of utmost importance. The amount of keratinized tissue firmly attached to the underlying bone in the denture bearing area should be distinguished from poorly keratinized or freely movable tissue. Palpation discloses hypermobile fibrous tissue inadequate for a stable denture base

Tissue at the depth of the vestibule should be supple and without irregularities for maximal peripheral seal of the denture. Assessment of the vestibular depth should include manual palpation of the adjacent muscle attachments. By tensing the soft tissue adjacent to the area of the alveolar ridge, one can note the muscle or soft tissue attachments, which approximate the crest of the alveolar ridge and are often responsible for the loss of the peripheral seal of the denture during speech and mastication.

The lingual aspect of the mandible should be inspected with a mouth mirror in the lingual vestibule area to determine the level of attachment of the mylohyoid muscle in relation to the crest of the mandibular ridge and the attachment of the genioglossus muscle in the anterior mandible. The lingual vestibular depth should be evaluated with the tongue in several positions, since movement of the tongue accompanied by elevation of the mylohyoid and genioglossus muscles is a common cause of movement and displacement of the lower denture.

TREATMENT PLANNING

Before any surgical intervention, treatment plan addressing the patient's identified oral problems should be formulated. Maintenance of the redundant soft tissue may be found necessary to improve the results of the grafting procedure. If this tissue were removed without any consideration of the long-term benefits of a grafting procedure, both the opportunity for improved immediate function and the opportunity for long-term maintenance of bone tissue and soft tissue would be lost.

Preprosthetic surgical preparation of the denture supporting areas begins early in the treatment sequence. It may be necessary to delay definitive soft tissue procedures until underlying bony problems have been adequately resolved. However, when bone or alloplastic grafting or other more complex treatment of bony abnormalities is not required, both bony and soft tissue preparation can be completed simultaneously.

PERIOPERATIVE CARE

1. The patient should be encouraged to maintain oral hygiene.
2. The diet of the patient should be such that it should not cause disturbance to the wound but at the same time the health of the patient should also be maintained.
3. Antibiotics and analgesics should be prescribed to prevent the wound from getting infected.
4. If a surgical splint has been prepared the patient should be instructed to maintain the hygiene of the prosthesis.
5. Periodic follow-up of the patient along with serial radiographs is essential to study the healing of the wound.

REFERENCE AND BIBLIOGRAPHY

1. *Contemporary Oral and Maxillofacial Surgery*, 4th edn; Larry J. Peterson, Edward Ellis, James R. Hupp, Myron R. Tucker.

Chapter 12

Implantology

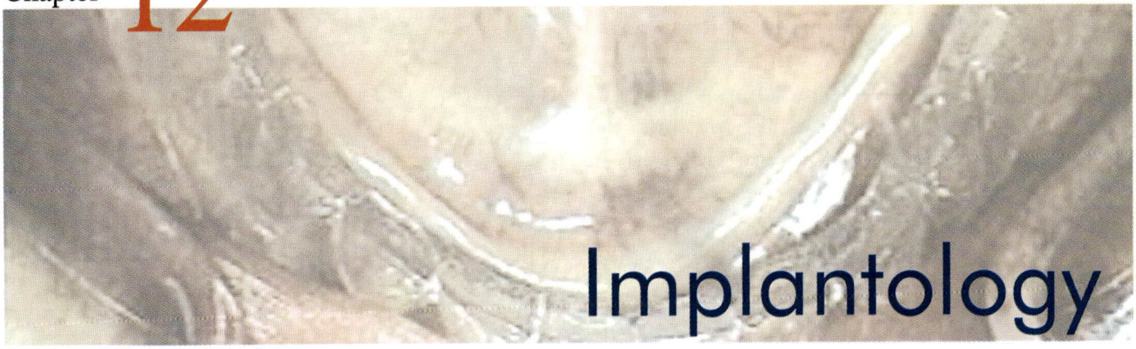

The success of newer implant systems is presently revolutionizing dentistry. Although some dentists have not participated in this revolution yet, it will occur and dentistry will never be the same. Compared to other dental innovations, implantology has enjoyed a rapid and progressive development. The quantum leap made in implant dentistry has been the result of tireless work by contemporary dentists who have pioneered the surgical and prosthetic procedures to which all of us today owe a debt of gratitude. Preceding this clinical advance is a solid foundation of research that definitively supports dental implantology as a viable alternative to conventional dentistry. Included in this framework of bioscience are a myriad of advances in new implant systems, implant biomaterials and new, improved diagnostic procedures to guide our surgical techniques. Added to this are advances in manufacturing of precision fit components which allow accurate dental restoration in concert with state of the art manufactured dental implants.

Today over 200 different dental implant systems are on the global market. Fifty different systems with FDA approval are available in the United States. Some of the newer systems incorporate technological advances which continue to improve the long-term survivability of dental implants and the restorative dental appliances placed upon them.

HISTORICAL PERSPECTIVE

The first attempts by man to replace lost teeth with implants dates to the 18th century when it was common practice to replace lost teeth with the teeth of other individuals. These individuals were usually young boys or girls who were paid for their donation. The implantation of other individuals teeth met with resounding failure as the body's immune system quickly attacked the foreign tissue leading to infection and rejection of the tooth.

Early pioneers in implantology quickly realized that other inert material such as ivory or gold were not rejected as quickly. Even though these materials were an abhorrent failure as well, it took longer for the body to reject them. Implantologists went back to work experimenting with different metals. In 1891 a physician named Hartman proposed that dentures be fixed to the jaws using metal screws. Although a great number of failures quickly led to the demise of this procedure as well, the foundation was laid for the first crude, potentially successful dental implant system. In 1939 a dental clinician by the name of Stock attempted to alter the shape of the dental implant to resemble a wood screw. This ushered in a new era of dental implantology with multiple variations of Stock's initial work.

In spite of new materials and shapes, implant success was fleeting. Although the implant site healed, loading of the dental implant with a crown or bridge quickly led to loosening of the fixture, with infection and failure.

It was during the early 1950's and 1960's that Per Ingvar' Branemark, beginning at the University of Lund and continuing at the University of Gottenburg in Sweden began researching the healing capabilities of the human body. One of his experiments involved the incorporation of two different types of metal cylinders into the jaw bone of rabbits. These metal cylinders were implanted in the bones of the rabbits to determine how the body healed after injury. Dr. Branemark theorized that the only way to observe the healing process was to place small optical chambers inside the metal cylinders directly in the bone. He observed that, at the end of the experiment, the optical chambers housed in titanium metal would not come out. They had "fused to the bone". He coined the term for this fusion "osseointegration". He used this term to describe the reaction of the titanium to the bone. This term is still used today and describes the successful placement of the dental implant into the jaw.

On the basis of these experiments other trials followed. This culminated with the development of an implant system that could be surgically placed in the jaws, allowed to osseointegrate and then be restored with metal connectors to artificial teeth and modified dentures.

With a few modifications, Branemark's system of dental implants has evolved into the most successful implant system in use today (Fig 12.1). New sizes and better and more user

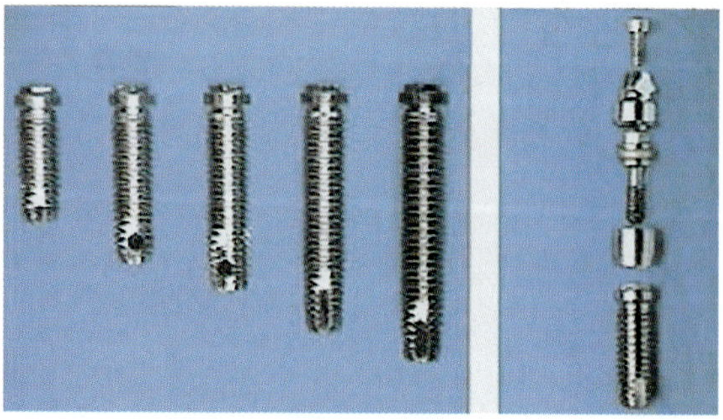

Fig. 12.1: Branemark implant system.

friendly components for the attachment teeth have been forthcoming.

IMPLANT TYPES (Figs 12.2 to 12.4)

Who is a candidate for Dental Implants?

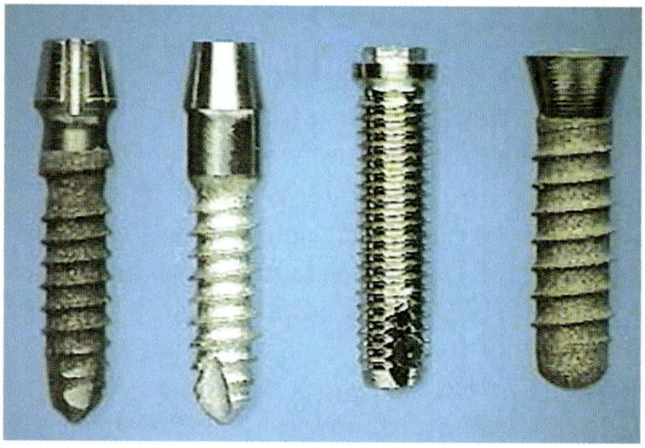

Fig. 12.2: Screw implants (Left to Right: TPS screw, Ledermann screw, Branemark screw, ITI Bonefit screw).

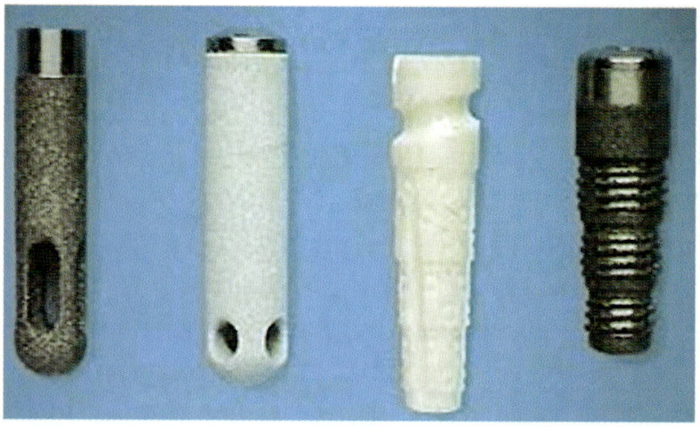

Fig. 12.3: Cylinder implants (Left to Right: IMZ, Integral, Frialit-1 step-cylinder, Frialit-2 step-cylinder).

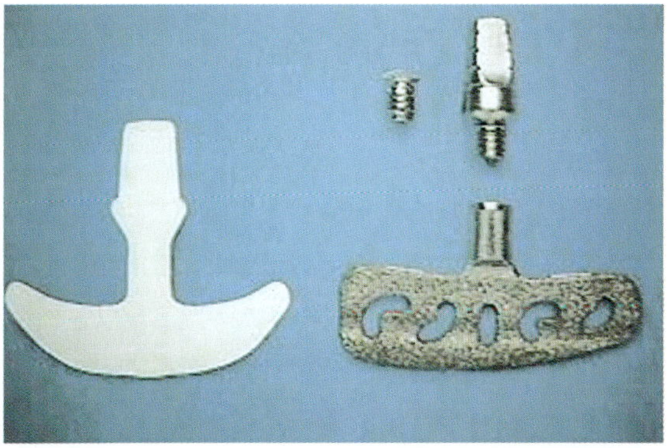

Fig. 12.4: Blade implants (Left: Single-post Biolox implant, Right: Single-post, two-stage titanium blade implant).

A great deal of information must be assimilated by the general dentist and oral surgeon to determine if you are a candidate for dental implants. Not all patients are candidates. In some cases more traditional, less expensive dental restorations will suffice to return the patient to good chewing function. Function is the key word. What is good chewing function for one patient may be inadequate function for another. Therefore, who is and who is not a candidate for dental implants requires a lengthy work-up to include x-rays, plaster molds of the occlusion and a detailed analysis of the patient's functional needs.

Just as important as the physical findings are the psychological needs of the patient. Losing ones teeth and replacing them with false teeth is not easily accepted by many patients. Those who find it emotionally traumatic are most appreciative of the dentist's ability to replace natural teeth with appliances that are firmly anchored to the jaws. Some of the questions that must be answered by the initial work-up are as follows:

- Do the upper and lower jaws align well enough to allow proper orientation of the implants and the appliances that fix to them?
- Are the sinus cavities in the upper jaw or the nerve running through the lower jaw in such a position as to limit the size and orientation of the implants?
- Does the patient have enough thickness of bone to hold the implants?
- Can the patient physically care for and clean the dental appliances that connect to the implants?

In addition to these questions which must be answered, there are many medical conditions which contraindicate implant placement.

- Pathologic conditions of the jaw.
- Diseases of the salivary glands.
- Past surgeries in the face and neck region.
- Radiation therapy for treatment of cancer.
- Patient's age and nutritional status.
- Metabolic diseases, i.e. diabetes, hyper-thyroidism.
- Blood disorders, i.e. anemias, blood clotting disorders.
- Severe heart or lung diseases.
- Bone disorders, i.e. severe osteoporosis.
- Collagen disorders, i.e. scleroderma.

PREREQUISITES FOR SUCCESS

Dental implantology demands that the oral surgeon and restorative dentist have a profound grasp of the biological, physical and engineering principals which govern the placement of implants. In addition, the specialist's office must be structured and organized to stress the art of implantology. What is needed?

- Adequate equipment, instruments, and inventory of implants and components.
- High level of surgical skill.
- Highly trained and skilled auxiliary personnel.
- A modern and well equipped surgical facility.
- A II systematic method of documentation using x-rays and photographs.
- A systematic recall program to confirm long term success of the implants placed.

- An adequate number of patients per month who require implant surgery in order to insure a smooth surgical routine and the maintenance of the surgical skills of the doctor and his or her staff.

DIAGNOSIS AND TREATMENT PLANNING

The first step in successful implant reconstruction is the hardest; diagnosis and treatment planning. Before attempting any implants several steps must be completed.

- Analysis of x-rays and mounted plaster casts.
- Determination of the quality and amount of bone available for implant placement.
- Determination of the exact location for the implants through a wax pattern.
- Determination of the type of implant restoration to be built upon the dental implants.

ANALYSIS OF X-RAYS

X-rays of the jaws help to quantify and qualify the amount of bone available to support the dental implants. Implants come in various diameters and lengths. With few exceptions,

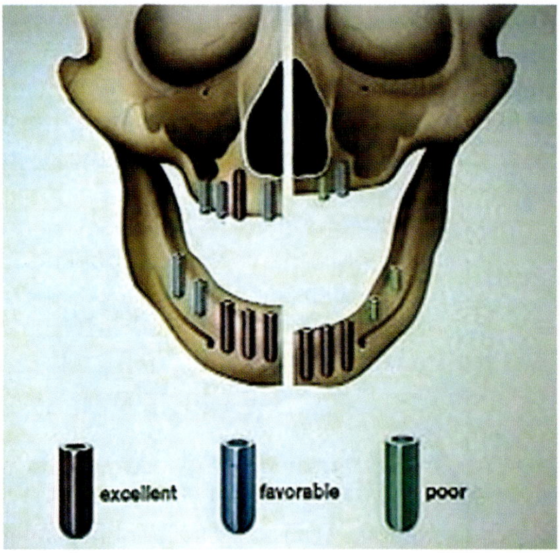

Fig. 12.5: Position of the maxillary sinus in the upper jaw.

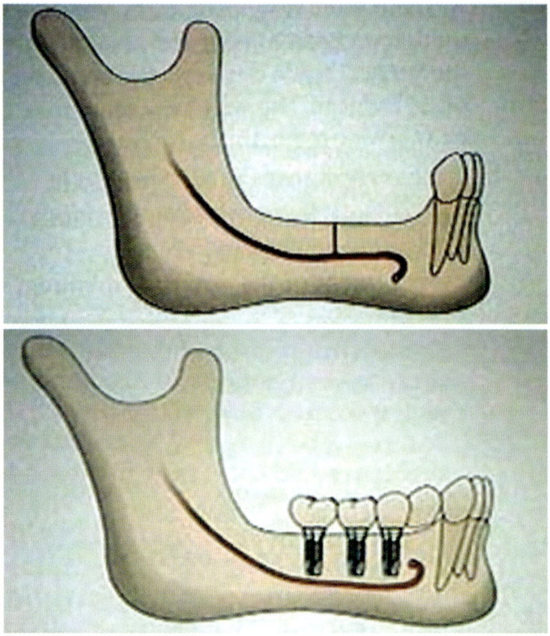

Fig. 12.6: Position of the mandibular nerve.

the longest and widest diameter implant that is possible to place in the jaw is the size favored. Many physical variables must be taken into consideration when determining the best size and shape of the implant (Figs 12.5, 12.6).

Thickness of Jawbone

Mounted plaster casts are important diagnostic tools because they allow the oral surgeon to

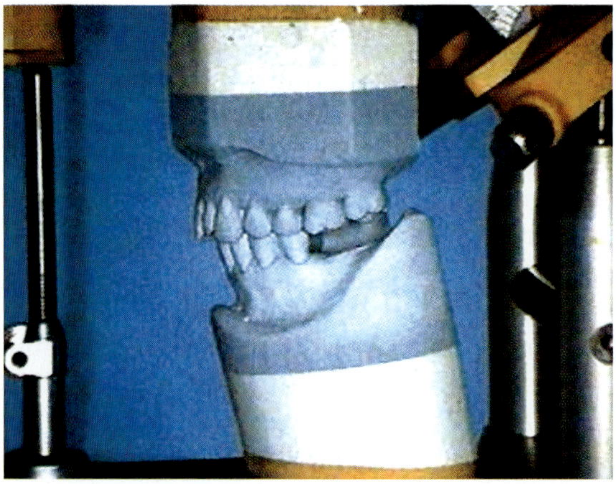

Fig. 12.7: Mounted plaster casts.

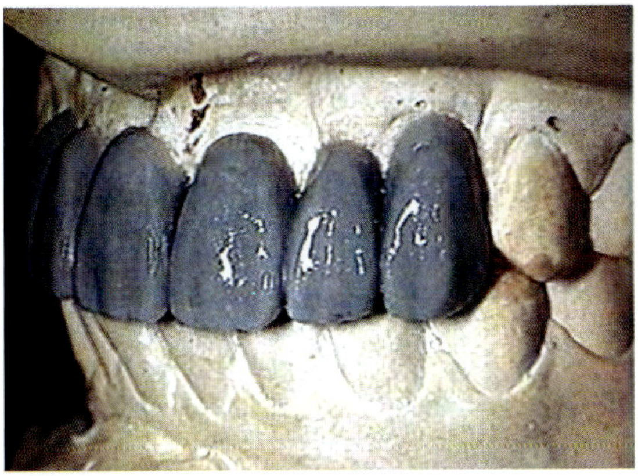

Fig. 12.8

accurately plan the placement of the implants (Fig. 12.7). They also allow the dentist to prepare a WAX MODEL of the anticipated final restoration before the implants have been placed in the bone (Fig. 12.8). Any changes in the position of the implants to achieve the most stable restoration can be made in the plaster and wax model first.

WAX MODEL DETERMINING THE AMOUNT OF BONE AND QUALITY OF BONE

Successful implants require good bone and plenty of it. Determining the amount of bone available and its quality is part science and part radiographic interpretation. The thickness of bone and the height of bone available is easily measured on CT DentaScan. The quality of bone, however, is harder to determine. The success of the implant is partly determined by how much surface area of the implant is embedded in and in intimate contact with the patient's bone. Denser bone, more calcified bone, provides a better interface for implant stabilization. Several classifications systems attempt to rate bone quality. These are beyond the scope of this Website. Suffice it to say that quality is as important as quantity. This becomes very apparent when one compares the success rate of upper jaw implants to lower jaw implants. The upper jaw is less dense. How long the implants will last is affected by this fact and is reflected in the increased success rate seen in lower jaw implants. Quality of the bone is one of the variables that, unfortunately, cannot be accurately determined prior to the placement of the implant.

DETERMINING THE EXACT LOCATION FOR THE IMPLANT

Successful reconstruction with dental implants requires accurate placement into good quality bone. The placement of the implant at the exact angle and position is paramount to success. As little as a few degrees error in placement or a

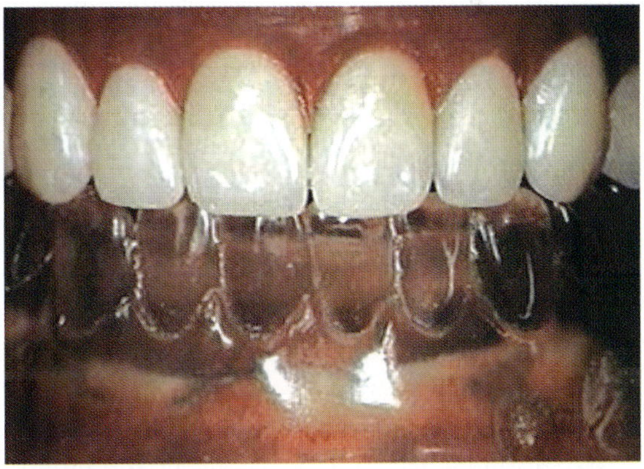

Fig. 12.9: Diagnostic plastic lower denture.

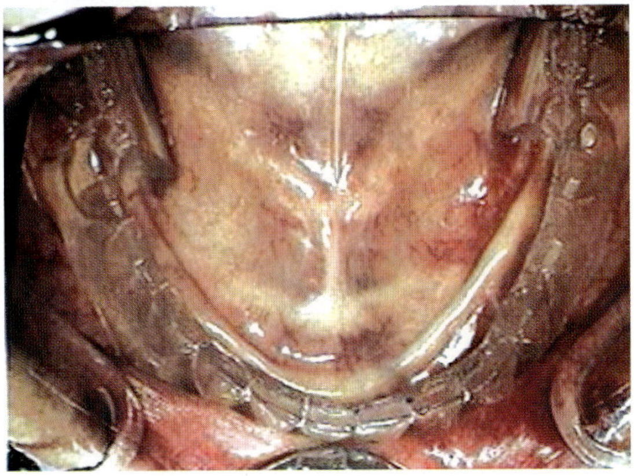

Fig. 12.10: View of same plastic denture from above.

few millimeters of error in position can limit success. Just like the foundation of a building or a bridge across a river, placement of the foundation is necessary for stability.

Cantilever and *poor angular positions* are to be minimized at all costs. To accurately place the implant requires a dental work-up that includes x-rays, preparing a wax model and mounted plaster casts. From the casts, the dentist will fabricate a surgical template to guide the placement of the implants into the bone (Figs 12.9, 12.10).

SUCCESS OF IMPLANTS

Long-term success of the dental implant requires a concerted effort on the part of the surgeon, the restoring dentist and the patient. Successful implant dentistry requires the following.

- Proper placement of the implant by the dental surgeon.
- Proper restoration of the implant by the restoring dentist.
- Proper care of the implant system by the patient.
- Proper placement, proper restoration and proper care ensures success. In spite of achieving these three requirements implants do not last forever. Success is measured in years of service. It is not measured by forever. All implants must be maintained and ultimately revised and replaced.

OBTAINING AND MAINTAINING A SUCCESSFUL IMPLANT

To obtain and maintain a successful implants, the oral surgeon must do the following.

- Accurately determine functional and aesthetic needs of the patient.
- Diagnose the dental health of the patient.
- Formulate the proper treatment plan.
- Select the best implant system.
- Treatment plan for the exact placement of the implant into the bone.
- Flawlessly execute the surgical placement of the implant.
- Prepare a dental restorative treatment plan which evenly and progressively loads the implants and avoids adverse forces on them.
- Prepare a dental restorative plan which accomplishes the aesthetic goals of the patient.
- Demand excellent oral hygiene and excellent oral care for the implant by the patient.

To define success of implant systems, the United States Department of Health and Human Services convened a conference on dental implants at Harvard University in 1980. At that conference success was defined as a 75% five-year survival rate of an implant. Today success rates surpass those defined by the 1980 Harvard conference. Today 90% 15-year success rates are commonplace for some implants.

A recent article in the *International Journal of Oral and Maxillofacial Implants*, entitled "Osseointegrated Implants for Single Tooth Replacement: A Five-year Multi-Center Study" sited a 96%, five-year survival rate of single tooth implants placed in the upper jaw. Success rates were even better in the lower jaw. How long your implants will last is impossible to predict. However, many clinicians agree that dental implants can be one of the most successful dental procedures done today.

REFERENCES AND BIBLIOGRAPHY

1. *Contemporary Oral and Maxillofacial Surgery*, 4th edn; Larry J. Peterson, Edward Ellis, James R. Hupp, Myron R. Tucker.

Chapter 13

AIDS and Its Oral Manifestations

Acquired Immunodeficiency Syndrome (AIDS) poses a significant challenge for health care institutions, care givers, patients and the community. The discovery of HIV and the development of HIV antibody screening tests have clarified many concerns regarding the disease. Every individual who is tested for HIV should receive pre- and post-test counselling and if found positive for HIV antibodies should continue to have psychological support, counselling on nutrition and regular medical checkup, etc. They should be encouraged to join self help groups to meet others in a similar situation. No HIV testing should be done without the individuals consent.

COUNSELLING IN HIV/AIDS

Education and counselling continue to be the main weapons for reducing the risk of infection and controlling the spread of HIV.

Counselling should be a face to face interaction. It should include discussion of the medical, psychological, social, ethical and legal implication of HIV. It is a continuous process from the day the HIV test turns positive to the very end. The needs of people living with HIV/AIDS vary at different times of their life and also for different individuals, depending on their emotional make up, cultural background and the community around them.

Essential elements of counselling include the following.

1. Being compassionate and nonjudgemental.
2. Allowing the patient to ask questions and to express feelings, concerns and reaction.
3. Helping the patient cope through further counselling or through referral for specialized services as necessary.

Counselling requires good interpersonal skills to establish rapport, which is particularly important.

Counselling at Various Points of Time

Pre- and Post-Test Counselling

When a dentist/physician suspects HIV infection, an informed consent is needed before HIV blood test is undertaken. Patient confidentiality is essential. Patient counselling includes providing information about HIV and the test, risk assessment, risk reduction and prevention of HIV transmission. A discussion on false positives and indeterminate results should be included.

If the patient is HIV positive, post test counselling is given. This includes help on how to inform his/her spouse and other close relatives, maintain the quality of life, reduce risk behaviour and avoid infecting others. Proper counselling will prevent two important issues at the ends of the spectrum - suicide and vengeance to spread the virus.

Well-being Counselling

It is essential especially in a country like India where majority of patients cannot afford antiretroviral drugs. High protein, high calorie diet at low cost with plenty of multivitamins, micronutrients, exercise, sleep, non-stressful activities, meditation and stress reduction protocols should be discussed.

Marriage Counselling

In addition to other pre-nuptial verifications and arrangements, a couple counselling session is appropriate in the context of high HIV prevalence among young people in India. This would include discussion of possible risks for HIV and behavioral strategies for prevention.

Grief Counselling

Since AIDS has no cure, the disease is fatal. But one can have a good quality of life if he/she is counselled and has a good support system. Eventually the family has to be prepared for death and helped to cope not only emotionally but also with the economic, legal issues that may follow.

HIV AND ITS TRANSMISSION

HIV and Its Transmission Research has revealed a great deal of valuable medical, scientific, and public health information about the human immunodeficiency virus (HIV) and acquired immunodeficiency syndrome (AIDS). The ways in which HIV can be transmitted have been clearly identified. Unfortunately, false information or statements that are not supported by scientific findings continue to be shared widely through the Internet or popular press. Therefore, the Centers for Disease Control and Prevention (CDC) has prepared this fact sheet to correct a few misperceptions about HIV.

HIV in the Environment

Scientists and medical authorities agree that HIV does not survive well in the environment, making the possibility of environmental transmission remote.

Households

Although HIV has been transmitted between family members in a household setting, this type of transmission is very rare. These transmissions are believed to have resulted from contact between skin or mucous membranes and infected blood.

Businesses and other Settings

There is no known risk of HIV transmission to co-workers, clients, or consumers from contact in industries such as food-service establishments (see information on survival of HIV in the environment). Food-service workers known to be infected with HIV need not be restricted from work unless they have other infections or illnesses (such as diarrhea or hepatitis A) for which any food-service worker, regardless of HIV infection status, should be restricted. CDC recommends that all food-service workers follow recommended standards and practices of good personal hygiene and food sanitation.

In 1985, CDC issued routine precautions that all personal-service workers (such as hairdressers, barbers, cosmetologists, and massage therapists) should follow, even though there is no evidence of transmission from a personal-service worker to a client or vice versa. Instruments that are intended to penetrate the skin (such as tattooing and acupuncture needles, ear piercing devices) should be used once and disposed of or thoroughly cleaned and sterilized.

Kissing

Casual contact through closed-mouth or "social" kissing is not a risk for transmission of HIV. Because of the potential for contact with blood during "French" or open-mouth kissing, CDC recommends against engaging in this activity with a person known to be infected. However, the risk of acquiring HIV during open-mouth kissing is believed to be very low. CDC has investigated only one case of HIV infection that may be attributed to contact with blood during open-mouth kissing.

Biting

In 1997, CDC published findings from a state health department investigation of an incident that suggested blood-to-blood transmission of HIV by a human bite. There have been other reports in the medical literature in which HIV appeared to have been transmitted by a bite. Severe trauma with extensive tissue tearing and damage and presence of blood were reported in each of these instances. Biting is not a common way of transmitting HIV. In fact, there are numerous reports of bites that did not result in HIV infection.

Saliva, Tears and Sweat

HIV has been found in saliva and tears in very low quantities from some AIDS patients. It is important to understand that finding a small amount of HIV in a body fluid does not necessarily mean that HIV can be transmitted by that body fluid. HIV has not been recovered from the sweat of HIV-infected persons. Contact with saliva, tears, or sweat has never been shown to result in transmission of HIV.

Insects

From the onset of the HIV epidemic, there has been concern about transmission of the virus by biting and bloodsucking insects. However, studies conducted by researchers at CDC and elsewhere have shown no evidence of HIV transmission through insects—even in areas where there are many cases of AIDS and large populations of insects such as mosquitoes. Lack of such outbreaks, despite intense efforts to detect them, supports the conclusion that HIV is not transmitted by insects.

The results of experiments and observations of insect biting behavior indicate that when an insect bites a person, it does not inject its own or a previously bitten person's or animal's blood into the next person bitten. Rather, it injects saliva, which acts as a lubricant or anticoagulant so the insect can feed efficiently. Such diseases as yellow fever and malaria are transmitted through the saliva of specific species of mosquitoes. However, HIV lives for only a short time inside an insect and, unlike organisms that are transmitted via insect bites; HIV does not reproduce (and does not survive) in insects. Thus, even if the virus enters a mosquito or another sucking or biting insect, the insect does not become infected and cannot transmit HIV to the next human it feeds on or bites. HIV is not found in insect feces. There is also no reason to fear that a biting or bloodsucking insect, such as a mosquito, could transmit HIV from one person to another through HIV-infected blood left on its mouth parts. Two factors serve to explain why this is so—first, infected people do not have constant, high levels of HIV in their bloodstreams and, second, insect mouth parts do not retain large amounts of blood on their surfaces. Further, scientists who study insects have determined that biting insects normally do not travel from one person to the next immediately after ingesting blood. Rather, they fly to a resting place to digest this blood meal.

OCCUPATIONAL HAZARDS

Healthcare personnel are at risk for occupational exposure to blood borne pathogens, including hepatitis B virus (HBV), hepatitis C virus (HCV), and human immunodeficiency virus (HIV). Exposures occur through needle sticks or cuts from other sharp instruments contaminated with an infected patient's blood or through contact of the eye, nose, mouth, or skin with a patient's blood. Important factors that influence the overall risk for occupational exposures to blood borne pathogens include the number of infected individuals in the patient population and the type and number of blood contacts. Most exposures do not result in infection. Following a specific exposure, the risk of infection may vary with factors such as these:

- The pathogen involved
- The type of exposure
- The amount of blood involved in the exposure
- The amount of virus in the patient's blood at the time of exposure

Your employer should have in place a system for reporting exposures in order to quickly evaluate the risk of infection, inform you about treatments available to help prevent infection, monitor you for side effects of treatments, and determine if infection occurs. This may involve testing your blood and that of the source patient and offering appropriate postexposure treatment.

How Can Occupational Exposures be Prevented?

Many needle sticks and other cuts can be prevented by using safer techniques (for example, not recapping needles by hand), disposing of used needles in appropriate sharp disposal containers, and using medical devices with safety features designed to prevent injuries. Using appropriate barriers such as gloves, eye and face protection, or gowns when contact with blood is expected can prevent many exposures to the eyes, nose, mouth, or skin.

IF AN EXPOSURE OCCURS

What should I do if I am Exposed to the Blood of a Patient?

1. Immediately following an exposure to blood
   - Wash needlesticks and cuts with soap and water.
   - Flush splashes to the nose, mouth, or skin with water.
   - Irrigate eyes with clean water, saline, or sterile irrigants.

   No scientific evidence shows that using antiseptics or squeezing the wound will reduce the risk of transmission of a blood borne pathogen. Using a caustic agent such as bleach is not recommended.
2. Report the exposure to the department (e.g. occupational health, infection control) responsible for managing exposures. Prompt reporting is essential because, in some cases, postexposure treatment may be recommended and it should be started as soon as possible. Discuss the possible risks of acquiring HBV, HCV, and HIV and the need for postexposure treatment with the provider managing your exposure. You should have already received hepatitis B vaccine, which is extremely safe and effective in preventing HBV infection.

RISK OF INFECTION AFTER EXPOSURE

What is the Risk of Infection after an Occupational Exposure?

HBV

Healthcare personnel who have received hepatitis B vaccine and developed immunity to the virus are at virtually no risk for infection. For a susceptible person, the risk from a single needlestick or cut exposure to HBV-infected blood ranges from 6–30% and depends on the hepatitis Be antigen (HBeAg) status of the source individual. Hepatitis B surface antigen (HBsAg)-positive individuals who are HBeAg positive have more virus in their blood and are more likely to transmit HBV than those who are HBeAg negative. While there is a risk for HBV infection from exposures of mucous membranes or nonintact skin, there is no known risk for HBV infection from exposure to intact skin.

HCV

The average risk for infection after a needlestick or cut exposure to HCV infected blood is approximately 1.8%. The risk following a blood exposure to the eye, nose or mouth is unknown, but is believed to be very small; however, HCV infection from blood splash to the eye has been reported. There also has been a report of HCV transmission that may have resulted from exposure to nonintact skin, but no known risk from exposure to intact skin.

HIV

- The average risk of HIV infection after a needlestick or cut exposure to HIV-infected blood is 0.3% (i.e. three-tenths of one percent, or about 1 in 300). Stated another way, 99.7% of needlestick/cut exposures do not lead to infection.
- The risk after exposure of the eye, nose, or mouth to HIV-infected blood is estimated to be, on average, 0.1% (1 in 1,000).
- The risk after exposure of non-intact skin to HIV-infected blood is estimated to be less than 0.1%. A small amount of blood on intact skin probably poses no risk at all. There have been no documented cases of HIV transmission due to an exposure involving a small amount of blood on intact skin (a few drops of blood on skin for a short period of time). How many healthcare personnel have been infected with blood borne pathogens?

TREATMENT FOR THE EXPOSURE

Is Vaccine or Treatment Available to Prevent Infections with Blood Borne Pathogens?

HBV

As mentioned above, hepatitis B vaccine has been available since 1982 to prevent.

HBV infection: All healthcare personnel who have a reasonable chance of exposure to blood or body fluids should receive hepatitis B vaccine. Vaccination ideally should occur during the healthcare worker's training period. Workers should be tested 1–2 months after the vaccine series is complete to make sure that vaccination has provided immunity to HBV infection. Hepatitis B immune globulin (HBIG) alone or in combination with vaccine (if not previously vaccinated) is effective in preventing HBV infection after an exposure. The decision to begin treatment is based on several factors, such as:

- Whether the source individual is positive for hepatitis B surface antigen?
- Whether you have been vaccinated?
- Whether the vaccine provided you immunity?

HCV

There is no vaccine against hepatitis C and no treatment after an exposure that will prevent infection. Neither immune globulin nor antiviral therapy is recommended after exposure. For these reasons, following recommended infection control practices to prevent percutaneous injuries is imperative.

HIV

There is no vaccine against HIV. However, results from a small number of studies suggest that the use of some antiretroviral drugs after certain occupational exposures may reduce the chance of HIV transmission. Postexposure prophylaxis (PEP) is recommended for certain occupational exposures that pose a risk of transmission. However, for those exposures without risk of HIV infection, PEP is not recommended because the drugs used to prevent infection may have serious side effects. You should discuss the risks and side effects with your healthcare provider before starting PEP for HIV.

How are Exposures to Blood from An Individual Whose Infection Status is Unknown Handled?

HBV–HCV–HIV

If the source individual cannot be identified or tested, decisions regarding follow-up should be based on the exposure risk and whether the source is likely to be infected with a blood borne pathogen. Follow-up testing should be available to all personnel who are concerned about possible infection through occupational exposure.

What Specific Drugs are Recommended for Post-Exposure Treatment?

HBV

If you have not been vaccinated, then hepatitis B vaccination is recommended for any exposure regardless of the source person's HBV status. HBIG and/or hepatitis B vaccine may be recommended depending on the source person's infection status, your vaccination status and, if vaccinated, your response to the vaccine.

HCV

There is no post exposure treatment that will prevent HCV infection.

HIV

The Public Health Service recommends a 4-week course of a combination of either two antiretroviral drugs for most HIV exposures, or three antiretroviral drugs for exposures that may pose a greater risk for transmitting HIV (such as those involving a larger volume of blood with a larger amount of HIV or a concern about drug-resistant HIV). Differences in side effects associated with the use of these drugs may influence which drugs are selected in a specific situation. These recommendations are intended to provide guidance to clinicians and may be modified on a case-by-case basis. Determining which drugs and how many drugs to use or when to change a treatment regimen is largely a matter of judgment. Whenever possible, consulting an expert with experience in the use of antiviral drugs is advised, especially if a recommended drug is not available, if the source patient's virus is likely to be resistant to one or more recommended drugs, or if the drugs are poorly tolerated.

How Soon After Exposure to a Blood Borne Pathogen should Treatment Start?

HBV

Post exposure treatment should begin as soon as possible after exposure, preferably within 24 hours, and no later than 7 days.

HIV

Treatment should be started as soon as possible, preferably within hours as opposed to days, after the exposure. Although animal studies suggest that treatment is less effective when started more than 24–36 hours after exposure, the time frame after which no benefit is gained in humans is not known. Starting treatment after a longer period (e.g. 1 week) may be considered for exposures that represent an increased risk of transmission.

Has the FDA Approved these Drugs to Prevent Blood Borne Virus Infection following an Occupational Exposure?

HBV

Yes. Both hepatitis B vaccine and HBIG are approved for this use.

HIV

No. The FDA has approved these drugs only for the treatment of existing HIV infection, but not as a treatment to prevent infection. However, physicians may prescribe any approved drug when, in their professional judgment, the use of the drug is warranted.

What is known about the Safety and Side Effects of these Drugs?

HBV

Hepatitis B vaccine and HBIG are very safe. There is no information that the vaccine causes any chronic illnesses. Most illnesses reported after a hepatitis B vaccination are related to other causes and not the vaccine. However, you should report to your healthcare provider any unusual reaction after a hepatitis B vaccination.

HIV

All of the antiviral drugs for treatment of HIV have been associated with side effects. The most common side effects include upset stomach (nausea, vomiting, diarrhoea), tiredness, or headache. The few serious side effects that have been reported in healthcare personnel using combinations of antiviral drugs after exposure have included kidney stones, hepatitis, and suppressed blood cell production. Protease inhibitors (e.g. indinavir and nelfinavir) may interact with other medicines and cause serious side effects and should not be taken in combination with certain other drugs, such as non-sedating antihistamines, e.g. Claritin®. If you need to take antiviral drugs for an HIV exposure, it is important to tell the healthcare provider managing your exposure about any medications you are currently taking.

Can Pregnant Healthcare Personnel take the Drugs Recommended for Post Exposure Treatment?

HBV

Yes. Women who are pregnant or breast-feeding can receive the hepatitis B vaccine and/or HBIG. Pregnant women who are exposed to blood should be vaccinated against HBV infection, because infection during pregnancy can cause severe illness in the mother and a chronic infection in the newborn. The vaccine does not harm the fetus.

HIV

Pregnancy should not rule out the use of postexposure treatment when it is warranted. If you are pregnant you should understand what is known and not known regarding the potential benefits and risks associated with the use of antiviral drugs in order to make an informed decision about treatment.

FOLLOW-UP AFTER AN EXPOSURE

What follow-up should be Done after an Exposure?

HBV

Because post exposure treatment is highly effective in preventing HBV infection, CDC does not recommend routine follow-up after treatment. However, any symptoms suggesting hepatitis (e.g. yellow eyes or skin, loss of appetite, nausea, vomiting, fever, stomach or joint pain, extreme tiredness) should be reported to your healthcare provider. If you receive hepatitis B vaccine, you should be tested 1–2 months after completing the vaccine series to determine if you have responded to the vaccine and are protected against HBV infection.

HCV

You should be tested for HCV antibody and liver enzyme levels (alanine aminotransferase or ALT) as soon as possible after the exposure (baseline) and at 4–6 months after the exposure. To check for infection earlier, you can be tested for the virus (HCV RNA) 4–6 weeks after the exposure. Report any symptoms suggesting hepatitis (mentioned above) to your healthcare provider.

HIV

You should be tested for HIV antibody as soon as possible after exposure (baseline) and periodically for at least 6 months after the exposure (e.g. at 6 weeks, 12 weeks, and 6 months). If you take antiviral drugs for postexposure treatment, you should be checked for drug toxicity by having a complete blood count and kidney and liver function tests just before starting treatment and 2 weeks after starting treatment. You should report any sudden or severe flu-like illness that occurs during the follow-up period, especially if it involves fever, rash, muscle aches, tiredness, malaise, or swollen glands. Any of these may suggest HIV infection, drug reaction, or other medical conditions. You should contact the healthcare provider managing your exposure if you have any questions or problems during the follow-up period.

What Precautions should be taken during the follow-up Period?

HBV

If you are exposed to HBV and receive post exposure treatment, it is unlikely that you will become infected and pass the infection on to others. No precautions are recommended.

HCV

Because the risk of becoming infected and passing the infection on to others after an exposure to HCV is low, no precautions are recommended.

HIV

During the follow-up period, especially the first 6–12 weeks when most infected persons are expected to show signs of infection, you should follow recommendations for preventing transmission of HIV. These include not donating blood, semen, or organs and not having sexual intercourse. If you choose to have sexual intercourse, using a condom consistently and correctly may reduce the risk of HIV transmission. In addition, women should consider not breast-feeding infants during the follow-up period to prevent the possibility of exposing their infants to HIV that may be in breast milk.

PREVENTING NEEDLESTICK INJURIES IN HEALTH CARE SETTINGS

The National Institute for Occupational Safety and Health (NIOSH) requests assistance in preventing needlestick injuries among health care workers. These injuries are caused by needles such as hypodermic needles, blood collection needles, intravenous (IV) stylets, and needles used to connect parts of IV delivery systems. These injuries may cause a number of serious and potentially fatal infections with blood borne pathogens such as hepatitis B virus (HBV), hepatitis C virus (HCV), or human immunodeficiency virus (HIV)—the virus that causes acquired immunodeficiency syndrome (AIDS). These injuries can be avoided by eliminating the unnecessary use of needles, using devices with safety features, and promoting education and safe work practices for handling needles and related systems. These measures should be part of a comprehensive program to prevent the transmission of blood borne pathogens. This alert provides current scientific information about the risk of needlestick injury and the transmission of blood borne pathogens to health care workers. The document focuses on needlestick injuries as a key element in a broader effort to prevent all sharps related injuries and associated blood borne infections.

DEVICES ASSOCIATED WITH NEEDLESTICK INJURIES

Health care workers use many types of needles and other sharp devices to provide patient care. However, data from hospitals participating in the CDC National Surveillance System for Hospital Health Care Workers (NaSH) and from hospitals included in the EPINet research database show that only a few needles and other sharp devices are associated with the majority of injuries (International Health Care Worker Safety Center 1997; EPINet 1999; CDC unpublished data 1999). Of nearly 5,000 percutaneous injuries reported by hospitals participating in NaSH between June 1995 and July 1999, 62% were associated with hollow-bore needles—primarily hypodermic needles attached to disposable syringes (29%) and winged-steel (butterfly-type) needles (13%).

ACTIVITIES ASSOCIATED WITH NEEDLESTICK INJURIES

Whenever a needle or other sharp device is exposed, injuries can occur. Data from NaSH show that approximately 38% of percutaneous injuries occur during use and 42% occur after use and before disposal. The circumstances leading to a Needlestick injury depend partly on the type and design of the device used. For example, needle devices that must be taken apart or manipulated after use (e.g. prefilled cartridge syringes and phlebotomy needle/ vacuum tube assemblies) are an obvious hazard and have been associated with increased injury rates [Jagger et al, 1988]. In addition, needles attached to a length of flexible tubing (e.g. winged-steel needles and needles attached to IV tubing) are sometimes difficult to place in sharps containers and thus present another injury hazard. Injuries involving needles attached to IV tubing may occur when a health care worker inserts or withdraws a needle from an IV port or tries to temporarily remove the needlestick hazard by inserting the needle into a drip chamber, IV port or bag, or even bedding. In addition to risks related to device characteristics, needlestick injuries have been related to certain work practices such as

- Recapping,
- Transferring a body fluid between containers, and
- Failing to properly dispose of used needles in puncture-resistant sharps containers.

Past studies of needlestick injuries have shown that 10–25% occurred when recapping a used needle (Ruben et al, 1983; Krasinski et al, 1987; McCormick and Maki, 1981; McCormick et al, 1991; Yassi and McGill, 1991). Although recapping by hand has been discouraged for some time and is prohibited under the OSHA blood borne pathogens standard (29 CFR 1910.1030) unless no alternative exists, 5% of Needlestick injuries in NaSH hospitals are still related to this practice. Injury may occur when a health care worker attempts to transfer blood or other body fluids from a syringe to a specimen container (such as a vacuum tube) and misses the target. Also, if used needles or other sharps are left in the work area or are discarded in a sharps container that is not puncture resistant, a needlestick injury may result.

USE OF IMPROVED ENGINEERING CONTROLS IN A PREVENTION STRATEGY

Safety and health issues can best be addressed in the setting of a comprehensive prevention program that considers all aspects of the work environment and that has employee involvement as well as management commitment. Implementing the use of improved engineering controls is one component of such a comprehensive program.

Desirable Characteristics of Devices with Safety Features

Improved engineering controls are often among the most effective approaches to reducing occupational hazards and therefore are an important element of a needlestick prevention program. Such controls include eliminating the unnecessary use of needles and implementing devices with safety features. A number of sources have identified the desirable characteristics of safety devices (OSHA, 1999c; FDA, 1992; Jagger et al, 1988; Chiarello,1995; Quebbeman and Short, 1995; Pugliese, 1998; Fisher, 1999; ECRI, 1999). These characteristics include the following.

- The device is needleless.
- The safety feature is an integral part of the device.
- The device preferably works passively (i.e. it requires no activation by the user). If user activation is necessary, the safety feature can be engaged with a single-handed technique and allows the workers hands to remain behind the exposed sharp.
- The user can easily tell whether the safety feature is activated.
- The safety feature cannot be deactivated and remains protective through disposal.
- The device performs reliably.
- The device is easy to use and practical.
- The device is safe and effective for patient care.

Examples of Safety Device Designs

Examples of safety device designs are listed as follows.

- Needleless connectors for IV delivery systems (e.g. blunt cannula for use with prepierced ports and valved connectors that accept tapered or luer ends of IV tubing)
- Protected needle IV connectors (e.g. the IV connector needle is permanently recessed in a rigid plastic housing that fits over IV ports)
- Needles that retract into a syringe or vacuum tube holder
- Hinged or sliding shields attached to phlebotomy needles, winged-steel needles, and blood gas needles
- Protective encasements to receive an IV stylet as it is withdrawn from the catheter
- Sliding needle shields attached to disposable syringes and vacuum tube holders
- Self-blunting phlebotomy and winged steel needles (a blunt cannula seated inside the phlebotomy needle is advanced beyond the needle tip before the needle is withdrawn from the vein.
- Retractable finger/heel-stick lancets

SELECTING AND EVALUATING NEEDLE DEVICES WITH SAFETY FEATURES

An increasing number and variety of needle devices with safety features are now available, but many of these devices have had only limited use in the workplace. Thus health care organizations and workers may find it difficult to select appropriate devices. Although these devices are designed to enhance the safety of health care workers, they should be evaluated to ensure that:

- the safety feature works effectively and reliably,
- the device is acceptable to the health care worker, and
- the device does not adversely affect patient care.

Recommendations for Employers

To protect health care workers from needlestick injuries, employers must provide a safe working environment that includes safer needle devices and effective safety programs. Many types of needle devices are associated with needlestick injuries, and these injuries can occur in many ways. Thus a combination of prevention strategies must be considered. Employers should take the following steps to implement a program for reducing needlestick injuries and to involve workers in this effort.

1. Employers of health care workers should implement the use of improved engineering controls to reduce needlestick injuries.
2. Needlestick injury reduction can best be accomplished when the use of improved engineering controls is incorporated into a comprehensive program involving workers.

Recommendations for Workers

To protect themselves and their coworkers, health care workers should be aware of the hazards posed by needlestick injuries and should use safety devices and improved work practices as follows:

1. Avoid the use of needles where safe and effective alternatives are available.
2. Help your employer select and evaluate devices with safety features.
3. Use devices with safety features provided by your employer.
4. Avoid recapping needles.
5. Plan safe handling and disposal before beginning any procedure using needles.
6. Dispose of used needle devices promptly in appropriate sharps disposal containers.
7. Report all needlestick and other sharps related injuries promptly to ensure that you receive appropriate follow-up care.
8. Tell your employer about hazards from needles that you observe in your work environment.
9. Participate in blood-borne pathogen training and follow recommended infection prevention practices, including hepatitis B vaccination.

UNIVERSAL PRECAUTIONS FOR PREVENTION OF TRANSMISSION OF HUMAN IMMUNODEFICIENCY VIRUS, HEPATITIS B VIRUS, AND OTHER BLOOD-BORNE PATHOGENS IN HEALTH-CARE SETTINGS

In 1983, CDC published a document entitled "Guideline for Isolation Precautions in Hospitals" that contained a section entitled "Blood and Body Fluid Precautions." The recommendations in this section called for blood and body fluid precautions when a patient was known or suspected to be infected with bloodborne pathogens. In August 1987, CDC published a document entitled "Recommendations for Prevention of HIV Transmission in Health-Care Settings" (1). In contrast to the 1983 document, the 1987 document recommended that blood and body fluid precautions be consistently used for all patients regardless of their bloodborne infection status. This extension of blood and body fluid precautions to all patients is referred to as "Universal Blood and Body Fluid Precautions" or "Universal Precautions." Under universal precautions, blood and certain body fluids of all patients are considered potentially infectious for human immunodeficiency virus (HIV), hepatitis B virus (HBV), and other bloodborne pathogens.

Universal precautions are intended to prevent parenteral, mucous membrane, and nonintact skin exposures of health-care workers to bloodborne pathogens. In addition, immunization with HBV vaccine is recommended as an important adjunct to universal precautions for health-care workers who have exposures to blood. Since the recommendations for universal precautions were published in August 1987, CDC and the Food and Drug Administration (FDA) have received requests for clarification of the following issues: (i) Body fluids to which universal precautions apply, (ii) use of protective barriers, (iii) use of gloves for phlebotomy, (iv) selection of gloves for use while observing universal precautions, and (v) need for making changes in waste management programs as a result of adopting universal precautions.

Body Fluids to Which Universal Precautions Apply

Universal precautions apply to blood and to other body fluids containing visible blood. Occupational transmission of HIV and HBV to health-care workers by blood is documented. Blood is the single most important source of HIV, HBV, and other bloodborne pathogens in the occupational setting. Infection control efforts for HIV, HBV, and other bloodborne pathogens must focus on preventing exposures to blood as well as on delivery of HBV immunization.

Universal precautions also apply to semen and vaginal secretions. Although both of these fluids have been implicated in the sexual transmission of HIV and HBV, they have not been implicated in occupational transmission from patient to health-care worker. This observation is not unexpected, since exposure to semen in the usual health-care setting is limited, and the routine practice of wearing gloves for performing vaginal examinations protects health-care workers from exposure to potentially infectious vaginal secretions.

Universal precautions also apply to tissues and to the following fluids: cerebrospinal fluid (CSF), synovial fluid, pleural fluid, peritoneal fluid, pericardial fluid, and amniotic fluid. The risk of transmission of HIV and HBV from these fluids is unknown; epidemiologic studies in the health-care and community setting are currently inadequate to assess the potential risk to health-care workers from occupational exposures to them. However, HIV has been isolated from CSF, synovial, and amniotic fluid, and HBsAg has been detected in synovial fluid, amniotic fluid, and peritoneal fluid. One case of HIV transmission was reported after a percutaneous exposure to bloody pleural fluid obtained by needle aspiration. Whereas aseptic procedures used to obtain these fluids for diagnostic or therapeutic purposes protect health-care workers from skin exposures, they cannot prevent penetrating injuries due to contaminated needles or other sharp instruments.

Body Fluids to Which Universal Precautions Do Not Apply

Universal precautions do not apply to feces, nasal secretions, sputum, sweat, tears, urine, and vomitus unless they contain visible blood. The risk of transmission of HIV and HBV from these fluids and materials is extremely low or nonexistent. HIV has been isolated and HBsAg has been demonstrated in some of these fluids; however, epidemiologic studies in the health-care and community setting have not implicated these fluids or materials in the transmission of HIV and HBV infections. Some of the above fluids and excretions represent a potential source for nosocomial and community-acquired infections with other pathogens and recommendations for preventing the transmission of nonbloodborne pathogens have been published.

Precautions for Other Body Fluids in Special Settings

Human breast milk has been implicated in perinatal transmission of HIV, and HBsAg has been found in the milk of mothers infected with HBV. However, occupational exposure to human breast milk has not been implicated in the transmission of HIV nor HBV infection to health-care workers. Moreover, the health-care worker will not have the same type of intensive exposure to breast milk as the nursing neonate. Whereas universal precautions do not apply to human breast milk, gloves may be worn by health-care workers in situations where exposures to breast milk might be frequent, for example, in breast milk banking.

Universal precautions do not apply to saliva. Special precautions, however, are recommended for dentistry. Occupationally acquired infection with HBV in dental workers has been documented, and possible cases of occupationally acquired HIV infection involving dentists have been reported. During dental procedures, contamination of saliva with blood is predictable, trauma to health-care workers' hands is common, and blood spattering may occur. Infection control precautions for dentistry minimize the potential for nonintact skin and mucous membrane contact of dental health-care workers to blood-contaminated saliva of patients. In addition, the use of gloves for oral examinations and treatment in the dental setting may also protect the patient's oral mucous membranes from exposures to blood, which may occur from breaks in the skin of dental workers' hands.

Use of Protective Barriers

Protective barriers reduce the risk of exposure of the health-care worker's skin or mucous membranes to potentially infective materials. For universal precautions, protective barriers reduce the risk of exposure to blood, body fluids containing visible blood, and other fluids to which universal precautions apply. Examples of protective barriers include gloves, gowns, masks, and protective eyewear. Gloves should reduce the incidence of contamination of hands, but they cannot prevent penetrating injuries due to needles or other sharp instruments. Masks and protective eyewear or face shields should reduce the incidence of contamination of mucous membranes of the mouth, nose, and eyes.

Universal precautions are intended to supplement rather than replace recommendations for routine infection control, such as handwashing and using gloves to prevent gross microbial contamination of hands. Because specifying the types of barriers needed for every possible clinical situation is impractical, some judgment must be exercised.

The following general guidelines are recommended:

1. Use sterile gloves for procedures involving contact with normally sterile areas of the body.
2. Use examination gloves for procedures involving contact with mucous membranes, unless otherwise indicated, and for other patient care or diagnostic procedures that do not require the use of sterile gloves.
3. Change gloves between patient contacts.
4. Do not wash or disinfect surgical or examination gloves for reuse. Washing with surfactants may cause "wicking," i.e., the enhanced penetration of liquids through undetected holes in the glove. Disinfecting agents may cause deterioration.
5. Use general-purpose utility gloves (e.g. rubber household gloves) for housekeeping chores involving potential blood contact and for instrument cleaning and decontamination procedures. Utility gloves may be decontaminated and reused but should be discarded if they are peeling, cracked, or discolored, or if they have punctures, tears, or other evidence of deterioration.

LABORATORY DIAGNOSIS OF HIV INFECTION

HIV serological testing is the most common approach for identifying HIV infected individuals or HIV contaminated blood products. HIV antibody testing has gained popularity because anti-HIV antibodies usually occur relatively early in the disease process and normally persists through out the course of HIV disease progression. Also, these assays are relatively inexpensive and most can be easily adapted to accommodate screening large test volumes.

Basic types of HIV Screening tests

ELISA/EIA (Enzyme linked immunosorbent assay)

Principle of ELISA

HIV antigens are attached to a solid support allowing HIV antibodies in the sample to bind, which are subsequently detected by enzyme-labelled anti-human immunoglobulin. A specific substrate is then added to produce a color reaction when HIV antibody is present in the test serum.

Advantages

a. Easy to perform
b. Large number of samples can be done at a time
c. Highly sensitive
d. Highly specific.

Disadvantages

a. False positives may occur
b. Needs to be read in an ELISA reader.

Rapid Assays

a. Dot blot
b. PAT (Particle agglutination test).

Advantages

a. These assays were developed as alternatives to ELISA for HIV screening.
b. Generally require < 30 minutes to perform.
c. Do not require sophisticated laboratory equipment and usually are easy to perform.
d. Positive results must be confirmed by standard HIV screening and confirmatory tests.

Confirmatory Test

1. Western blot
2. IFA (Indirect fluorescent antibody assay)
3. RIPA (Radioimmuno precipitation assay)
4. Line immunoassays.

Western Blot Principle

Confirmatory assays must be highly specific to ensure that individuals who test reactive in screening assays are correctly identified as being HIV infected. Western Blot (WB) is the most commonly used confirmatory test.

PCR (Polymerase Chain Reaction) Principle

A variety of techniques have been developed to amplify the nucleic acid target sequence of the molecular probe attached to the target sequence to improve the sensitivity of nucleic acid detection.

HIV TESTING STRATEGIES FOR INDIA

WHO recommends three testing strategies or algorithms to maximize accuracy and minimize cost. These strategies are delineated in the following algorithms.

Strategy I

All serum is tested with one ELISA or Rapid/Simple assay. Serum that is reactive is considered HIV antibody positive. Serum that is non-reactive is considered HIV antibody negative.

Strategy II

All serum is tested with one ELISA or Rapid/Simple assay. Any serum found reactive on the first assay is retested with a second ELISA or Rapid/Simple assay based on a different antigen preparation and/or different test principle (e.g. indirect versus competitive). Serum that is reactive on both tests is considered HIV antibody positive. Serum that is non-reactive on the first test is considered HIV antibody negative. Any serum that is reactive on the first test but non-reactive on the second test is also considered antibody negative.

Strategy III

As in Strategy II, all serum is first tested with one ELISA or rapid/simple, assay, and any reactive samples are retested using a different assay. Strategy III, however requires a third test if serum is found reactive on the second assay. The 3 tests in this strategy should be based on different antigen preparation and/or different test principles. Serum reactive on all 3 tests is considered HIV antibody positive. Serum that is non-reactive on the first test is considered HIV antibody negative as is serum that is reactive in the first test but non-reactive in the second. Serum that is reactive in the first and second tests but non-reactive in the third test is considered to be equivocal.

BASIC AND EXPANDED HIV POST-EXPOSURE PROPHYLAXIS REGIMENS

Basic Regimen

- **Zidovudine (Retrovir™; ZDV; AZT) + lamivudine (Epivir®; 3TC); available as Combivir™**

Preferred dosing

— ZDV: 300 mg twice daily or 200 mg three times daily, with food; total: 600 mg daily.

— 3TC: 300 mg once daily or 150 mg twice daily

— Combivir: one tablet twice daily.

Dosage forms

— ZDV: 100 mg capsule, 300 mg tablet

— 3TC: 150 or 300 mg tablet.

— Combivir: tablet, 300 mg ZDV + 150 mg 3TC.

Advantages

— ZDV associated with decreased risk for HIV transmission

— ZDV used more often than other drugs for PEP for health-care personnel (HCP)

— Serious toxicity rare when used for PEP

— Side effects predictable and manageable with antimotility and antiemetic agents

— Can be used by pregnant HCP

— Can be given as a single tablet (COMBIVIR™) twice daily.

Disadvantages

— Side effects (especially nausea and fatigue) common and might result in low adherence

— Source-patient virus resistance to this regimen possible

— Potential for delayed toxicity (oncogenic/teratogenic) unknown.

- **Zidovudine (Retrovir®; ZDV; AZT) + emtricitabine (Emtriva™; FTC).**

Preferred dosing

— ZDV: 300 mg twice daily or 200 mg three times daily, with food; total: 600 mg/day, in 2–3 divided doses

— FTC: 200 mg (one capsule) once daily.

Dosage forms

— ZDV: see above

— FTC: 200 mg capsule.

FTC general comments

— Nucleoside analogue; same structure as 3TC, except fluoride residue at position 5 on pyrimidine ring

— Same resistance and safety profile as 3TC

— No apparent advantage over 3TC; tolerability and virologic response rates appear better than regimens containing ddI + d4T.

Advantages

— ZDV: see above.

— FTC

- Convenient (once daily)
- Well tolerated
- Long intracellular half-life (~40 hours).

Disadvantages

— ZDV: see above.

— FTC

- Rash perhaps more frequent than with 3TC
- No long-term experience with this drug
- Cross resistance to 3TC
- Hyperpigmentation among non-Caucasians with long-term use: 3%

- **Tenofovir DF (Viread®; TDF) + lamivudine (Epivir®; 3TC).**

Preferred dosing

— TDF: 300 mg once daily

— 3TC: 300 mg once daily or 150 mg twice daily.

Dosage forms

— TDF: 300 mg tablet

— 3TC: see above.

Advantages

— 3TC: see above

— TDF

- Convenient dosing (single pill once daily)
- Resistance profile activity against certain thymidine analogue mutations
- Well tolerated.

Disadvantages

— TDF

- Same class warnings as nucleoside reverse transcriptase inhibitors (NRTIs)
- Drug interactions
- Increased TDF concentrations among persons taking atazanavir and lopinavir/ritonavir; need to monitor patients for TDF-associated toxicities

— Preferred dosage of atazanavir if used with TDF: 300 mg + ritonavir 100 mg once daily + TDF 300 mg once daily

- **Tenofovir DF (Viread®; TDF) + emtricitabine (Emtriva™; FTC); available as Truvada™**

Preferred dosing

— TDF: 300 mg once daily

— FTC: 200 mg once daily

— As Truvada™: one tablet daily

Dosage forms

— TDF: 300 mg tablet

— FTC: see FTC

— Truvada™ (TDF 300 mg plus FTC 200 mg)

Advantages

— FTC: see above

— TDF

- Convenient dosing (single pill once daily)
- Resistance profile activity against certain thymidine analogue mutations
- Well tolerated

Disadvantages

— TDF

- Same class warnings as NRTIs
- Drug interactions
- Increased TDF concentrations among persons taking atazanavir and lopinavir/ritonavir; need to monitor patients for TDF-associated toxicities
- Preferred dosing of atazanavir if used with TDF: 300 mg + ritonavir 100 mg once daily + TDF 300 mg once daily

Alternate Basic Regimens

- **Lamivudine (Epivir®; 3TC) + stavudine (Zerit®; d4T)**

Preferred dosing

— 3TC: 300 mg once daily or 150 mg twice daily

— d4T: 40 mg twice daily (can use lower doses of 20–30 mg twice daily if toxicity occurs; equally effective but less toxic among HIV-infected patients with peripheral neuropathy); 30 mg twice daily if body weight is <60 kg.

Dosage forms

— 3TC: see above
— d4T: 15, 20, 30, and 40 mg tablet

Advantages

— 3TC: see above
— d4T: gastrointestinal (GI) side effects rare

Disadvantages

— Possibility that source-patient virus is resistant to this regimen
— Potential for delayed toxicity (oncogenic/teratogenic) unknown.

- **Emtricitabine (Emtriva™; FTC) + stavudine (Zerit®;d4T)**

Preferred dosing

— FTC: 200 mg daily
— d4T: 40 mg twice daily (can use lower doses of 20–30 mg twice daily if toxicity occurs; equally effective but less toxic among HIV-infected patients who developed peripheral neuropathy); if body weight is <60 kg, 30 mg twice daily.

Dosage forms

— FTC: see above
— d4T: see above.

Advantages

— 3TC and FTC: see above; d4T's GI side effects rare.

Disadvantages

— Potential that source-patient virus is resistant to this regimen
— Unknown potential for delayed toxicity (oncogenic/ teratogenic) unknown.

- **Lamivudine (Epivir®; 3TC) + didanosine (Videx®; ddI)**

Preferred dosing

— 3TC: 300 mg once daily or 150 mg twice daily.
— ddI: Videx® chewable/dispersible buffered tablets can be administered on an empty stomach as either 200 mg twice daily or 400 mg once daily. Patients must take at least two of the appropriate strength tablets at each dose to provide adequate buffering and prevent gastric acid degradation of ddI. Because of the need for adequate buffering, the 200 mg strength tablet should be used only as a component of a once-daily regimen. The dose is either 200 mg twice daily or 400 mg once daily for patients weighing >60 kg and 125 mg twice daily or 250 mg once daily for patients weighing >60 kg.

Dosage forms

— 3TC: 150 or 300 mg tablets
— ddI: 25, 50, 100, 150, or 200 mg buffered white tablets.

Advantages

— ddI: once daily dosing option
— 3TC: see above.

Disadvantages

— Tolerability: diarrhea more common with buffered preparation than with enteric-coated preparation
— Associated with toxicity: peripheral neuropathy, pancreatitis, and lactic acidosis
— Must be taken on empty stomach except with TDF
— Drug interactions
— 3TC: see above.

- **Emtricitabine (Emtriva™; FTC) + didanosine (Videx®; ddI)**

Preferred dosing

— FTC: 200 mg once daily
— ddI: see above.

Dosage forms

— ddI: see above
— FTC: see above.

Advantages

— ddI: see above
— FTC: see above.

Disadvantages
- Tolerability: diarrhea more common with buffered than with enteric-coated preparation
- Associated with toxicity: peripheral neuropathy, pancreatitis, and lactic acidosis
- Must be taken on empty stomach except with TDF
- Drug interactions
- FTC: see above.

Preferred Expanded Regimen

Basic Regimen Plus
- **Lopinavir/ritonavir (Kaletra®; LPV/RTV)**

Preferred dosing
- LPV/RTV: 400/100 mg = 3 capsules twice daily with food.

Dosage form
- LPV/RTV: 133/33 mg capsules.

Advantages
- Potent HIV protease inhibitor
- Generally well-tolerated.

Disadvantages
- Potential for serious or life-threatening drug interactions
- Might accelerate clearance of certain drugs, including oral contraceptives (requiring alternative or additional contraceptive measures for women taking these drugs)
- Can cause severe hyperlipidemia, especially hypertriglyceridemia
- GI (e.g. diarrhea) events common.

Alternate Expanded Regimens

Basic regimen plus one of the following

- **Atazanavir (Reyataz®; ATV) + ritonavir (Norvir®; RTV)**

Preferred dosing
- ATV: 400 mg once daily, unless used in combination with TDF, in which case ATV should be boosted with RTV, preferred dosing of ATV 300 mg + RTV: 100 mg once daily

Dosage forms
- ATV: 100, 150, and 200 mg capsules
- RTV: 100 mg capsule

Advantages
- Potent HIV protease inhibitor
- Convenient dosing—once daily
- Generally well tolerated

Disadvantages
- Hyperbilirubinemia and jaundice common
- Potential for serious or life-threatening drug interactions
- Avoid co administration with proton pump inhibitors
- Separate antacids and buffered medications by 2 hours and H2-receptor antagonists by 12 hours to avoid decreasing ATV levels
- Caution should be used with ATV and products known to induce PR prolongation (e.g. diltiazem)

- **Fosamprenavir (Lexiva®; FOSAPV) + ritonavir (Norvir®; RTV)**

Preferred dosing
- FOSAPV: 1400 mg twice daily (without RTV)
- FOSAPV: 1400 mg once daily + RTV 200 mg once daily
- FOSAPV: 700 mg twice daily + RTV 100 mg twice daily

Dosage form
- FOSAPV: 700 mg tablets
- RTV: 100 mg capsule.

Advantages
- Once daily dosing when given with ritonavir

Disadvantages
- Tolerability: GI side effects common
- Multiple drug interactions. Oral contraceptives decrease fosamprenavir concentrations.

— Incidence of rash in healthy volunteers, especially when used with low doses of ritonavir. Differentiating between early drug-associated rash and acute seroconversion can be difficult and cause extraordinary concern for the exposed person

- **Indinavir (Crixivan®; IDV) + ritonavir (Norvir®; RTV).**

Preferred dosing
— IDV 800 mg + RTV 100 mg twice daily without regard to food.

Alternative dosing
— IDV: 800 mg every 8 hours, on an empty stomach.

Dosage forms
— IDV: 200 mg, 333, and 400 mg capsule
— RTV: 100 mg capsule.

Advantages
— Potent HIV inhibitor.

Disadvantages
— Potential for serious or life-threatening drug interactions
— Serious toxicity (e.g. nephrolithiasis) possible; consumption of 8 glasses of fluid/day required
— Hyperbilirubinemia common; must avoid this drug during late pregnancy
— Requires acid for absorption and cannot be taken simultaneously with ddI, chewable/dispersible buffered tablet formulation (doses must be separated by >1 hour).

- **Saquinavir (Invirase®; 3SQV) + ritonavir (Norvir®; RTV).**

Preferred dosing
— SQV: 1,000 mg (given as Invirase) + RTV 100 mg, twice daily
— SQV: five capsules twice daily + RTV: one capsule twice daily.

Dosage forms
— SQV (Invirase): 200 mg capsule
— RTV: 100 mg capsule

Advantages
— Generally well-tolerated, although GI events common.

Disadvantages
— Potential for serious or life-threatening drug interactions
— Substantial pill burden.

- **Nelfinavir (Viracept®; NFV)**

Preferred dosing
— NFV: 1,250 mg (2 x 625 mg or 5 x 250 mg tablets), twice daily with a meal.

Dosage forms
— NFV: 250 or 625 mg tablet.

Advantages
— Generally well-tolerated.

Disadvantages
— Diarrhea or other GI events common
— Potential for serious and/or life-threatening drug interactions.

- **Efavirenz (Sustiva®; EFV)**

Preferred dosing
— EFV: 600 mg daily, at bedtime.

Dosage forms
— EFV: 50, 100, 200 capsules
— EFV: 600 mg tablet.

Advantages
— Does not require phosphorylation before activation and might be active earlier than other antiretroviral agents (a theoretic advantage of no demonstrated clinical benefit)
— Once daily dosing.

Disadvantages
— Drug associated with rash (early onset) that can be severe and might rarely progress to Stevens-Johnson syndrome
— Differentiating between early drug-associated rash and acute seroconversion can be difficult and cause extraordinary concern for the exposed person

— Central nervous system side effects (e.g., dizziness, somnolence, insomnia, or abnormal dreaming) common; severe psychiatric symptoms possible (dosing before bedtime might minimize these side effects)
— Teratogen; should not be used during pregnancy
— Potential for serious or life-threatening drug interactions.

ANTIRETROVIRAL AGENTS GENERALLY NOT RECOMMENDED FOR USE AS PEP

- **Nevirapine (Viramune®; NVP)**

Disadvantages
— Associated with severe hepatotoxicity (including at least one case of liver failure requiring liver transplantation in an exposed person taking PEP)
— Associated with rash (early onset) that can be severe and progress to Stevens-Johnson syndrome
— Differentiating between early drug-associated rash and acute seroconversion can be difficult and cause extraordinary concern for the exposed person
— Drug interactions can lower effectiveness of certain antiretroviral agents and other commonly used medicines.

- **Delavirdine (Rescriptor®; DLV)**

Disadvantages
— Drug associated with rash (early onset) that can be severe and progress to Stevens-Johnson syndrome
— Multiple drug interactions.

- **Abacavir (Ziagen®; ABC)**

Disadvantages
— Severe hypersensitivity reactions can occur, usually within the first 6 weeks
— Differentiating between early drug-associated rash/hypersensitivity and acute seroconversion can be difficult.

- **Zalcitabine (Hivid®; ddC)**

Disadvantages
— Three times a day dosing
— Tolerability
— Weakest antiretroviral agent.

ANTIRETROVIRAL AGENT FOR USE AS PEP ONLY WITH EXPERT CONSULTATION

- **Enfuvirtide (Fuzeon™; T20)**

Preferred dosing
— T20: 90 mg (1 ml) twice daily by subcutaneous injection

Dosage forms
— T20: Single-dose vial, reconstituted to 90 mg/ml

Advantages
— New class
— Unique viral target; to block cell entry
— Prevalence of resistance low.

Disadvantages
— Twice-daily injection
— Safety profile: local injection site reactions
— Never studied among antiretroviral-naïve or HIV negative patients
— False-positive EIA HIV antibody tests might result from formation of anti-T20 antibodies that cross-react with anti-gp41 antibodies.

ORAL MANIFESTATIONS OF AIDS

Classification

Group 1: Lesions strongly associated with HIV infection

Candidiasis (erythematous, pseudomembranous)
Hairy leukoplakia
Kaposi's sarcoma
Non-Hodgkin's lymphoma
Periodontal disease (linear gingival erythema, Necrotising (ulcerative) gingivitis, necrotising (ulcerative) periodontitis).

Group 2: Lesions less commonly associated with HIV infection.

Bacterial infections
Mycobacterium avium-intracellulare
Mycobacterium tuberculosis
Melanotic hyperpigmentation
Necrotising (ulcerative) stomatitis
Salivary gland disease
Dry mouth due to decreased salivary flow rate
Unilateral or bilateral swelling of major salivary glands
Thrombocytopenic purpura
Ulceration NOS (not otherwise specified)
Viral infections
Herpes simplex virus
Human papilloma virus (warty-like lesions)
Condyloma acuminatum
Focal epithelial hyperplasia
Verruca vulgaris
Varicella-zoster virus
Herpes zoster
Varicella.

Group 3: Lesions seen in HIV infection

Bacterial infection:
Actinomyces israelii
Escherichia coli
Klebsiella pneumoniae
Cat—scratch disease (also bacterial)
Epithelioid (bacillary) angiomatosis
Drug reactions (ulcerative, erythema multiforme, lichenoid, toxic epidermolysis)
Fungal infections other than candidiasis
Cryptococcus neoformans
Geotrichum candidum
Histoplasma capsulatum
Mucoraceae (mucormycosis, zygomycosis)
Aspergillus flafus
Neurologic disturbances
Facial palsy
Trigeminal neuralgia
Recurrent aphthous stomatitis
Viral infections
Cytomegalo virus
Molluscum contagiosum.

ORAL CANDIDIASIS

Candidiasis, an opportunistic fungal infection is the oral condition most strongly associated with HIV infection. The most common species is *Candida albicans*. It has been reported that HIV patients with oro-oesophageal candidiasis may develop full blown AIDS within two years.

It is diagnosed by:

i. Clinical appearance (see below)
ii. By taking a smear and staining for candidal hyphae
iii. By culturing the fungus on Sabaroud's agar medium. (Takes 48 hours at room temperature, easy to perform and very specific.)

Four clinical patterns are seen:

1. Pseudomembranous
2. Erythematous
3. Hyperplastic
4. Angular cheilitis.

PSEUDOMEMBRANOUS CANDIDIASIS

Clinically appears as white to yellowish white plaques which can be easily scraped off leaving red areas. In HIV disease the lesions tend to be extensive involving almost all the sites in the oral cavity. It may also extend to involve the oro-pharynx and esophagus. See the figure below showing Pseudomembranous candidiasis of the tongue (Fig. 13.1).

ERYTHEMATOUS CANDIDIASIS

Erythematous candidiasis appears as a red lesion commonly located on the dorsum of the tongue, palate and buccal mucosa. Tongue lesions have also been called as:

i. Central papillary atrophy
ii. Median rhomboid glossitis (Fig. 13.2).

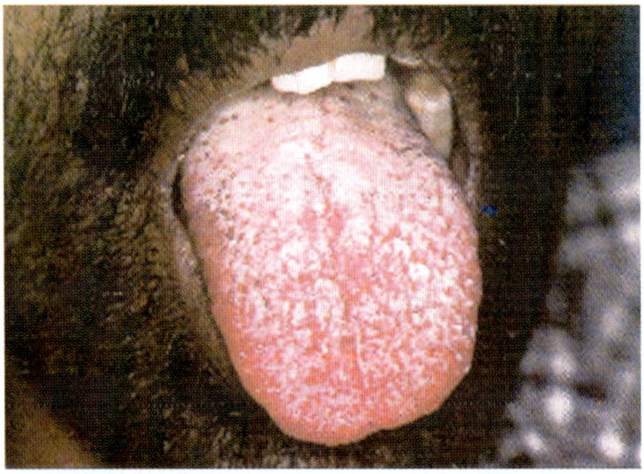

Fig. 13.1: Pseudomembraneous candidiasis.

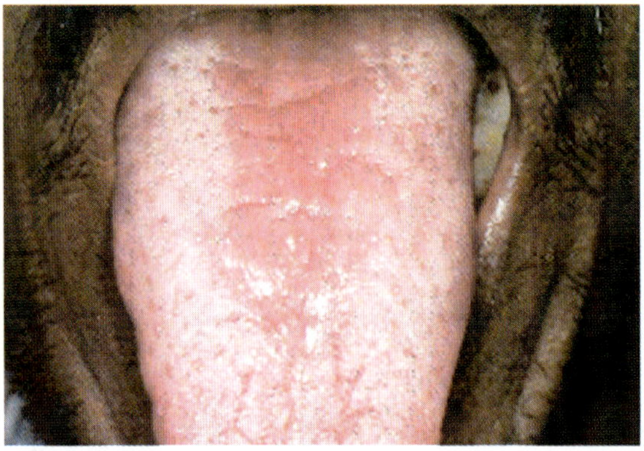

Fig. 13.2: Median rhomboid glossitis.

HYPERPLASTIC CANDIDIASIS

Hyperplastic candidiasis is characterised by white plaques which cannot be removed by scraping. They can be differentiated from many other forms of oral white lesions by resolution after treatment with topical/systemic anti-fungal therapy (our patients responded well to orally administered fluconazole). Diagnosis can be confirmed by biopsy, which shows the fungal hyphae invading the superficial cornified layers of the epithelium. This is the least common variant of candida infection present in HIV patients. (Fig. 13.3)

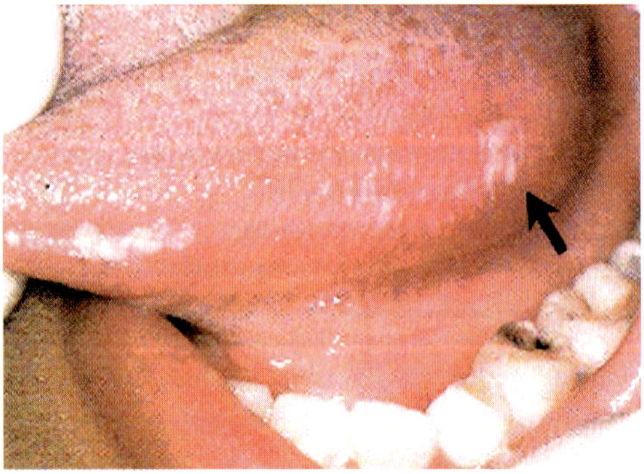

Fig. 13.3: Hyperplastic candidiasis of tongue.

ANGULAR CHEILITIS

This is characterised by erythema and/or fissuring and/or scaling of the angles of the mouth. Microbiological studies in the United States of America have indicated that 20% of these cases are caused by candida albicans alone, 60% are due to a combined infection with candida albicans and staphylococcus aureus, and 20% are associated with staphylococcus alone (Fig. 13.4). The arrows point at the lesions.

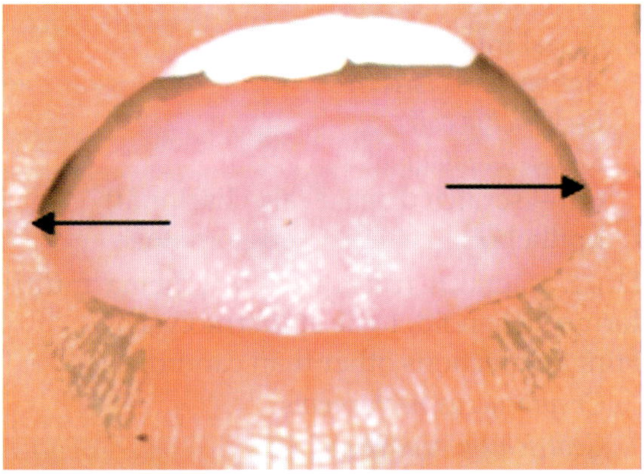

Fig. 13.4: Angular cheilitis.

REFERENCES AND BIBLIOGRAPHY

1. Preventing Needlestick Injuries in Health Care Settings; DHHS (NIOSH) Publication No. 2000-108, November 1999.

2. Exposure to Blood What Healthcare Personnel Need to Know; Information from the Centers for Disease Control and Prevention National Center for Infectious Diseases Division of Healthcare Quality Promotion and Division of Viral Hepatitis; Updated July 2003.
3. Updated U.S. Public Health Service Guidelines for the Management of Occupational Exposures to HIV and Recommendations for Post exposure Prophylaxis; Recommendations and Reports September 30, 2005/Vol. 54/No. RR-9.
4. HIV and it's Transmission, July 1999; CDC National Prevention Information Network; P.O. Box 6003 Rockville, Maryland 20849-6003; 1-800-458-5231 NPIN: Internet Resources DHAP: http://www.cdc.gov/hiv NCHSTP: http://www.cdc.gov/nchstp/od/nchstp.html
5. Perspectives in Disease Prevention and Health Promotion Update: Universal Precautions for Prevention of Transmission of Human Immunodeficiency Virus, Hepatitis B Virus, and Other Blood borne Pathogens in Health-Care Settings.; MMWR HTML documents.

Chapter 14

Oral Manifestations of Systemic Diseases

There are a number of systemic diseases that can become important factors in oral and maxillofacial surgery by complicating the operation or retarding healing. Even a simple tooth extraction, usually performed in the office without great inconvenience or danger to the patient's life, becomes a formidable and serious undertaking if the patient has uncontrolled diabetes, cardiovascular disease, liver dysfunction, or a blood dyscrasia. It is, therefore, important to be aware of the oral manifestations of systemic diseases.

Besides the presence of unusual changes in the mouth, a careful history of previous illnesses and operations may yield important information. Complications that attended former operations or even the administration of anesthetics may be illuminating. Unless a patient is under the care of a physician from whom information may be obtained, a thorough physical examination is indicated whenever systemic conditions are suspected. In some cases, evaluation and treatment by a consultant internist may also be required. The oral and maxillofacial surgeon, however, should be familiar with the nature of such diseases, especially with the signs and symptoms they produce in the oral region and with the effect they may have on the course of surgical operations.

BLOOD DISEASES

Blood diseases very often produce signs in the oral cavity that can lead to their diagnosis. Serious complications may develop if the causes of these conditions are not recognized before an operation is performed. Primary or secondary uncontrollable hemorrhage may occur that can lead to exsanguination and result in death. Oral manifestations or even a suspicious history is an indication for laboratory tests and possible examination by an internist or hematologist.

1. Hypochromic Anemia

Many patients, especially middle-aged women, suffer from hypochromic anemia. This results in a diminished oxygen-carrying capacity of the blood. General anesthesia in adults is contraindicated if the hemoglobin is below 9 gm% (in children, 11–12 gm%). When general anesthesia is used, adequate oxygenation must be ensured.

Oral Signs and Symptoms

The oral tissues, especially the lips, are very pale. The tongue may be smooth on the side and dorsum, or there may be only small areas affected by desquamation of the filiform papillae. In addition, muscular atrophy may cause a decrease in the size of the tongue. There is a predisposition to wound infection and ulceration. Septicemia has been reported to occur after extraction of infected teeth.

Plummer-Vinson Syndrome

Vinson described the Plummer-Vinson syndrome in 1922 and named it hysterical dysphagia. However, Plummer-Vinson syndrome is the name commonly used. It is also known as sideropenic dysphagia, a name suggested by Waldenstrom (1939) because the outstanding symptoms are iron deficiency, anemia, and dysphagia. Many patients also suffer from achlorhydria. The precancerous nature of the disease, however, must also be recognized (Watts, 1961).

Oral Signs and Symptoms

The lips are thin with a narrow vermilion border. The oral as well as the pharyngeal mucosa is pale and atrophied, and the tongue is smooth because of atrophy of the filiform papillae (Fig. 14.1).

Occasionally, leukoplakia develops on the tongue, and angular cheilosis may be present.

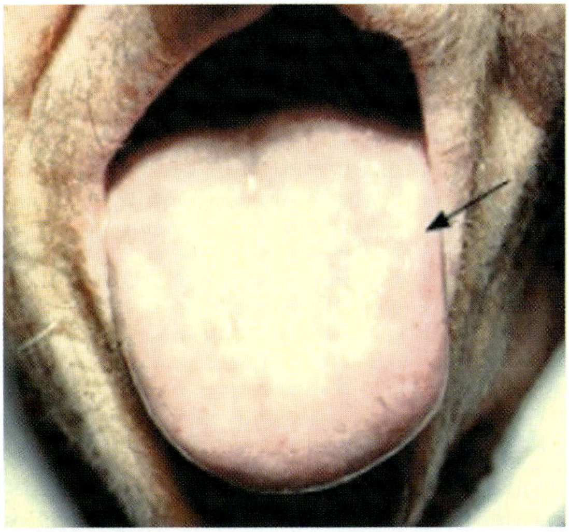

Fig. 14.1: Oral lesions in Plummer-Vinson syndrome.

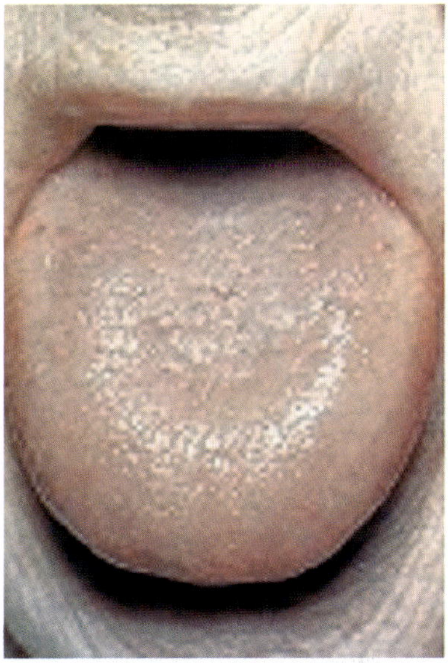

Fig. 14.2: Tongue in Pernicious anaemia.

Carcinoma may develop on the posterior part of the tongue or pharynx and esophagus in the late stages of the syndrome.

Pernicious Anemia

This macrocytic, hyperchromic anemia usually occurs between the ages of 45 and 60 years. It is caused by a deficiency of an intrinsic factor secreted by the parietal cells of the fundus of the stomach.

Oral Signs and Symptoms

At first the tongue is red in contrast to the yellowish color of the rest of the mucosa. Later, atrophy of the filiform papillae causes a characteristic smooth, waxy appearance. The tongue is never coated and therefore has a very clean appearance (Fig. 14.2).

The subjective oral symptoms are often distressing; the patient complains of an unbearable burning and sometimes of numbness. The condition is aggravated by extreme temperatures of food as well as salty and highly seasoned meals.

Aplastic Anemia (Pancytopenia)

This disease is characterized by a great diminution of all the blood elements caused by failure of the bone marrow to produce hematopoietic cells. Besides the idiopathic type there is a secondary form that is caused by toxic chemicals, irradiation, and radioactive substances. Among chemical substances, the injudicious use of chloramphenicol (chloromycetin), especially in children, should be mentioned. Aplastic anemia also occurs in osteosclerosis, marble bone disease (Albers-Schonberg disease), and with extensive bone metastases, all caused by reduction or elimination of bone marrow.

Oral Signs and Symptoms

The tongue is only rarely atrophic but is smooth and either burns or feels numb. Secondary mouth infections develop toward the end of the disease. Gingival bleeding may occur because of the associated thrombocytopenia.

Thrombocytopenic Purpura

Both idiopathic and secondary purpura can occur. The main clinical manifestation is extravasation of blood beneath the skin. Petechial hemorrhages also are seen, especially in the moving parts such as the eyelids.

Oral Signs and Symptoms

Slight trauma causes bleeding and petechial hemorrhages in the mouth. Areas of ecchymosis on the palate or the buccal mucosa are common and often the first signs of the disease. Occasionally large hematomas may form on the palate and buccal mucosa; on the ventral part of the tongue, and on the gingivae.

Haemophilia

Hemophilia A, *true hemophilia,* is a sex-linked, recessive, hereditary disease transmitted by females to male descendants. It is caused by a deficiency of antihaemophilic globulin (AHG; factor VIII).

Aggeler *et al* (1952) and White, Aggeler, and Glendenning (1953) described *plasma thromboplastin component (PTC) deficiency,* which is also a sex-linked recessive trait. All patients with factor IX deficiency are males. They have normal quantities of antihaemophilic globulin. This variety is also known as hemophilia B or Christmas disease (Biggs and Douglas, 1953).

Rosenthal, Dreskin, and Rosenthal (1953) described *plasma thromboplastin antecedent (PTA; factor XI) deficiency (hemophilia C).* This type of hemophilia is not sex-linked; it is transmitted to both male and female descendants by female and probably male carriers.

Oral Signs and Symptoms

The patient may complain of bleeding from slight causes such as use of the toothbrush and large clots may develop around the teeth. In other instances the shedding and eruption of teeth may be associated with oozing of blood for days or weeks. Tooth extraction may give the first indication of the disease; exsanguination is possible if proper treatment is not available.

Leukemias

Leukemia is a fatal disease that arises in the blood forming organs and is characterized by an abnormal proliferation of the white blood cells and their precursors, with infiltration into the various tissues of the body. At some time during the course of the disease, abnormal white blood cells, sometimes in great numbers appear in the circulating blood.

Myelogenous Leukemia

This form of leukemia is characterized by a widespread hyperplasia of the leukopoietic tissue. Both primitive myelocytes and adult neutrophilic, eosinophilic, and basophilic leukocytes may be increased in number, but the myelocyte is the main feature of the blood picture. Myeloblasts are more abundant than mature cells in acute leukemia, and in the terminal stage of the disease the white cell count may be as high as 400,000 to 500,000/cu mm of blood, with 95–99% of the cells of myeloid origin.

Oral Signs and Symptoms

The interdental papillae and later the gingivae become so greatly enlarged that they may cover the teeth almost completely. In the acute form there is a tendency for hemorrhage, and the mucosa shows a deep red or purplish discoloration. The teeth may he covered with blood clots. Ulcerations are common. The loose gingival margin allows the establishment of periodontal infection and causes loosening of the teeth. There is severe fetor oris.

Lymphatic Leukemia

In lymphatic leukemia the lymphoid cells proliferate in the bloodstream and accumulate in the tissues. The white cell count may be 100,000 or more, with 90–99% lymphoid cells.

Oral Signs and Symptoms

In chronic lymphatic leukemia one may find extreme hypertrophy of the gingiva, whereas in acute cases ulcerations may be the main feature. The patient is especially susceptible to Vincent's infection.

Monocytic Leukemia

This form of leukemia is comparatively rare. The leukocytes are only moderately increased (15,000–45,000); the primary feature is a marked increase in monocytes to about 70% to 90%.

Oral Signs and Symptoms

It produces hyperplasia and ulceration in the mouth and haemorrhages from the gums.

Agranulocytopenia

Agranulocytopenia, also called agranulocytosis or pernicious leukopenia, is characterized by fever and an almost complete absence of granular leukocytes; it is accompanied by a drop in the total white cell count. Drug therapy may be a causative factor, but there is also a recurrent type found in children. The mortality rate is 50–95%.

Oral Signs and Symptoms

Great variety of oral lesions occur. The only common characteristic is an absence of any local cause. Spontaneous hemorrhage is not uncommon. Necrosis may be a feature and produces a nonspecific ulcerating stomatitis. Gangrenous lesions may involve the periodontium and bone. The lymph nodes may become enlarged. The patient may suffer considerable pain and have difficulty in swallowing. Lesions in the throat give rise to agranulocytic angina.

Hodgkin's Disease

Hodgkin's disease was first described by Thomas Hodgkin in 1832. It is associated with loss of weight, weakness, pallor, and an enlarged spleen and liver. A continuous fever is common. Painless swellings appear in the neck or other sites where lymph nodes are present; these generally increase in size. Although there is no characteristic blood picture, leukocytosis is usually present, often with slight anemia and eosinophilia.

Oral Signs and Symptoms

A patient with enlarged lymph nodes in the neck may be referred to the oral and maxillofacial surgeon. When there is a single node, a differential diagnosis from a branchial cleft cyst or submandibular gland enlargement must be made, generally by biopsy or excision. Multiple and bilateral enlargement is easier to recognize.

Cardiovascular Diseases

Certain heart diseases can account for unexpected death during an operation. If nephritis is also present, an increase in the risk is noted. This risk may he greatly diminished by careful preoperative study and judicious selection and expert administration of anesthetic agents. The added risk caused by heart disease is generally proportional to the degree of decrease in the cardiac reserve. The degree of cardiac reserve may be determined by the amount of fatigue on moderate exertion or the experience of breathlessness or cardiac pain after exercise, the occurrence of dependent edema, and the complaint of nocturnal dyspnea.

Oral Signs and Symptoms

The color of the lips and oral mucosa may be changed significantly. Jacoby (1960) states that in early cases cyanosis may cause a bluish discoloration. Reduced blood circulation in cardiac insufficiency also produces a cyanotic, reddish violet color of the tongue as well as an increase in size. Dilation of the lingual veins may also be noted. Right-sided cardiac failure can cause distention of the cervical veins.

Liver Disease

Patients with serious liver damage, such as occurs in advanced cirrhosis, often bleed spontaneously and excessively after operations. Such bleeding in the presence of vomiting may represent ruptured oesophageal varices.

Oral Signs and Symptoms

In severe liver disease the tongue is dark red, smooth on the dorsal surface and has no coating. The red colour of the tongue contrasts with the yellow coloured soft palate and gingiva. Rhagades of the lip are sometimes prominent. If prothrombin deficiency occurs, petechial haemorrhages and ecchymotic areas as well as spontaneous gingival bleeding may be noted (Fig. 14.3).

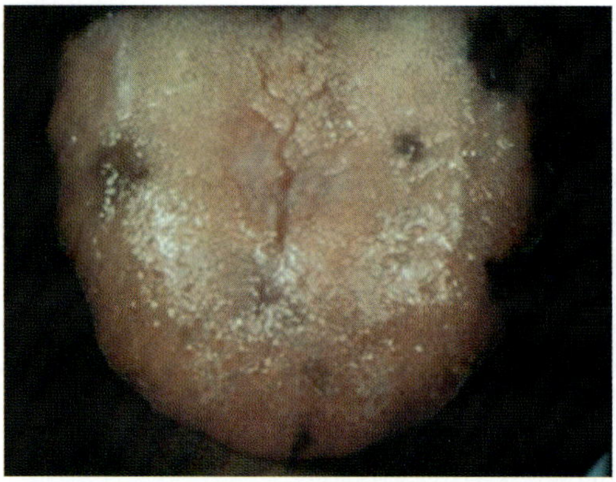

Fig. 14.3: Lesions in liver disease.

Kidney Disease

Renal disease is often associated with a disturbance in fluid and electrolyte balance; and impaired renal function limits or eliminates the ability to excrete waste products. Kidney disease requires a careful selection of anaesthetic agents and drugs. Generally those agents that are excreted through the kidneys should not be used especially when the non-protein nitrogen is high.

Oral Signs and Symptoms

In uraemic stomatitis the oral mucosa is red and swollen and often covered by a pseudomembrane that can be detached, leaving a dry red surface. An offending fetor oris, the so-called ammonia breath, is a characteristic feature (Fig. 14.4).

Diabetes Mellitus

In diabetes mellitus the ability to utilize carbohydrate is diminished or lost because

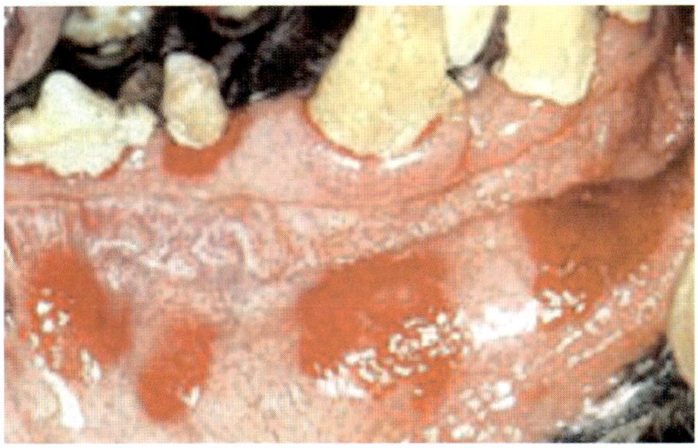

Fig. 14.4: Uraemic stomatitis.

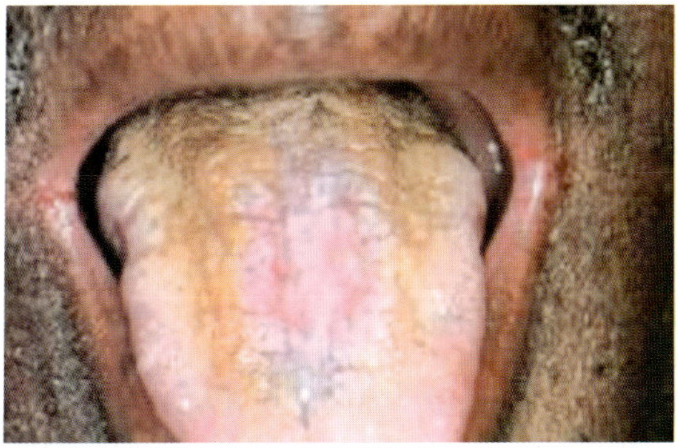

Fig. 14.5: Oral lesions in diabetes mellitus.

of faulty pancreatic activity. This produces hyperglycemia with glycosuria and polyuria, producing symptoms of thirst, hunger, emaciation and weakness. There is also a lowered resistance to pyogenic infections.

Oral Signs and Symptoms

The oral signs and symptoms of diabetes are not remarkable in the early stages. Severe gingival and periodontal disease is one of the most common findings. Gottsegen (1963) associated some cases of denturesore mouths and denture intolerance with diabetes. Lowered resistance to infection is likely the cause of gingival abscesses. Healing of wounds is slow and often complicated. Ulcers and angular cheilosis may not heal until the diabetes is controlled. Belting, Hiniker, and Dummett (1964) stated that vascular occlusive disorders increase the severity of periodontal disease. Xerostomia is common and often the patient complains of burning of the tongue, but the red beefy tongue of diabetes is not often seen today. A sweet, fruity (acetone) breath is another characteristic occurring mostly in the advanced stages of the disease (Fig. 14.5).

Amyloidosis

Amyloidosis is a degenerative disease affecting various tissues and organs of the body. In most cases the spleen, kidneys, liver, and adrenal glands are principally affected.

Oral Signs and Symptoms

Amyloidosis is a difficult disease to diagnose. Gingival biopsy is of considerable value in this regard. The most common findings are related to the tongue, which may show firm ridges and nodules. The buccal mucosa may also be involved (Fig. 14.6).

Systemic Reactions to Heavy Metals

A number of the heavy metals can cause systemic reactions frequently associated with oral findings. In the mouth, the deposition of the metallic salts in the tissues can interfere with circulation, and· the reduced resistance permits

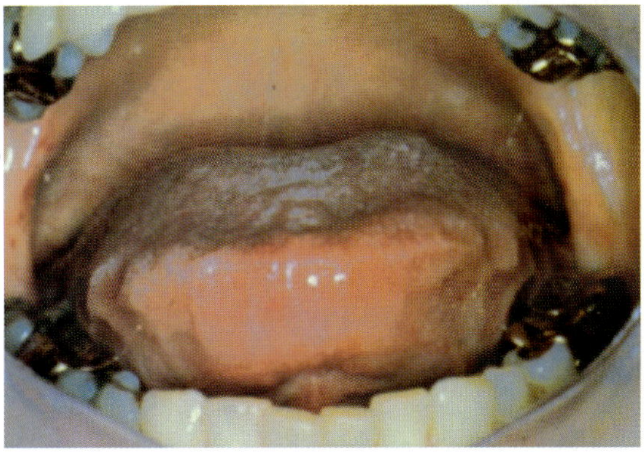

Fig. 14.6: Oral lesions in amyloidosis.

secondary invasion by bacteria. Secretion of some of the metals in saliva increases salivary flow and produces a metallic taste. The secreted metals may also be directly irritating to the tissues.

Lead Poisoning

Lead poisoning is due to absorption of lead through the skin or respiratory or gastrointestinal tract. Painters are frequently affected as well as children who chew on painted objects. The characteristic black-blue lead line along the gingival margin (halo saturninus) and the so-called lead breath (halitus saturninus) are common oral findings. The patients frequently complain of a sweet metallic taste and excessive salivation.

Bismuth Poisoning

Bismuth may, if used over a long period of time, produce deposits in the gingival margins that cause a bluish black line, especially if gingivitis is present. Similar deposits may occur on the cheeks and at the junction of the papillated dorsum of the tongue with the smooth ventral surface.

Argyria

Silver compounds are found in some nasal drops and sprays, and in former years were used to treat syphilis and gastric ulcer. Absorption of silver can cause permanent discoloration of the skin. The tissues have a gray color and the appearance can be confused with cyanosis. The sclera and conjunctiva may also be involved.

Orally, the mucous membranes will also have a uniform gray color owing to the even distribution of the silver throughout the tissues. Despite the patient's appearance, there are few, if any, subjective symptoms.

Mercurialism (ptyalism)

Mercurialism can develop as a result of occupational contact or self-medication with mercury-containing drugs. The general symptoms include intestinal colic, diarrhoea, headache, and insomnia. Renal symptoms may also develop. The lips are dry, cracked, and swollen. Oral ulceration may develop and the tongue can become enlarged and painful. There is an excessive production of a viscid saliva and a metallic taste. The oral tissues may have a burning sensation. Enlargement of the salivary glands is not uncommon.

Aurism

Gold salts used in treating rheumatoid arthritis and some dermatologic diseases can cause systemic reactions in from 10–40% of patients. The usual findings are dermatitis and stomatitis. Auric stomatitis is characterized by vesiculation and ulceration of the mucous membranes. Purpura and neutropenia have also been reported.

Erythema multiforme is an inflammatory disease characterized by red macules, papules, and occasionally vesicles or bullae, which are likely to recur. In the mouth, vesiculobullous lesions form with rapid onset, followed by necrosis of epithelium, ulceration, bleeding, and crust formation after a few hrs (Fig. 14.7).

The causes are viral conditions, systemic infections, malignant disease, and ingestion of drugs. The result of the last is known as stomatitis medicamentosa. The most common sites are the lips, cheeks, and tongue. Differential diagnosis should include benign mucous membrane pemphigoid and pemphigus.

Generally, the oral lesions in stomatitis medicamentosa are not pathognomonic. A few drugs, however, produce symptoms that can be recognized. Among these are the granulomatous lesions resulting from iodides and the noninflammatory gingival hyperplasia seen in epileptic patients who have been given diphenytoin (Dilantin) sodium over a long period of time.

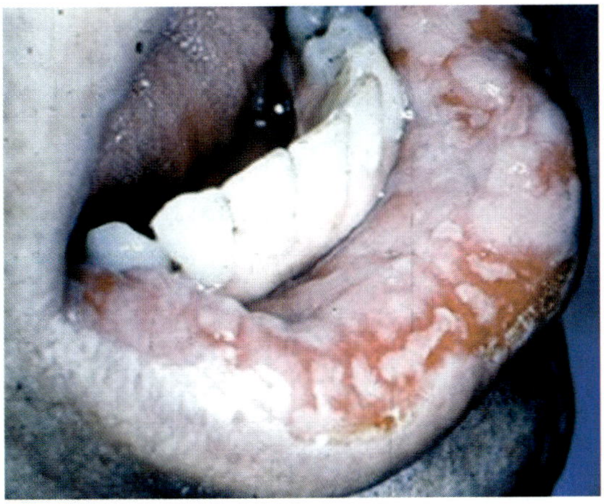

Fig. 14.7: Oral lesions in erythema multiforme.

Allergy

Susceptible people may become sensitized by foreign substances and develop specific antibodies against them; the antibodies combine with a body protein, which then produces a histamine-like reaction. In most instances the allergic reactions occur on the skin and mucosae of the body.

Some well-known allergies are to foods such as fish, lobsters, oysters, eggs, nuts, strawberries, and cheese. Food allergies, however, are sometimes actually drug allergies caused by contamination or additives. Milk, for example, may contain penicillin used to treat mastitis in cows. Honey may be contaminated with sulfa drugs the apiarist gives in sugar syrup to prevent or cure diseases of bees.

Drug allergies have become quite common. They are frequently produced by the antibiotics but also by other drugs. A careful history may reveal similar reactions to the drug when taken previously. A sudden appearance of the systemic symptoms after its use is characteristic. Withdrawal of the drug and replacement by another may confirm the diagnosis. In some cases the drug causing the allergic reaction may be a component of a combined medication. An example is a patient sensitive to procaine who was given procaine penicillin G by his dentist because of an infection and immediately went into anaphylactic shock.

Oral Signs and Symptoms

The oral mucosa may have a generalized redness or sometimes only reddish spots may occur. Vesicles, blebs, and ulcerations may form, often in asymmetric distribution (Fig. 14.8).

There is no itching, as on the skin, but a burning sensation is frequently felt. The association with dermal urticaria and itching of the skin is significant. Angioneurotic edema is the most frequent oral symptom. Edematous, circumscribed, painless swellings may affect the lips or cheeks. The swelling is not symmetric and must be distinguished from that associated with submandibular or other dental abscesses.

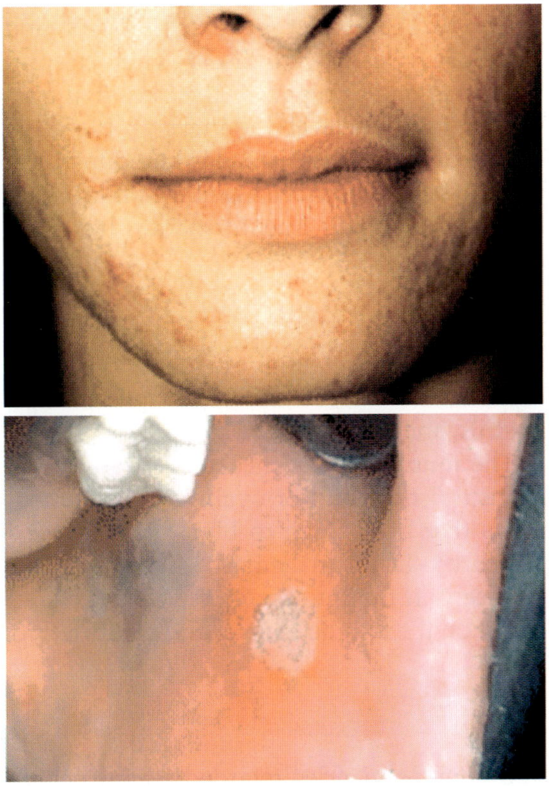

Fig. 14.8: Manifestations of allergic reactions.

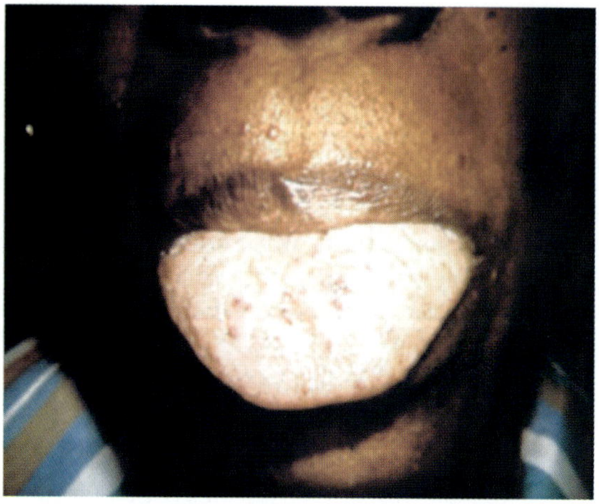

Fig. 14.9: Oral manifestations in Peutz-Jeghers.

The tongue, soft palate, and epiglottis may be involved.

Peutz-Jeghers Syndrome

Peutz (1921) and later Jeghers, Mc-Usick, and Katz (1949) described a disease characterized by formation of polyps in the intestinal tract that may give rise to abdominal pain, bleeding, and peritonitis. The disease is hereditary and the polyps are described as being hamartomas, though malignant transformation has been reported.

Oral Signs and Symptoms

Melanotic pigmentations are found in the face and mouth. Fine spots develop around the lips, nostrils, and eyes.

The mucosa of the cheeks is covered with characteristic round or oval, rarely confluent spots that are brown to black in color and measure 1–12 mm in diameter. Sometimes they are seen on the mucosa of the lips but only rarely on the tongue, palate, and gingiva (Fig. 14.9).

Vitamin Deficiencies

In vitamin deficiencies, retarded healing of both bone and soft tissues may result. In addition, the deficiencies can lower the resistance to infection so that secondary infections may occur, and often various mouth diseases develop that resist the accepted therapeutic measures.

Deficiencies rarely occur singly but manifest their presence in groups, such as the B-complex group and the fat-soluble vitamin group. They arise from inadequate intake, diminished absorption, increased need (as in pregnancy and infection with fever), increased destruction, and diminished utilization. Poor selection of food and destruction of the gastrointestinal flora by oral antibiotics are common causes of vitamin deficiency.

Vitamin C Deficiency

In the severest form of ascorbic acid deficiency, scurvy results which is rather a rare disease at present. In the past scurvy was caused by the lack of available fresh vegetables and fruits that contain vitamin C. Ascorbic acid deficiency produces hemorrhagic manifestations that are caused by failure of the intercellular material to bind the vascular endothelial cells. Clinically, the patient loses weight and develops secondary albuminuria and anemia. Hemorrhages into the skin and joints are common.

Oral Signs and Symptoms

Scorbutic stomatitis is characterized by gingival inflammation and classic enlargement of the gingival margins and interdental papillae. The gingivae have a purplish appearance and bleed easily. They become enlarged and cover the teeth almost completely (Fig. 14.10).

Later, necrosis and infection may cause severe destruction involving the periosteum and periodontal tissues (Boyle, Bessey, and Wolbach 1937), and the teeth loosen because of the breakdown of the collagen fibers of the periodontal ligament. Occasionally large hematomas may form and gingival bleeding from slight trauma is common. Vincent's infection often complicates the disease.

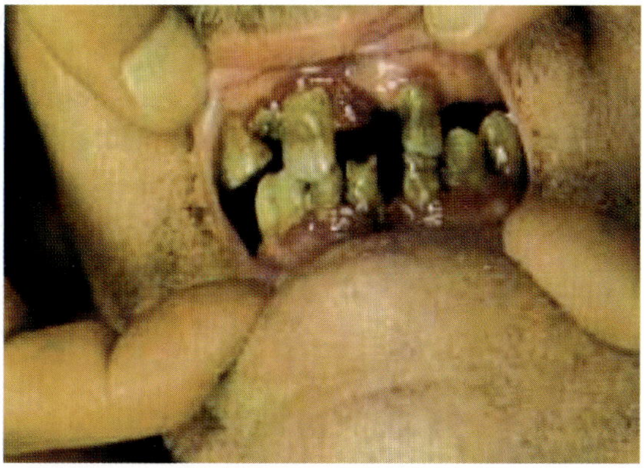

Fig. 14.10: Scorbutic gingivitis.

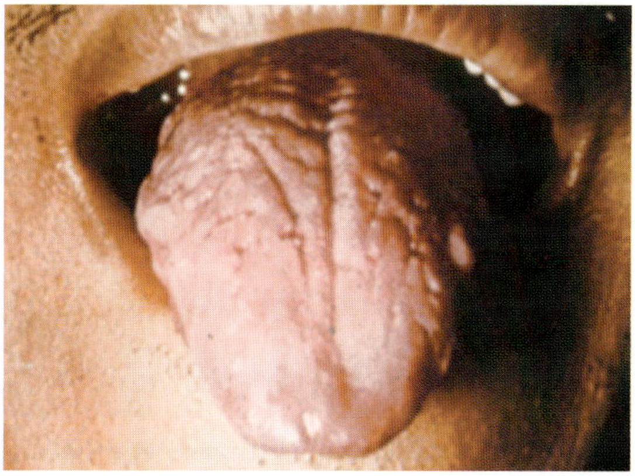

Fig. 14.11: Oral lesions in niacin deficiency.

Vitamin B Complex Deficiency

An effort has been made to find specific symptoms for each component of the vitamin B complex, but even in well-established deficiencies there are almost always concomitant deficiencies in some of the other components present, even deficiencies of other types, such as iron.

Niacin Deficiency

In its full-blown state niacin deficiency produces pellagra. Patients complain of sleeplessness, tiredness, absence of appetite, and loss of weight.

Oral Signs and Symptoms

Gingivitis and stomatitis are seen in niacin deficiency; often ulcers form on the mucosa. The lips are reddened and cracked, and the mouth feels as if it were scalded. The ulcers may contain Vincent's organisms in enormous numbers. The tongue shows the most characteristic changes, resulting in the so-called Sandwith's bald tongue (Fig. 14.11).

This is caused by desquamation of the lingual papillae. In the beginning only the tip or sides of the tongue may be affected. Later, the entire tongue becomes fiery red and swollen and shows an eroded, beef-red surface; for this reason it is also spoken of as beefy tongue. In the chronic stage the tongue shows fissuring and loss of substance caused by muscular atrophy.

Thiamine Deficiency

Thiamine or vitamin B_1 deficiency results in beriberi with polyneuritis and bradycardia

Oral Signs and Symptoms

The mouth lesions in thiamine deficiency are not distinctive. Gingivitis and oedema of the oral mucosa may be accompanied by atypical types of facial neuralgia. The tongue and gingival tissues may have a satiny appearance and a rose colour. Enlargement of the fungiform papillae and indentation markings along the periphery of the tongue are common. Vesicles may develop at the vermillion border and small cracks in the lips may also be present (Fig. 14.12).

Riboflavin Deficiency

Riboflavin or vitamin B_2 deficiency is often a secondary manifestation occurring with other vitamin B deficiencies.

Oral Signs and Symptoms

Cracks develop at the corner of the mouth. Candida albicans is a common secondary

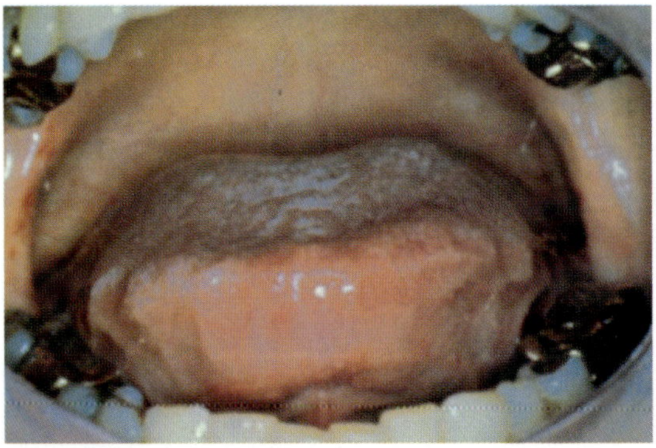

Fig. 14.12: Enlarged tongue in thiamine deficiency.

invader. The tongue may be enlarged and red with slight enlargement of the fungiform papillae and loss of muscle tone (Fig. 14.13). This may be accompanied by glossodynia.

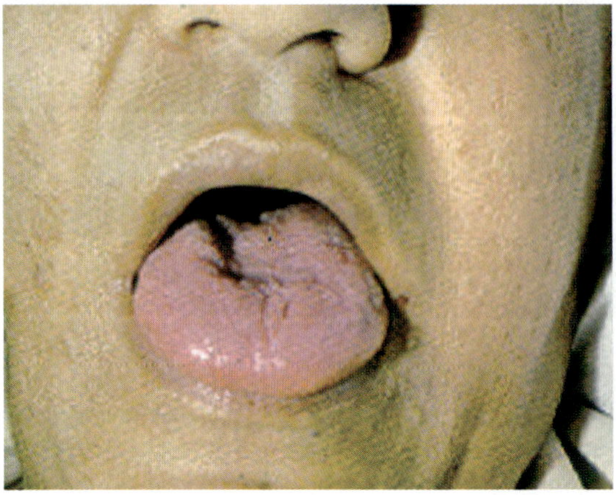

Fig. 14.13: Tongue lesions in riboflavin deficiency.

Pyridoxine Deficiency

Pyridoxine or vitamin B_6 deficiency produces weakness, nervousness and irritability. Seborrheic skin lesions about the eyes, nose and mouth occur as well as erosions resembling the cheilosis seen in riboflavin deficiency.

Oral Signs and Symptoms

Glossitis and stomatitis may also be seen.

Vitamin B_{12} Deficiency

This macrocytic, hyperchromic anemia usually occurs between the ages of 45 and 60 years. It is caused by a deficiency of an intrinsic factor secreted by the parietal cells of the fundus of the stomach.

Oral Signs and Symptoms

At first the tongue is red in contrast to the yellowish color of the rest of the mucosa. Later, atrophy of the filiform papillae causes a characteristic smooth, waxy appearance. The tongue is never coated and therefore has a very clean appearance (Fig. 14.14).

The subjective oral symptoms are often distressing; the patient complains of an unbearable burning and sometimes of numbness. The condition is aggravated by extreme temperatures of food as well as salty and highly seasoned meals.

Vitamin K Deficiency

Antibiotics, especially if administered orally, may bring about a vitamin K deficiency through the elimination of the gastrointestinal bacteria that are involved in the formation of vitamin K. Secondary deficiency can also occur from malabsorption.

Oral Signs and Symptoms

Spontaneous gingival bleeding or ecchymosis can occur with vitamin K deficiency. Excessive bleeding during an operation, with ecchymosis and the development of hematomas, is also characteristic.

SPECIFIC INFECTIONS

Specific diseases that can involve the jaws and oral tissues include tuberculosis, sarcoidosis, syphilis, granuloma inguinale, candidiasis, actinomycosis, aspergillosis, and leprosy, as well as some of the South American diseases that are now occasionally seen in other countries.

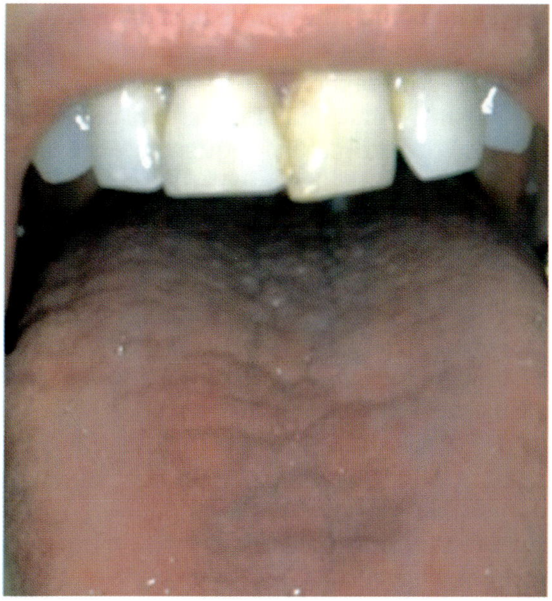

Fig. 14.14: Tongue lesions in vitamin B_{12} deficiency.

Tuberculosis

Tuberculosis of Soft Tissue

Tubercle bacilli that occur in the sputum of patients affected by pulmonary tuberculosis may invade a wound in the oral mucosa and produce a variety of lesions. Some are hypertrophic and are called tuberculomas, others appear as ulcers with ragged edges and undermined borders. The tongue is frequently affected because of injury by sharp, decayed teeth. The gingival tissues may also become infected.

Tuberculous Bone Infection

The jaw bone may be involved via a superficial ulcer or from the bacillus entering through a carious tooth or extraction wound. Two locations in the mandible have great affinity for the tuberculous infection—the alveolar process and the angle of the jaw. If the infection enters through a root canal, caseous foci develop that appear on the radiograph as radiolucent areas. These are often surrounded by a zone of sclerotic bone.

Sarcoidosis

Sarcoidosis was first described by Hutchinson in 1898 and become known as Mortimer's malady, the name of his patient. Schaumann (1914) was the first to describe its generalized nature; he named the disease lupus pernio. It is also known as maladie Besnier-Boeck. Boeck (1899) himself suggested the name sarcoid or sarcoidosis.

Oral Signs and Symptoms

Bhaskar (1977) cited evidence of sarcoid in the parotid gland, soft palate, and cheek.

Syphilis

This disease may be divided into congenital or acquired forms (primary, secondary, and tertiary stages). Except in the congenital form, the initial lesion is the so called chancre. All other lesions follow chancre formation and involve many parts of the body. The disease is caused by infection with *Treponema pallidum.* Accidental infection is rare but may occur in the office, laboratory, or necropsy room.

Congenital Syphilis

The teeth show characteristic abnormalities: severe hypoplasia of the deciduous teeth, as well as the screwdriver permanent incisors and mulberry molars (Hutchinson's teeth), are pathognomonic.

Primary Syphilis

Chancres in the oral region are found mostly on the lip and tongue. The lesions are almost always solitary and have the appearance of an ulcer or tumefaction covered by thick, adherent, dark crusts. No pain is caused by the lesion, but the regional lymph nodes become enlarged.

Secondary Syphilis

The secondary lesions occur 6–12 weeks after the onset of the disease. Multiple, discrete, oval, grayish white, or reddish pink patches form on the buccal mucosa and tongue. They are surrounded by a slightly raised, reddish, inflammatory halo. These lesions are known as mucous patches. They are highly infective. Usually the patient develops generalized enlargement of the lymph nodes.

Diffuse glossitis is common in the early stages of the disease and causes atrophy of the lingual papillae. Hyperkeratosis may develop, which gives the tongue a glazed appearance and produces the so called bald or glass tongue.

Tertiary Syphilis

Gummas usually develop within 3–10 years after the onset of the disease. They are deeply seated and often involve the underlying bone.

The solitary gumma produces a painless swelling most frequently found on the tongue, palatal mucosa, and uvula. Later central necrosis and ulceration develop. The deeply excavated lesion often is difficult to differentiate from carcinoma. The hard palate is one of the frequent sites of a solitary gumma.

Diffuse involvement of the tongue often results in interstitial fibrosis and papillary atrophy. Leukoplakia frequently occurs in association with this type of glossitis. The incidence of carcinomatous change in these leukoplakic areas is relatively high.

In the mandible the gummatous process may resemble acute pyogenic osteomyelitis. The process may be so extensive that the teeth become loose. Large areas of the alveolar and basilar bone can become destroyed.

Candidiasis (Moniliasis)

Candidiasis may be generalized, causing widespread infections not only of the skin but also of the respiratory passages and gastrointestinal tract. Localized lesions may also occur in various parts of the body, especially the axillary, submammary, and inguinal regions, and there is a vulvovaginal variety.

In the oral cavity the fungus produces candidal stomatitis, often spoken of as thrush.

REFERENCE AND BIBLIOGRAPHY

1. *Oral and Maxillofacial Surgery*; Daniel M. Laskin.

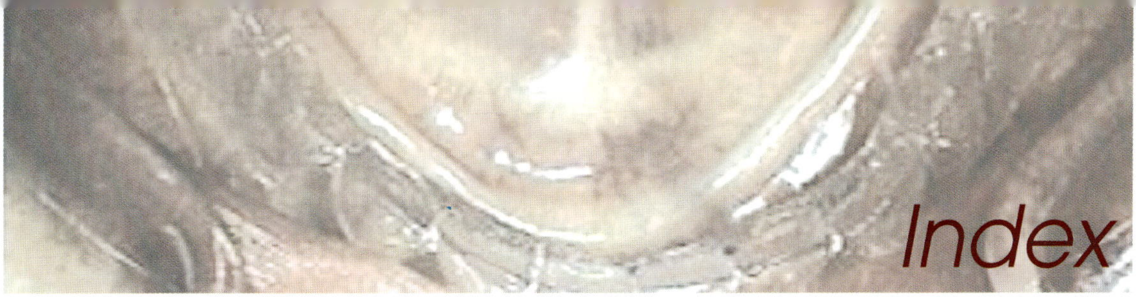

Index